Edited by Nancy Waxler-Morrison, Joan M. Anderson, Elizabeth Richardson, and Natalie A. Chambers

Cross-Cultural Caring
A Handbook for Health Professionals

Second Edition

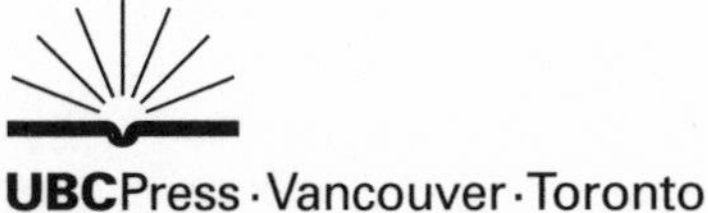

UBCPress · Vancouver · Toronto

15 14 13 12 11 10 09 08 07 06 05 5 4 3 2 1

Printed in Canada on acid-free paper

Library and Archives Canada Cataloguing in Publication

Cross-cultural caring : a handbook for health professionals / edited by Nancy Waxler-Morrison ... [et al.]. – 2nd ed.

Includes bibliographical references and index.
ISBN-13: 978-0-7748-1255-9 (bound); 978-0-7748-1025-8 (pbk.)
ISBN-10: 0-7748-1255-9 (bound); 0-7748-1025-4 (pbk.)

1. Minorities – Medical care – Canada. 2. Medical anthropology – Canada. 3. Medical personnel and patient – Canada. 4. Health attitudes – Canada – Cross-cultural studies. 5. Minorities – Health and hygiene – Canada. I. Waxler-Morrison, Nancy, 1931-

RA563.M56C76 2005 362.1'089'00971 C2005-903357-6

Canada

UBC Press gratefully acknowledges the financial support for our publishing program of the Government of Canada through the Book Publishing Industry Development Program (BPIDP), and of the Canada Council for the Arts, and the British Columbia Arts Council.

This book has been published with the help of a grant from the Canadian Federation for the Humanities and Social Sciences, through the Aid to Scholarly Publications Programme, using funds provided by the Social Sciences and Humanities Research Council of Canada, and with the help of the K.D. Srivastava Fund.

UBC Press
The University of British Columbia
2029 West Mall
Vancouver, BC V6T 1Z2
604-822-5959 / Fax: 604-822-6083
www.ubcpress.ca

Cross-Cultural Caring

Contents

Acknowledgments

We are grateful to the University of British Columbia's School of Nursing and Department of Anthropology and Sociology for their support, and, especially, to Mary Sun for her administrative assistance.

We are pleased to acknowledge, with thanks, the generous financial grant from the (then) Ministry for Children and Families of British Columbia. Special thanks to Dr. Barbara Herringer and her staff at the ministry for their encouragement, support, and assistance.

The staff at UBC Press has always provided knowledgeable and efficient assistance, and we are especially grateful to Larry MacDonald for copy editing our manuscript with care and intelligence. Over the years that it took to complete this second edition, Jean Wilson's understanding, encouragement, and patience were most important to us. Thanks to Jean and to everyone at the Press.

Many members of the immigrant communities as well as many health professionals provided us with invaluable information that could be obtained in no other way. Their names appear at the end of each chapter. Here we wish to thank them for their help and to join with them in the hope that this book will contribute to a form of health care that is both more effective and more acceptable to all Canadians.

Nancy Waxler-Morrison
Joan M. Anderson
Elizabeth Richardson
Natalie A. Chambers

Cross-Cultural Caring

INTRODUCTION
The Need for Culturally Sensitive Health Care
Nancy Waxler-Morrison and Joan M. Anderson

Mrs. L., a social worker at the public health department in a small town in western Canada, received a call from Dr. N., a local physician, who said, "I've just examined a two-year-old child from one of those Vietnamese families living out north of town. He's got bruises all over his back and I think you had better make a home visit because it looks like a case of child abuse to me. We'll probably have to report it." Mrs. L. discovered that the family lived in a trailer park full of Vietnamese refugees. The mother worked as a cleaner in the local hospital; the father was unemployed and stayed at home with their four young children. The two-year-old had had a severe cold and trouble breathing, which led the parents to take him to the doctor. When Mrs. L. looked at the child she saw the bruise marks down his back. The child's mother looked somewhat embarrassed as she explained that they were short of money so they hadn't taken him to the doctor right away but instead tried a treatment everyone used in Vietnam – "spooning." A silver spoon was pressed firmly up and down the child's back as a way to remove the illness. That's where the bruises had come from. They had done this for about five days, but when it didn't seem to work they finally took the child to the doctor.

Purpose of This Book

The potential "problem" in the Vietnamese family described above arises not simply from the use of a traditional healing practice that many Western practitioners would think useless or even harmful because it delays good treatment. It arises also from the Western practitioner's assumptions that parents may harm children and that the government may or should intervene. Thus both Vietnamese parents and Western-trained family doctors have different ways of understanding and treating illness that derive from their own cultures. These "cultures of medicine" are often incongruent and in conflict. It is to avert this "clash of cultures" and the resulting dissatisfaction and poor health care that we have written this book. We hope to inform health professionals about the social background, beliefs, and practices of particular cultural groups in order to ease patient management. We hope also to provide guidelines to members of various immigrant groups in Canada which will ensure that their expectations, needs, and interests are attended to when they require health care.

How are ethnic and cultural factors associated with health and health care? First, some diseases are associated with ethnic group membership. These diseases may be genetically linked to the group, or prevalent in the home country because it is poorly served by preventive medicine, or linked to diet or other cultural practices. Because these culturally linked diseases are often unusual and not a central part of Western medical training, learning about them is obviously useful to professionals dealing with patients from that culture. Second, ethnic membership often means that family structure, religion, medical beliefs, and practices are incongruent with Western society or its health beliefs, thus leading to unfulfilled expectations and dissatisfied health professionals and patients. Third, these incongruencies often result in ineffective health care, to patient non-compliance from the point of view of the practitioner, and to continued illness, alienation, and feelings of being discriminated against from the point of view of the immigrant patient.

This handbook provides the health practitioner with basic information on medically relevant cultural practices in some immigrant groups in Canada. The contents of this second edition have been brought up to date to represent the situations of these immigrants at the beginning of the new millennium. Close attention is paid to the social contexts in which these patients live: why they came to Canada, where and how they may live, what sorts of family situations are common, who provides support, who makes decisions, what medical practices and beliefs they may have brought from their home countries, and what problems they may experience in obtaining health care in Canada. The focus is on information that may aid professionals in providing more culturally sensitive health care.

Perspective

A distinctive "culture of health" is not found only among recent immigrants to Canada. Immigrants do indeed bring with them beliefs about what causes symptoms – from the "evil eye" to "too much bile gone to the head" to "germs" – and about suitable treatments, ranging from talismans to aspirin to coriander tea. But Western-trained health professionals equally have a distinctive culture of health, often taken for granted and thus unrecognized. For example, Western-educated health professionals tend to attribute disease to individual behaviour, such as exposing oneself to germs or eating improperly and not exercising, and to regard the individual as thus largely responsible for getting well. Moreover, to a Western doctor getting well usually means cooperation with technical procedures applied to the body, such as medicines and surgery.

Health care is a social process to which each party – the professional and the patient – brings a set of beliefs, expectations, and practices. Their common task is to negotiate an understanding of the problem, or diagnosis, and decide what to do about it. Health practitioners usually do not think of their day-to-day work in terms of cultural transactions. Instead, they use phrases like "taking the history," "physical examination," or "management" to describe medical work as a technical task to which they apply their expertise and training. It is easy to think in technical terms when the health practitioner and the patient share very basic assumptions about illness and treatment. If both are members of the Canadian cultural majority, it is likely that they both believe, for example, that bacteria and viruses cause disease, that the patient should provide concise and relevant information about symptoms, and that the technical recommendations of the health professional should be followed if the illness is to be cured. Negotiations between a health professional and a patient who share the medical culture can be smooth and satisfying to both parties.

However, when the same health professional treats a patient with a different culture of medicine, the negotiations are often ineffective and unsatisfactory to both. The professional may regard medical care as largely a technical task requiring the individual cooperation of the patient. The patient may not see it that way. For example, in some non-Western cultures the patient is expected to wait passively for the doctor's diagnosis since "the doctor should know" what the problem is. Western-style taking of histories is not part of the patient's experience. Or, in some cultures, whether or not a prescribed medicine is taken is not the sick person's decision but the prerogative of the family head, who is often the grandfather or grandmother. Instructions or recommendations by health professional to patient, stemming from a Western assumption of individual responsibility, are thus ineffective.

The culture of medicine of most Canadian health professionals and the differing culture of an immigrant or minority patient are both legitimate perspectives. In the eyes of the latter, the Western medical system does not have a monopoly on wisdom about how a sick person should behave, the kinds of recommendations a health professional should make, or even the causes and proper description of disease. It is unrealistic and unhelpful to ignore cultural differences and expect that Western medical practices will work smoothly and immigrant patients will simply adapt to them. Instead, the professional who is alert to cultural differences will more easily find a mutually satisfactory way to achieve "compliance" or effective treatment with a patient who is more likely to recover and feel satisfied.

Cross-Cultural Caring provides a basic introduction to the social background and culture of a number of immigrant groups in Canada. Comprehensive knowledge about every ethnic group is impossible and unnecessary, and we have not attempted to furnish it. Moreover, people differ individually even though they share a culture. What we have done is to alert health practitioners and other professionals to some of the important cultural and social characteristics that have been described to us by members of these groups as possibly affecting health care. These can be explored in more detail with an individual patient or family. In the last chapter, we suggest culturally sensitive ways of obtaining important information from patients and their families, of negotiating common understandings, and of agreeing upon care plans that are consistent with the cultures of both health practitioner and patient.

Problems Common to Ethnic and Cultural Minorities in Canada

Although each cultural minority group has a distinct history, social situation, and set of beliefs, they have some experiences and problems in common. These are often reflected in their use of health services, their experiences with health professionals, and their common illnesses. Some of these problems appear repeatedly in the chapters that follow.

Many of the cultural minorities described are relatively recent migrants to Canada. The disruption of life associated with migration affects many people from different cultures in similar ways. Much has been lost: family ties, familiar language, community support, and the comfort that comes from the general predictability of life. Some migrants, too, have not lost the familiar life by choice; though some have come to Canada to better their lives, others have come as refugees who have been forced against their will to leave their home countries. Recent migrants have lost a great deal and need strength to reintegrate and begin again.

Migration also requires adaptation to a new society. Many migrants must learn a new language, find new supports, and change how they eat, live, and relate to their own children. They must also learn new jobs, and create new visions of the future. Dealing with adaptation, like dealing with loss, takes time and energy.

Three problems are felt by almost all cultural groups, most strongly soon after arriving in Canada. The first is lack of English or French. Many are eager to learn and do so quickly, but lack of a Canadian language makes health service encounters frustrating and unrewarding for everyone, and the help available for this problem in no way meets the need. The second problem is lack of money. Some immigrants have or can bring funds to cover living expenses; others rely on relatives in Canada. The majority live at a basic subsistence level and find it difficult, for example, to buy medicine or pay for bus fares to the hospital. A third problem for many is posed by the health, social service, and immigration bureaucracies, which they find difficult to understand and utilize. Many newcomers spend scarce time and money going from one office to another to obtain clarification of status and medical insurance. Immigrants may not be familiar with social workers, for example, and may be understandably reluctant to discuss family problems with a stranger.

Other issues affect immigrants as family members. Crucial for many immigrant women is learning to balance housework and a paid job without the support of the family network that they once had at home. Immigrant women who are not employed are often the last to learn the new language, enduring social isolation and deprived of what help is available. Men, too, experience loss of status and self-esteem when jobs for which they were trained in their home countries are closed to them in Canada; doctors may work as hospital orderlies and teachers as store clerks. Family relationships change. Children usually learn English or French sooner and tend to become intermediaries between parents and the outside world; doing so may displace their father from his former role. Moreover, children may adopt Western dress, behaviour, and aspirations that are believed by their parents to be bad, immoral, or disrespectful. The resulting personal and family stresses can lead to physical and mental health problems.

Members of these cultural minority groups frequently experience problems with hospitals and health professionals that represent, in microcosm, the general difficulties they have in the new society. They feel frustrated and insecure because few health professionals can communicate in the family's language and translators are not readily available. Even if someone in the family can speak English or French, the family's lack of understanding of how the Canadian health system works and how it differs from such services in their home country creates difficulties. This problem is often compounded by the health professional's neglect of the need for explanation. Such confusions may waste time and energy which working family members can ill afford. Members of cultural minorities often feel that health professionals do not understand them and simply assume that they feel and think about health just as other Canadians do. Some experience their contact with health professionals as "stereotyping," such as behaving towards them as if "all South Asians are the same." Some immigrants report encounters in hospitals and clinics in terms of discrimination, prejudice, or racism.

Health professionals in turn report problems in working with cultural minority groups. Patients may not follow instructions with medications, or medicines are given to another family member with a different disease.

Families may not abide by hospital policies and instead visit in large numbers, bringing small children and forbidden food. Parents may not dress their small children "properly" or provide nutritious food or may send sick children to school. Appointments may be missed, advice not followed. Health professionals often see real problems in completing the provision of good care to immigrant and minority group patients.

Some of these "problems," as seen by minority group members or by health professionals, are linked to differences in cultures of health. The parties often have distinctly different understandings of illness, beliefs about appropriate behaviour for doctors and sick people, and ideas about proper treatment. But the cultural differences are accentuated by the fact that health professionals, mostly members of the majority culture, also seem very powerful to their patients. Professionals have, or seem to have, the expertise that the patient lacks, and they regard their expertise as the reason the patient seeks professional care in the first place. When the professional also belongs to the majority culture, it is extremely difficult for the immigrant patient or family to ask questions, seek a second opinion, or disagree with the proposed treatment. Relative differences in power between professional and patient compound the cultural differences hindering collaboration between ethnic minority members and health professionals.

Immigrant Groups Described

We have not tried to describe all immigrant groups in Canada, nor do we focus on the largest groups or the most recent arrivals. Instead, we have selected the people who report that they have problems in obtaining satisfactory health care and those cultural groups believed by health professionals to be difficult to work with. In short, we describe people who have "problems" with health care.

Reported problems with health care can certainly be found in every segment of the Canadian population. Our selection, necessarily somewhat arbitrary and subjective, does not imply that all is well in health care with other cultural groups, including the cultural majority. For example, Aboriginal peoples sometimes express dissatisfaction with mainstream health care, but they are not discussed in this book because they are not immigrants. Also not covered are the predominant Anglo- and French-Canadian groups, which have their own "culture of health." Other groups like these deserve attention in further publications. The immigrant groups we have chosen to discuss are those that provide useful insights into the variety of cross-cultural problems in health care and possible solutions to them.

The immigrant groups we describe represent minority cultures in Canada: Central Americans, Chinese, Cambodians and Laotians, Iranians, Japanese,

South Asians, and Vietnamese. We describe them in terms of their country or area of origin. Many members of these groups in Canada are Canadian citizens or will become so. In the chapter on refugees we also mention other recent migrants, such as those from Afghanistan and Somalia.

A "cultural minority" is a distinctive and identifiable subgroup in the Canadian population that sees itself as having origins, beliefs, and values that contrast with the culture of the homogeneous, most-dominant, subgroup of the Canadian population, the white, largely European, culture. Underlying this contrast is an imbalance in economic and political power that favours the dominant group. Therefore, "minority" cultures often imply both distinctive cultural beliefs and less powerful social and economic positions – at least within Canada. Both characteristics are reflected in the problems facing subgroups and health professionals in devising mutually satisfactory health care.

When describing a cultural group, there is always the danger of stereotyping, of implying that all group members are the same. Yet if one takes the opposite position – that the group is only a collection of unique individuals – one would deny the reality of the common culture by which the group expresses and maintains its distinctiveness. In practice, we know that people of South Asian descent widely believe that imbalance in the body humours can cause illness and that a diet of hot and cool foods may relieve the symptoms. Yet we also know that some South Asians who come to Canada have adopted Western concepts of illness and no longer believe in this traditional concept of bodily imbalance. Immigrant cultures are filled with change and adaptation. Thus, to recognize diversity and avoid stereotyping, we attempt to point out important variations within each cultural minority group.

One must also beware of generalizing about cultural minorities across different countries. Each country receiving immigrants has unique policies and services that can profoundly affect the experiences of new residents. In Canada, for example, all immigrants and asylum seekers receive government-funded health care and so have fewer worries about the cost of basic health services. Moreover, the bureaucratic procedures for confirming refugee status in Canada cause most asylum seekers high anxiety at certain points in the screening procedures. Historical and political events usually mean that a country receives immigrants representing specific subgroups of persons from other countries. For example, the Hmong people, a tribal group from Laos, were taken in mainly by the United States, while Laotians who came to Canada were often professionals and government servants from urban areas.

For such reasons, professionals must be very cautious about generalizing from situations in other countries. The policies and social contexts of their own country and the characteristics of specific cultural minorities will determine how to work successfully with immigrants and refugees. And in any case, it will always be up to the health professional to investigate carefully each patient's particular circumstances so as to understand that individual's "culture of health."

How This Book Was Written

We have asked members of cultural minority groups to speak for themselves, through the authors of each chapter. In most cases, our authors are members of the cultural groups they describe. Yet most are also health or social service professionals with day-to-day experience with patients and families from that group. They have drawn upon their own experiences as well as their cultural knowledge. We also asked professionals who work with, but do not belong to, that cultural group to read and comment on the work. Thus each chapter is the work of one or more authors who were helped by a number of contributors. All the contributors besides the authors are listed at the end of each chapter.

New Information in This Second Edition

All chapters have been completely revised and updated using information obtained from interviews of practitioners and immigrants themselves. Some very significant changes have occurred since 1988-89 when the first edition was completed. For example, by 2000 the majority of immigrants of Chinese background came from mainland China, not from Hong Kong or Taiwan as in the 1980s. The Vietnamese who arrived in Canada as refugees in the latter part of the 1970s are now, in the early part of the new century, sponsoring mostly elderly family members as well as new young wives. The first wave of Iranians, mostly from the upper middle class, is now being joined by working-class families. All of the shifts in these and other immigrant populations mean different settlement problems and new issues for health professionals.

By the turn of the century, about 30,000 refugees were arriving in Canada every year. We have recognized the special circumstances of refugees with a new chapter that provides an overview of the formal definitions of different types of refugees and the health and other services available to them, along with some of the social, physical, and mental problems many of them face. This new information highlights the need for professionals to know whether their clients are immigrants who chose to come to Canada or refugees who were forced out of their home countries. The experiences and problems of these two groups are often radically different.

We have included a few short immigrant and refugee stories, set in boxes, to bring to life some of the experiences and problems that people from other cultures bring when they settle in Canada and seek health care. These vignettes are based on real-life experiences and have been disguised to protect privacy. The subtle implications of a story can be more fully understood by reading the chapter in which it appears.

How To Use This Book

A problem identified in the first edition of this book was the potential for stereotyping different groups of people. We take this concern seriously, because it assumes the opposite of our intention. We suggest ways in which the book can be used to see through the casual assumption that all members of a particular cultural group share certain characteristics. We want our book to help health professionals recognize how ethnic stereotypes may prevent them from understanding the individual patients they are seeking to help.

Use the Book as a Starting Point in Work with a Client

We provide concrete information about the backgrounds from which different groups of people come. For example, we have included histories of different groups, political and economic factors that influence decisions to migrate, and the experiences people have had with physicians and hospitals in their home countries that may have an impact on their experiences in Canada. Although chapter authors discuss beliefs and practices at the group level, obviously there are individual variations within each group, differences based on social class, length of time in Canada, and so on. Moreover, cultures are continually changing. Therefore, each chapter should be regarded not as a portrayal of a foreign way of life but rather as a resource for clues and indications about where to begin learning about a client as a person living in Canadian society.

Get To Know the Individual Client

The information in this book is meant to encourage interaction, not replace it. The professional should get to know his or her clients by inquiring about their past experiences with health care, their beliefs and current practices, the circumstances under which they live and work, and the obligations they carry – which often have a profound effect on how they manage health and illness. For example, since the first edition of this book, major changes in the Canadian health care system often require patients and families to take on a more central role in caregiving. Hospital stays are shorter, and clients usually go home while they still experience significant symptoms and require complex treatments. In these circumstances it is imperative to learn about the client's home situation. Background information in the relevant chapter will point to important issues a professional might follow up.

Know Yourself

We professionals, no less than our clients, have personal values that are deeply embedded in our own histories, in our upbringing, and in the cultures that continue to shape us. These personal values influence our professional identities and how we use professional knowledge. As professionals, therefore, we ought to be self-reflective about the personal values we bring to each health care encounter, how our personal values may affect what we hear and see, and how we interact with people. We are not just passive observers, objectively viewing the "Other," but active participants in interactions with clients.

We have to find a way to connect with each person regardless of how different we might at first perceive that person to be from ourselves. Professional and client may find themselves sharing the discovery that neither fits the other's cultural stereotype. A client sensing such sharing and connections will begin to participate more openly in the meeting. For the professional this implies more than "knowing the right questions to ask." It means establishing a relationship of mutual respect, opening up a space where differences in perspective can be recognized and managed.

It is in the spirit of a common humanity that we invite you to engage with *Cross-Cultural Caring*. The book provides background information that may offer clues to a client's experiences, perspectives, and values. Your ability to connect at a human level with clients from all cultures and backgrounds remains central to professional practice.

1
People of Central American Descent

Danica Gleave, Natalie A. Chambers, and Arturo S. Manes

Since 1980, Canada has experienced a marked increase in the number of immigrants from the region that extends from Southern Mexico to Colombia, many of whom have come as refugees. In the 1980s, El Salvador, Guatemala, Honduras, and Nicaragua were the most important countries of origin, with most immigrants arriving as refugees and many coming to Canada via Mexico or the United States. By the year 2000, Colombia, Mexico, and Costa Rica had become the most significant countries of origin, with a small number from Honduras. Most have come as refugees. By 2001, 304,650 people in Canada had been born in Central America. While historical conditions in each country are important in understanding why people have left for Canada, the countries in the region have similar histories, and most now have similar social conditions.

Spanish, English, French, and Dutch explorers began arriving in the region some four hundred years ago and exerted a lasting impact on the resident indigenous population. The violent introduction of Christianity, foreign languages such as Spanish, the Spanish semi-feudal landownership patterns, as well as a host of foreign goods caused major cultural shifts for peoples native to the region. Many indigenous communities were ravaged by disease, dehumanized by the aggression or beliefs of new settlers, or assimilated into Spanish culture. Other communities survived and continue to speak their own languages and maintain their own unique knowledge systems, some blending European practices into their own cultures. Consequently, in Central America today one finds a wide spectrum of cultural diversity, from rural landlords descended from urban Westernized Europeans, to merchants of mixed ancestry, to Mayan agricultural workers. The implication for health professionals is that they must learn their Central American patients' backgrounds. Since every immigrant has a unique history and migration story, cultural stereotypes can lead to painful misunderstandings.

Situation in the Region

If one ignores political boundaries, it is easy to envisage the backbone of mountains that swings southeast from Mexico to join the Andean range in South America. North of the mountains are various minor ridges and flat plains, many covered in dense jungle. Lakes large and small are found throughout the diverse countryside, a source of pleasure and beauty to residents and visitors. The year-round tropical climate means that people coming to Canada are unfamiliar with snowy winter conditions. The mountainous and tropical terrains combine to limit the available agricultural land, while political and economic interests ensure that this arable land is used overwhelmingly for cash crop production and worked by landless labourers.

The farms are often huge, owned by international corporations or wealthy families. This regional pattern of landownership has helped to create a society where wide gulfs separate the very wealthy from the poor. While professional classes exist, they are small and relatively powerless compared to the wealthy above them, and are heavily outnumbered by the blue-collar workers, labourers, and unemployed or underemployed people beneath them. This imbalance in resource distribution has meant that, by Canadian standards, in most countries roads and communications are inadequate, education and health facilities are poor, and so on. In El Salvador, for example, it is a legal requirement that every child attend school between the ages of seven and twelve, but there are not enough schools to accommodate the nation's children. Dysfunctions such as this, accompanied by an all-encompassing poverty, have been a primary source of the political unrest and civil war endemic in the region for a century. A second factor has been ongoing political turmoil. Nations in the region have tended to be ruled by military dictators, most of whom have used armed force to restrain public debate and civil uprisings. Guerrilla resistance movements have countered with violence of their own. By 2000, new refugees continued to arrive, as well as family members of former refugees coming to join relatives already in Canada. The largest group was immigrating from Mexico, Colombia, and Costa Rica, for a mix of economic and security reasons.

El Salvador

El Salvador (whose name translates as "The Saviour") is the smallest and most densely populated of the Central American countries. Until recently, it was the source of most refugees coming to Canada from the region. Although more industrialized and with a healthier economy than its neighbours, El Salvador suffers high unemployment, especially in rural areas, and a large disparity between rich and poor. Most people are descendants of the Spanish and indigenous peoples, and Spanish is the national language. Approximately 20 percent of the people are illiterate. Life expectancy is seventy years. Women have an average of 2.9 children, in contrast to Canada's fertility rate of 1.5 children. These factors result in a young population and a heavy demand for jobs and arable farmland. The coffee crop has fuelled the economy, although there are other export commodities, including cotton and sugar. Beans, corn, and rice are the dietary staples for most, and dairy products and meat are enjoyed when possible. Fresh vegetables and fruits are relatively abundant, especially in rural areas.

Politically, El Salvador has a history of military dictatorships, fraudulent elections (1972, 1976, and 1982), and state-sanctioned terror. In the early 1980s members of the extreme right formed the Frente Marti para la Liberacion Nacional (FMLN) and embarked on campaigns of organized terror against the civilian population. In 1981 US military aid was used to strengthen anti-guerrilla efforts. The ensuing violence, combined with crippling poverty, forced more than 850,000 rural and urban refugees to flee to the United States, Mexico, other Central American countries, and Canada (Garcia and Rodriguez 1989, 73). Another 500,000 refugees were internally displaced within El Salvador. While the national government turned a blind eye, over 70,000 civilians were murdered during "clean-up" campaigns and organized terror. During this period civilian attempts to organize and demonstrate were violently suppressed, resulting in more deaths. In 1982 alone, there were at least 3,059 political murders (UN Security Council 1993).

Civilians often could find no safe place except to try to leave. Rural communities were frequently the targets of both coercive FMLN forces and government-sponsored military death squads. Army forces massacred rural peasants, while large numbers of FMLN rebels (4,000-9,000) fought the army. Instability continued throughout the 1980s, finally achieving some resolution in 1992 with the signing of a peace accord between the warring sides. However, the underlying issues of poverty, underemployment, and corruption have continued to fuel outbreaks of violence. The combined natural disasters of Hurricane Mitch in 1998 and earthquakes in January and February 2001 were devastating blows with significant losses of life.

In 2001 El Salvador began using the American dollar for its currency. An important source of income for the country is money sent home by expatriates in the United States. Health care, as with other social services, varies greatly between rich and poor, and between urban and rural areas. Doctors and hospitals are rare in the countryside, while overcrowded and poorly supplied public clinics and hospitals are standard for the urban working class. The wealthy can have access to a good standard of care. People coming to

Canada from El Salvador are frequently victims of violence. Others are coming to join family members already here through the family reunification program.

Guatemala

While the circumstances and details of Guatemala are different from those of El Salvador, Guatemalans of Spanish descent face a very similar situation. Guatemala has been ruled by a succession of military dictators since 1838, except for a ten-year democratic respite from 1944 to 1954. A handful of wealthy families control most of the land and economic activities, leaving insufficient arable land to feed adequately the rest of the population. Meanwhile, landless agricultural labourers have been victims of tremendous human rights violations. Consequently, land reform is a key political issue. Coffee and bananas, the most important export crops, are grown in large plantations primarily, worked by Maya peoples.

About 30 percent of the population in Guatemala is illiterate, life expectancy is sixty-five years, and unemployment is chronic. Guatemala stands out from the other Latin American countries we describe with its very high birth rate of 4.3 births per woman. Like many developing countries, Guatemala has experienced major migrations from rural areas as people come to urban areas in search of jobs and services. The rise of evangelical Christianity has been significant, influencing communities and political candidates. Publicly funded hospitals, available only in the cities, are also overworked and understaffed; only 41 percent of births are attended by trained health workers. Guatemala was also affected by Hurricane Mitch in 1998, with loss of life as well as of crops and infrastructure such as bridges and roads.

The democratic period from 1944 to 1954 under an elected president, Juan Jose Arevalo, brought increased rights and freedoms, including recognition of the rights of women, freedom of speech, and the development of labour unions. However, land reforms that facilitated the seizure and redistribution of unused plantation land to landless labourers led to opposition from elitist groups, and particularly from the American-owned United Fruit Company. In 1954 a CIA-sponsored coup d'état ended ten years of democratic rule; civil liberties were curtailed, and social justice organizations were systematically dismantled.

As in El Salvador, state-sponsored violence has been rampant in Guatemala from the mid-1950s onward, and wealthy members of the elite have used the military to control and oppress the civilian population. Government efforts to suppress human rights and freedoms resulted in the emergence of the Guatemalan Revolutionary Unity (URNG) coalition of guerrillas.

Government death squads sought to curtail rebellion, more than 100,000 people were killed or "disappeared," and many more suffered violent abuses of their human rights, including torture.

Despite several attempts at democratically resolving the political tensions, it was only in 1996 that the civil war officially ended with the signing of a peace accord between the government and the guerrilla coalition. Although violence has definitely declined, it still occurs. In 1998, a Roman Catholic bishop was murdered after releasing a report on human rights abuses. This sparked a huge outcry and demands for justice, which resulted in the conviction of four men. His was the most prominent of an ongoing number of similar assassinations. However, there have been positive changes such as more freedom for the press and improved economic opportunities.

The Maya: The Indigenous People of Guatemala

Unlike other countries in Central America, Guatemala has a large indigenous population, the Mayan people, who in 2004 made up 80 percent of the population. Most contemporary Maya speak one or several of four main Mayan languages of which there are many dialects. Most Mayan people live and work in their own agricultural communities, do not speak Spanish, and are not active participants in mainstream Guatemalan urban culture.

In 2004 it is estimated that there are between four and five hundred Mayan people in Vancouver. Most arrived in the 1990s. They encountered special challenges when they came to Canada, usually as government- and group-sponsored refugees. Here in Canada they are routinely mistaken for Spanish-speaking Latin Americans. They struggle to raise awareness of who they are, fielding frustrating questions about their origins. Many Maya are mistaken for Spanish Guatemalans, and there is a widespread lack of knowledge or understanding of their experiences in their home country. As visible minorities with little or no English, Maya are also faced with racism and discrimination. All these factors create barriers to their use of the health care system. Here we will provide some information that may serve to raise awareness of Mayan people, their culture, and the circumstances that have brought them to Canada.

Mayan People and Culture

Mayan people have lived in parts of Mexico, Guatemala, El Salvador, Belize, and Honduras for thousands of years. Since the earliest times they have been agriculturists who also farm, hunt, and fish. After AD 300, Mayan society became extremely hierarchical, with kings ruling over a large population of farmers. The Maya are best known for developing complex trade networks, building great pyramids, and mastering mathematics, hieroglyphic writing, astronomy, and architecture.

In 2004 the Maya continue to practise agriculture. They grow their own corn, vegetables, and herbs and raise chickens and cows. This provides food for their families, and money is often scarce. Some Maya work as landless labourers for wealthy plantation owners, while others are merchants who sell traditional crafts. Many couples have large families, with up to ten children, who contribute to the household economy by helping their parents. Some boys may attend school for a short period of time where they learn Spanish as a second language, but few girls do so. Consequently, many people have poor reading or writing skills. Traditional remedies are used to treat illness; few Maya will have ever visited a medical doctor. Pregnancy is a normal, happy event, and women give birth in their homes with the help of experienced women in their own communities.

Colonization of the Mayan Region

The Maya have experienced significant persecution throughout their history of contact with Spanish and European peoples. When they were attacked and colonized by the Spanish in the early 1500s, they had already suffered considerable losses from civil wars and the new European diseases that had spread throughout the region from Mexico, preceding the invaders.

During the thirty-six years of civil war that ripped through Guatemala in the last century, Mayan men were drafted by the military and forced to fight against the URNG guerrilla coalition; some rebelled and joined the guerrillas to fight the army. Approximately 200,000 people died during the war, mostly Maya; others became political prisoners, were tortured, or were "disappeared" (*Economist* 2004). During this period entire Mayan villages were massacred, creating a flood of Mayan refugees into Chiapas in Mexico, the United States, and Canada. These refugees often arrived in a state of grief and shock, having lost their entire families in the conflict and leaving all their belongings in Guatemala.

In 1999 Guatemala held a referendum to amend the Constitution of Guatemala to recognize and uphold the unique indigenous languages, customs, and religions of Mayan people. Though the referendum failed and these amendments were not instituted, the changed political mood at the turn of the century promises hope for Mayan people. Following his 2004 inauguration, the new president of Guatemala has made moves that indicate some support for increased indigenous rights, for limited compensation to war victims, and for adherence to the United Nations peace accords. Canadian government sponsorship of Mayan refugees ceased in the late 1990s as the international community observed the improved political climate in Guatemala. However, in 2004 sporadic kidnappings, rapes, and murders of Maya persist, so that Mayan people continue to struggle towards self-determination and remain distrustful and uncertain about their future.

Contemporary Mayan women are the group in Guatemala most discriminated against. Unlike traditional Mayan women, who remain valued in their own communities, Mayan women trying to make their way within the dominant Spanish and mestizo society of Guatemala experience systemic sexism and racism. Repeated negative experiences of this kind over time diminish Mayan women's self-esteem and confidence and place enormous strain on their mental health. However, after large numbers of Mayan men were killed during the civil war years, many Mayan women whose traditional roles were centred on home and family took work outside of their homes and assumed positions of leadership in their communities. As a result Mayan women have emerged as powerful new actors in the national fight for social justice.

In 2004 the living conditions for the Maya in Guatemala are poor. Persistent health problems include malnutrition and infant mortality. Their diet is limited to corn-based food and vegetables because many families cannot afford to purchase meat except as an occasional luxury. Most Maya remain illiterate. Basic services such as running water and electricity are also uncommon in Mayan rural communities.

Special Challenges for Maya in Canada

In the 1990s Maya arrived in Canada both alone and in families with children. The Canadian government and humanitarian and religious groups sponsored these refugees. Many had spent years living in exile in Chiapas in Mexico before coming to Canada. Sponsored Maya usually arrived on flights that were paid for with government loans. In 2004 few Maya continue to arrive because government refugee sponsorship programs no longer assist this group; Mayans who come now are individuals who found their own way here as asylum seekers.

There are no agencies in Canada that provide services in Mayan languages. Since Maya are usually unable to speak English or French when they arrive here, they are often expected to communicate in Spanish, which many do not speak. Even those who do speak Spanish are mistrustful because of the persecution they have experienced at the hands of Spanish-speaking people and persons in authority. Mayan people tend not to mix voluntarily with the Spanish-descended Latin Americans in Canada, although they may find themselves being expected to trust and confide in health professionals and authorities of Spanish descent.

While the Mayan community in Canada is small and Mayan families tend to know one another, the group is fragmented by the anxiety and divisive loyalties formed during the civil war. Brothers in the same Mayan family may have joined opposing sides in the Guatemalan civil war, some fighting with the guerrillas, others with the army. Family members may have been murdered by one side or both. Consequently Mayan immigrants may not feel safe in their own community, even in Canada.

As with other immigrants and refugees having large families, Maya can experience problems finding housing, especially as some agencies will not provide housing unless there is a room for every child. Difficulties with language barriers can make it very hard for Maya to find gainful employment. For these reasons many Maya may find it difficult to survive in the urban centres of Canada; they may choose to settle in the BC interior, especially the Okanagan, where they can do familiar agricultural work.

The mental health of Mayan refugees may be fragile even many years after their arrival in Canada. Most people have suffered tremendously: loss and separation from close family members, kidnappings, torture, and exile. Many arrived in Canada engulfed in grief and continue to suffer from symptoms of post-traumatic stress syndrome. (More detailed information about these mental health issues can be found in Chapter 8: Refugees in Canada.)

Many Maya may continue to wear traditional clothing in Canada. However, their school-age children usually wear Western clothing and are fluent in English. Families may find it difficult to continue to eat their traditional diet of mostly corn-based and fresh produce. Women who do not have English may initially find that using the bus system is difficult; they may depend on corner stores that do not have familiar fresh vegetables or fruit. These unwelcome changes to their traditional diet may have some negative effects upon their physical and mental health.

Before coming to Canada, many Mayan people never sought help from a medical health professional, so they may be unsure of their role in this kind of encounter. In their country, people took care of their own families and used traditional medicine and spiritual healing. In Canada, Mayan women may prefer to visit female physicians, and the shortage of female doctors here can become a barrier to their use of the Canadian health system. Some women may tolerate illness and visit a male doctor only for great pain; diseases may go undetected, bringing, in the long term, more health complications for women. Only when a woman has established a trust-based relationship with a Canadian family doctor may it become possible for her to learn of the importance of regular preventive physical exams such as mammograms or Pap tests.

Like many refugees and immigrants, Mayan women may also be suspicious of the Western medical approach to pregnancy and labour. Women who arrive in Canada with five children may wonder why they are encouraged to have prenatal medical check-ups, attend prenatal classes, or give birth in the hospital. In particular, labour in the hospital can be a disturbing experience for women accustomed to giving birth in their own homes surrounded by loving and skilful community midwives. The impersonal atmosphere of

Liy, from Guatemala

Liy, sixteen, sat with her mother in the school office in Chilliwack, waiting to see the psychologist. The school counsellor was concerned that Liy often failed to come to school, and, when she did attend, her teachers found her very tired and unable to concentrate. Liy looked drawn. That morning again she had wakened exhausted and anxious. The psychologist asked her to talk about her home situation. When she refused to respond, her mother told their story in broken English.

They had finally begun to feel "settled" in Canada after three extremely stressful years. Liy's father worked six days a week on a farm outside Chilliwack where they lived. Although he was happy to be doing work he knew, the hours were long, from 5:00 a.m. to 7:00 p.m., and the work was exhausting. Two nights each week Liy's mother rushed off to ESL class at the local community centre. She was happy to have learned to communicate in basic English but felt constantly worn out attending to their six children. Neither parent had time to spend with Liy, their eldest daughter. In fact they relied on her to help care for the others.

They had arrived in Canada in 1995, still in shock, grieving for two of their children and many relatives who had died in a paramilitary raid on their village. Their small house had burned down, and they lost all their belongings. Fleeing for their lives, they walked across the border from Guatemala to Mexico and spent one year in a refugee camp.

When they arrived at the airport in Canada, an immigration officer called in a Spanish-speaking officer, who quickly realized that Liy understood some Spanish while her parents spoke only Mayan. Liy was terrified and confused. She had been taught never to answer Spanish-speaking officials to avoid endangering her family, and she was fearful of all authorities, including the Canadian official for the same reason. To this day she has great difficulty speaking to authorities such as the teachers and counsellors at school.

As the children in the family began to seem more settled, Liy, who had coped so well during their escape to Mexico and their journey to Canada, became increasingly withdrawn. She had learned English extremely quickly and became the parents' interpreter when they rented their house, enrolled a child in kindergarten, and went to parent-teacher conferences at school. She began sleeping late on school days and missing the school bus. But at home she was needed to care for the younger children while her mother did the household chores.

Liy hated going to school in Canada. Often she woke up exhausted, having had only about four hours of sleep. Her sleep was regularly broken by frightening dreams about that terrible day in Guatemala. Sometimes in class she thought of her two dead sisters and her heart would race, her hands would tremble, and she would feel nauseous. She tended to stay in bed late so that she could stay home where she was needed. Her school work was bad since she seldom had time to do homework in the evenings, and she felt ashamed being placed in the grade beneath her age group. When she was at school she was treated like a child, but at home she had adult responsibilities. The other girls at school seemed so childish; they just talked about their looks and boys, and they didn't even seem to care about their families. She could not fit in. Her accent was heavy; she was the only girl in her class with brown skin; and she looked "healthy," or by comparison with her classmates, "plump."

Liy thought, "Everything was going well until the school principal called in the psychologist to talk with my mother. Family counselling! How could I put my parents through this? If only I could tell them how afraid I was when I had been acting so brave all along." She thought of how hard her mother and father worked to improve their lives, of how successfully they had forgotten about the past; after all, they never talked with her about it. "My family needs me to be strong; they will be so disappointed in me. I mustn't think about being sad, my brothers and sisters need me and Mom will start crying again if I tell her how I really feel."

the hospital setting, the bright lighting, and the unnatural labour aids, such as epidurals or Caesarean sections, can be extremely intimidating.

Mayan women may arrive in Canada expecting to be subject to the kind of systemic discrimination they experienced in urban Guatemalan society. However, after a period of adjustment, some women will gain self-confidence as they learn their rights in Canada. It is challenging for women to find a balance between their traditional roles in Mayan culture, to unlearn negative self-beliefs born from racism in Guatemalan society, and to feel comfortable with their new rights and responsibilities in Canada. Making these adaptations to life in Canada can create challenges in their relationships with their husbands and children and in extreme cases may bring separation or divorce.

As with many refugees, it can be extremely hard for Mayan people to think of Canada as home because they did not voluntarily leave Guatemala behind. Since about 2000 it has been considered fairly safe for Mayan refugees to return to Guatemala to visit families and home communities. But atrocities occasionally still occur, and any refugee planning a visit back must seriously weigh the possible dangers. Many Mayan immigrants to Canada dream of being able one day to return home permanently with no fear for the lives of themselves or their families.

Nicaragua

The current situation in Nicaragua is somewhat different from those of Guatemala and El Salvador, although their histories share elements in common, such as governments by a wealthy elite backed by the military. From 1933 until 1979 the country was ruled by Anastasio Somoza, and later by his son. In 1979 the Sandinista National Liberation Front, a coalition group opposed to the Somoza reign, led and won a fight to topple the regime. The hope was that the new government would reduce economic disparity, corruption, and violence and improve living conditions. However, Marxist forces within the Sandinistas held majority power, and a combination of factors, including an ongoing civil war and an adherence to Communist principles, brought further hardships to the country. The development of allegiances with Cuba and the Soviet Union led to the drying up of American aid and the enactment of an American import embargo. Despite rising national debt and corruption, the Sandinistas did make strides in implementing health and education programs. The objective was to bring health professionals and facilities to the rural areas, and to integrate active and interested locals into a preventive health care system.

The country went on to have the lowest annual income of any nation in the Western Hemisphere. Many wealthy Nicaraguans left during the civil war, and many young men fled to escape military service and have not returned. Immigrants to Canada can be from widely different political backgrounds. The 1990s saw the election of right-of-centre presidents, who have brought more stability and some improvement in the economy. The development of a special free-trade zone for assembling garments and other products, the maquiladora, has helped somewhat with unemployment. Coffee is the biggest export crop, but the health of that industry depends on the international price, which has been low in recent years. Many producers are in debt. Hurricane Mitch in 1998 was devastating both to lives and to the economy.

Poverty remains the biggest social issue in Nicaragua. Many people are landless and compelled to work for landlords who do not pay enough money to live on. There is a strong international aid presence with many development projects such as Swedish- and Taiwanese-sponsored hospitals. Access to health care varies greatly depending on location and economic means. In 2004 there were 3.7 births per woman; the infant mortality rate was thirty-two per thousand live births, very high in contrast to the Canadian rate of five.

Honduras

Hondurans began to arrive in British Columbia in the 1990s. Honduras is a very poor nation, with the typical Central American history of Spanish colonization of indigenous people's land and resources, followed by centuries of rule by a small aristocratic landholding class (called *terra tenientes*) over a much larger land-poor peasant class. Fortunately, Honduras has not seen civil war, as was experienced in nearby countries. However, many struggles have arisen, and continue to rage, over landownership and ongoing poverty, resulting in murders and violence. Caught physically between Nicaragua and El Salvador, Honduras has received refugees from those countries and been used as a military staging place by American troops and others who wish to have influence in the region. For example, the Misquito Indians resident in the northwest corner of Nicaragua fled into Honduras as refugees following a violent effort by the Nicaraguan government to relocate their communities.

Honduras became a democracy in 1982, and has been politically stable since then, with right-of-centre governments. The economy has traditionally been based on bananas, grown on large American-owned farms. Recently coffee has become the primary crop. Peasants have limited access to arable land. In 1998, Hurricane Mitch hit Honduras hardest of all, and caused huge devastation to the national infrastructure, the reconstruction of which resulted in large increases in international debt.

In Honduras it is estimated that trained health workers attend 56 percent of births. Families are often large, with a fertility rate of 4.0 children per woman. The percentage of adults with HIV/AIDS is 1.67, the highest of all Central American countries.

Immigrants to British Columbia are mostly young single men, many of them minors. They have usually left Honduras in search of economic opportunities, many with the hope of returning to Honduras with enough money to establish their own business. Many send money home from Canada. However, once here they face unique problems. Since Honduras does not have a history of civil war, Hondurans are commonly perceived to be "economic refugees," thus making it almost impossible for them to become protected persons, and then permanent residents, in Canada. Land conflicts are not as easily recognized by the Immigration and Refugee Board, even though claimants may face murder if they are sent home.

The majority of Honduran asylum seekers are denied refugee status and ordered to return to their home country. Some of these individuals, having returned to Honduras, soon come back to Canada to make more money and again claim asylum. With this pattern, many young Honduran men perceive their stays in Canada as temporary. They head to large urban centres in Canada, hoping to make fast cash to take back home. With an illiteracy rate of about 40 percent (in Spanish, higher in English), uncertain legal status, and language barriers, young Honduran men usually have a hard time finding legitimate work in Canada, and some become involved in the drug trade with its offer of quick rewards.

For the most part, Hondurans are not considered by agencies that serve immigrants and refugees to be demanding on the system. It is estimated that Hondurans who decide to stay take only two years on average to settle into life in Canada, perhaps partly because of the extensive kin networks and large Latin American communities that provide social, financial, and emotional support to newcomers.

While most Honduran asylum seekers are men or male minors, some women may also leave Honduras, fleeing domestic violence.

Mexico

By 2004, more people are coming to Canada from Mexico than in the past. Mexico's political and economic history, like that of other countries in Central America, differs significantly from Canada's. However, Mexican immigrants overall will have experienced greater access to health care and education than those from other Central American countries. For example, 86 percent of births are attended by trained persons, and literacy is high, at

91 percent. The election of President Vicente Fox in 1997 ended more than a century of rule by one political party. With him came promises to decrease corruption and provide universal access to health care. Mexico has both a private and a public health care system, and many physicians work in both. Mexicans new to Canada may expect a system which gives better care to those who can pay privately, whereas the Canadian system gives universal access to good quality care.

Immigrants from Mexico may come from huge industrialized cities, such as Mexico City, or from rural areas. In general, the southern parts of the country experience more poverty than the north. The south is also home to many Maya, both native and refugees from neighbouring Guatemala. Southern Mexico has seen political violence throughout the 1990s, particularly in the state of Chiapas, prompting international agencies to investigate human rights abuses there. In the north, many people work in the factories bordering the United States. While wages and working conditions in these factories are lower than in North America, the jobs are attractive to local people because they are better than other available work. Many Mexicans have experienced violence related to drug cartels, especially along northern border areas. Layers of corruption in the police, judicial, and political systems have impeded control of the drug trade as well as created a culture of mistrust of legal and other authorities. A number of immigrants arrive as agricultural workers hoping to find temporary work such as fruit-picking in order to send money home. These workers are usually single and male. Settlement workers in Vancouver note that Mexicans generally assimilate into Canadian culture more quickly than Latin American peoples from more southern countries.

Costa Rica

Costa Rica, located south of Nicaragua, has had a stable political and economic history. Settled by the Spanish in the 1500s, the country has experienced prosperity, initially through coffee and bananas and more recently through high-tech assembly plants. Costa Ricans have a very high literacy rate of 96 percent and a much higher standard of living than other countries in the region. The country has 178 physicians per 100,000 people, compared to 186 in Canada. Political unrest in neighbouring Nicaragua saw the entry of refugees into Costa Rica and an increase in violent crime. Since tourism is a developing industry, crime reduction has become a major political goal. Costa Ricans who come to Canada are usually immigrating, though some Costa Ricans also claim asylum in Canada.

Colombia

Colombia is located at the northwest corner of South America, adjacent to Central America. Violence has characterized its political history from Spanish colonization to the twenty-first century. Spanish colonizers were met by strong resistance from the indigenous people who were already living there. In 2004 Colombia was one of the most dangerous places in the world to live, producing an estimated 70 percent of the world's kidnappings (Mennonite Committee Council 2004). Decades of civil war between the national liberal and conservative parties have fostered political corruption, improper elections, and violence. The civilian population has been ruled by dictators and terrorized by powerful, autonomous right-wing paramilitary and left-wing guerrilla groups. Since 2002 the elected president has introduced extraordinary military measures to crush guerrilla insurgencies, yet he has failed to implement United Nations recommendations to dismantle the paramilitary groups or to discipline the armed forces that commit human rights abuses against the civilian population.

The economic interests of international investors and members of the military continue to rely on the proliferation of the cocaine trade. One estimate is that 60 percent of Colombians are economically linked to the drug trade. Coca leaves from other Latin American countries are processed into cocaine in Colombia, which is then shipped to markets in North America and Europe, often through northern Mexico. This has resulted in tremendous, unregulated wealth in the hands of drug lords. Armed conflicts between the national army, the various drug cartels, and guerrilla groups who oppose the government have resulted in thousands of deaths. Violence is so pervasive that authorities (police, judges, and so on) who speak out against it are in real danger of being murdered. The cost of hiring someone to kill a targeted police officer or judge is a few thousand dollars, a trivial amount to wealthy drug lords. Complicating the situation are strong American anti-drug policies, which, for example, until recently, allowed foreign aid to counter only drug activities but not violence from other sources.

At the turn of the century the situation in Colombia worsened as paramilitary groups employed scorched earth tactics similar to those used in the genocide against Maya in Guatemala, "killing community leaders, burning entire villages, and driving inhabitants from their homes" (Amnesty International Canada 2004). Every year in Colombia 26,000 to 30,000 violent deaths and 3,000 kidnappings are reported (Mennonite Committee Council 2004). Most Colombians come to Canada as government-sponsored refugees under the "urgent protection" program (see Chapter 8: Refugees in Canada). Most will have experienced and witnessed repeated human rights violations, either personally or within their family. Many Colombian refugees to Canada are professionals who have been targeted for violence. These people often held respected positions with good incomes, and their change in status once in Canada can be very stressful.

Migration to Canada

Most permanent residents from Central America originally arrived in Canada as government-sponsored refugees or as asylum seekers. (For details about refugees, see Chapter 8: Refugees in Canada.) A refugee is someone who is compelled to leave home for reasons of pressing personal safety and well-being. The person concerned may have heard that he or she was on a new government "hit list," may have witnessed the abduction or murder of friends or family members, or may have had home and crops destroyed by the military or a rich landlord. He or she may also have experienced detention and torture.

Refugees from Central America usually fall into one of four groups. One group consists of politically active opponents of the current regime who are forced into exile in fear for their lives. Often middle-class professionals, these people may come to Canada as government-sponsored refugees or arrive independently as asylum seekers. They feel a strong bond with the home country and hope to return some day. A second group is the rural peasant population, whose homes may be under general attack and who flee to neighbouring countries or regions for shelter. Sometimes a whole village, consisting primarily of women, children, and the elderly, may move. These people also hope to return home, and are often sponsored to come to Canada by humanitarian or church organizations or the federal government, and they may be the beneficiaries of international resettlement schemes to establish them as subsistence agriculturalists in Canada.

Most refugees coming to Canada fall into a third group. These people have not been active politically, although they may have been members of a trade union or a similar organization. They are generally urban working-class people or labourers who are able to gather the means to move northwards to the United States or Canada. These people, often single men, may be nostalgic for the ways of home but wish to settle and become established in Canada. They usually make their own way to Canada and claim asylum once they arrive. A small number of urban working people who are not refugees may apply as skilled workers from their home country and be accepted into Canada in the normal way as permanent residents.

A fourth group, Mayan refugees from Guatemala, arrived predominantly during the 1990s when they were sponsored by the Canadian government. Since the signing of the peace accord in 1996, Mayan refugees must find their own way to come to Canada as asylum seekers, and they may apply for refugee status once here.

For many people the road to Canada is an indirect one, with lengthy stops in Mexico, Honduras, and, more commonly, the United States. Until February 1987 it was fairly easy for illegal residents in the United States to find jobs, and some people set up home and had children while there. For them, migration to Canada has meant not only leaving the original community in Central America, but also leaving the new home in the United States. These people have the advantage of at least having more exposure to North American customs, food, expectations, and so on and, most important, have had the chance to learn some English.

As Chapter 8 shows, the social, psychological and economic implications of being a refugee affect every individual deeply and uniquely. The acculturation process is an arduous one that is fraught with difficulties.

Settlement in Canada

In the early 1980s, when the first Central Americans began to come to Canada in any number, young working-class men who were single or who had left their wives behind were the most common. By 2000, there had been an increase in the number of families, most fairly young. Elderly people rarely come as immigrants or refugees. Both rural and urban people come, although the latter are the most common, and urban areas are more attractive as destinations in Canada. Many of these people have spent up to three or four years living and working in the United States, gaining experience and skills that are valuable when seeking work here. Like the Maya from Guatemala, a significant minority of refugees and immigrants from Latin America are illiterate in Spanish, which makes the task of learning written English very difficult.

The shock of being in Canada can last one to three years and often longer, as people learn the language, finalize their immigration status, establish a home in the new community, find jobs, and so on. While community and church groups, as well as concerned individuals, put tremendous amounts of time, energy, and money into sponsoring refugees or helping them to adjust to life in Canada, many refugees are bewildered by the refugee and immigration process.

Most immigrants worked hard at their jobs and were active in family and community life back in Central America and are extremely unhappy about accepting charity and being seen as burdens to Canada. The government settlement procedures for refugees can be humiliating for individuals who have a history of being exploited and abused by anonymous officials or professionals in their home country. The shame experienced can be particularly harmful to the health and well-being of some Latin American men.

For example, in Canada, Guatemalan men have described losing the gender privileges that they "deserve as" men, such as being the sole decision maker and breadwinner for the family. Back home, social, financial, and emotional needs were usually met within their own extended, well-known kin networks. Unlike in Canada, a family would find an apartment or house through social and family contacts. In a bank or other public office, one would deal only with staff known to the family. From such a background it is easy to believe that services provided by persons unconnected with the family are worthless or even dangerous. Although initial guidance about Canadian procedures may help alleviate these concerns, the patterns of seeking social support within kin networks usually continue within the large Latin American communities that have established themselves in the urban centres in Canada (Leslie 1992). In this respect, individuals from Central America may be slow to adapt to mainstream society.

Once a refugee finds a job, many initial adjustment problems begin to be resolved. Although lack of English fluency often means that jobs are low-paying or menial, self-esteem improves, in that the person no longer feels like an object of charity. Minors who have to come to Canada alone are especially vulnerable to being enticed into employment ventures or activities that promise fast cash. Both men and women look for work, and even though small children may prevent a mother from leaving home, the women are often more successful in finding initial employment. This can provoke extreme anxiety in husbands, who are accustomed to being the family breadwinner. Typical jobs for both sexes include housecleaning, dishwashing in restaurants, cutting and sewing in factories, and cleaning windows.

Middle-class professional refugees, while happy to work, may become bitter about the marked decline in income and social status associated with the available jobs. Highly skilled, and often very experienced, these people are suddenly no longer valuable and esteemed. For many there is little hope of resuming their careers in Canada. For example, immigrant physicians cannot receive the necessary residency training in hospitals even if they pass the qualifying exams. This is particularly frustrating, given the media reports about the lack of medical services in northern and rural Canada. They have the skills and the willingness to go to these areas but are prevented from doing so.

Language

For nearly all Central American immigrants, the primary obstacle to getting settled, finding jobs, and obtaining satisfactory medical care is the lack of ability in English, a difficulty exacerbated for Mayan refugees who speak only their own indigenous languages. Those accepted as protected persons outside of Canada through the sponsorship program are entitled to five months of free English classes through the LINC program (Language Instruction for Newcomers to Canada). But others (the great majority) who come independently to the border to seek refugee status are provided only with funding for food and shelter.

Church groups, school boards, concerned volunteers, community centres, and some public libraries offer free or very inexpensive language classes. But even after six months or so of instruction, many people still lack the confidence to accept jobs requiring English proficiency, or even to participate fully in the life of the larger Anglo-Canadian community. As one Guatemalan man explained, his difficulties speaking English harm his health and hinder his adaptation to Canada: "You are afraid to do something or to get something for yourself, because most of the time they will reject you because they don't understand you. Not all of the time of course, but most of the time people are rude and they don't really pay attention to what you are trying to say. And as I don't speak English very well, sometimes I get trapped in my own mumble because I am nervous" (Dunn 2000, 133). The fact that a subgroup of the refugee population is illiterate in their native language makes matters even worse, because their ability to learn is severely handicapped. For women with children, the pressures of having to go to classes and find child care on a very limited budget add to the stress, creating significant anxiety.

Experience with Canadians

Central American refugees overall are deeply grateful for the aid and shelter provided in Canada, but language difficulties and financial restrictions are the main obstacles to developing friendships with many non-Latin Canadians. In most Canadian urban centres there are large Latin communities of fellow Spanish-speaking immigrants to provide companionship and help. The overwhelming support given by the community to needy members speaks volumes for the group's generosity and compassion.

In terms of social life, the predominantly working-class Central Americans do not associate with the professionals who came as political refugees from Chile and Argentina in the 1970s. Despite their common language, the groups differ in socio-cultural aspects, and the professionals have adapted more easily and have become largely integrated into Canadian society.

Special Problems in Canada

Minors in Canada

In Central America, young males from very poor villages may decide to travel to Canada with dreams of making money to send back to their families. Some minors leave their homes in search of brothers or cousins who have already left for Canada. They may fail to inform anyone of their plans and simply travel overland, panhandling for money on the way. Having reached British Columbia, for example, as minors they fall under the jurisdiction of the Ministry for Children and Family Development. The ministry has a responsibility either to place these young asylum seekers, or "economic refugees," in a Spanish-speaking foster family or to offer minimal financial support for them to live independently. The latter option is more commonly chosen by young men who do not want their freedoms curtailed: financial assistance in Vancouver in 2001 included $325 per month allocated for rent and $185 for all other necessities. While these allowances may seem generous to youths who have come from poverty-stricken areas, they soon learn that the amounts are not sufficient in Canada to find safe accommodation and food.

As minors in Canada, these young men can become a burden on the limited resources of refugee-serving agencies because advocating for them with provincial social services and providing both language and cultural interpretation is time-consuming and complex. For example, refugee settlement workers may sometimes have to explain to a Canadian social worker that it is not possible simply to call and speak to a minor's family. Many parents do not have a telephone; many villages have only one telephone. In fact, many parents will not even know that their son is in Canada.

While some minors are drawn to Canada in order to participate in the illegal drug trade, most come with no prior experience of drug use. They tend to have naïve intentions of finding legitimate employment, despite their lack of English or a formal education. For these minors, it is their idealism that brings them and their youth that makes them vulnerable to predatory adults.

Racism and Discrimination

Latin Americans are visible minorities in Canada, and many individuals encounter racism and the negative stereotypes of involvement in drug dealing and prostitution. These images are frustrating for the majority of young Latin American men who are not even remotely involved in these activities. They may find themselves targeted by police for random body searches or wrongly accused of criminal activity.

Changes in Family Roles

As with many other immigrant peoples, the role changes between husbands and wives as they adjust to Canadian life can also be a problem for Central American families. In Central America the man traditionally has the responsibility of providing for his family's needs, usually as the sole breadwinner. Wives have the traditional responsibilities of keeping the home, bearing and raising children, cooking, cleaning, maintaining health, and so on. The opportunities in Canada for women to find work threaten the man's traditional status. When wives are the first to find work, husbands may experience depression. Some men discourage their wives from learning English or, in severe cases, resort to violence. In the latter instance, the woman's entitlement in Canada to police protection and legal redress may shock her husband even further and be seen as a direct challenge to his marital rights. Support, counselling, and an explanation of Canadian notions of basic human rights can help to resolve these difficulties.

Problems can also arise between generations. Some of the few elderly people who have come to Canada feel that they are no longer regarded as sources of family knowledge and no longer enjoy the deep respect they were accorded in Central America. Instead they may feel ill used, as if they had become mere live-in babysitters and house cleaners.

Raising teenagers in Canada presents a host of difficulties in addition to the normal stresses of adolescence. While boys in Central America are allowed considerable freedom and have few domestic responsibilities, girls are not permitted to stay out late, to date and associate with anyone they please, and so on. They also cook, clean, and care for younger siblings. Some parents are shocked by the behaviour and values of Canadian teenagers and think them a bad influence on their own children, especially the girls. Working out some kind of satisfactory compromise within the family therefore becomes difficult. Parents can feel betrayed by the government when children who have moved away from home receive welfare money for rent and food. They believe strongly that they know what is best for their children. During the early years of life in Canada, power struggles can also arise when children are the first to learn English and parents become dependent on them for translation and interactions with authorities.

The Central American Community

Central Americans in Canada often avoid discussing political issues amongst themselves. People with differing political views may avoid interaction, even if they belong to the same church. For example, while an upper-class family from Nicaragua may idealize their past life and enjoy visiting their home country and staying in luxurious resorts, another family of labourers from the countryside will undoubtedly have a contrasting perspective.

Religion

While the statistics from Central America indicate that nearly everyone is Roman Catholic, there is considerable religious diversity among Latin Americans in Canada. Many are active Catholics, who accept the church both as provider of social support and as a major participant in community life. (In Central America, religious festivals mark the calendar much more strongly than in Canada, with such events as Carnival being celebrated as festive holidays.) Others are non-practising members of the church, with varying degrees of commitment to Catholic belief and ritual. Some are Protestants, either by birth or conversion. The aid given by particular church groups to refugees has resulted in some immigrants joining those churches. Evangelization is also taking place with some success in Central America itself. The Mennonites, Jehovah's Witnesses, Mormons, and Baha'i are among the denominations which have Central American followers. Mayan refugees from Guatemala may combine their traditional spiritual beliefs with some Christian practices.

Family Structure

When a couple marries in Central America, they are expected to set up an independent household which is intimately, though not physically, tied to the extended families on both sides. The husband is head of the family, but important decisions, including those concerning health care, will generally be made in consultation with the wider family. The number of children in a family may range from four to six, but the high cost of living in Canada may cause some couples to practise family planning. Some of the social supports and services that were available and affordable in Central America are unattainable in Canada, such as having a maid to help with household chores or having relatives available to babysit or take over housekeeping during periods of family sickness.

The extended family is made up of blood relatives, kin, and godparents, creating a widespread net of social, business, professional, and bureaucratic connections. Assuming a role that comes from Christian tradition, godparents play an important and serious role in nearly all social aspects of a Latin American child's life. They have the right to offer advice to parents and are expected to care for the child in the event of the parents' death. Extra sets of godparents are added at communion and marriage, and will provide food and money for the celebrations. In El Salvador, for example, the bridal couple's godmother brings an elaborate, delicious cake, while the godfather gives the groom a pouch of silver coins with which to "buy" his bride. More importantly, godparents enlarge the communal links of trust and security for the couple and their children.

Marriage and Divorce

In many Latin American countries people tend to marry much younger than in Canada. Women will be between sixteen and nineteen years of age, while men are in their early twenties. Virginity is considered important for women though not for men. Common-law unions are rare and frowned upon, as marriage is seen to provide legal security for the wife and children.

The frequency of divorce varies greatly between classes and religious groups. Affluent urban residents are believed to have more divorces than others. Practising Catholics, especially those living in rural areas, are far less likely to divorce, even in extreme situations. For women, the stigma of divorce can be a heavy burden, but some are willing to risk this rather than live with a man who is abusive or keeps a mistress. After divorce, the most common method of obtaining support is for the woman and her children to return to her family's home. The husband's family may also take responsibility for raising a child, especially a son.

Women

When a baby is expected, the parents keenly anticipate the arrival of the child, although their expectations for a child of either sex are not necessarily the same. As in other areas of the world, a girl will grow up with the paramount objective of becoming wife, mother, and home-maker. Naturally, every individual interprets these ideas differently, and a small but active feminist community in Central America is beginning to voice its opposition to the traditional roles and inequalities.

Customarily and ideally, the woman's territory is the home, while men are responsible for activities away from the domestic sphere. For this work, women are theoretically esteemed and respected, but this can often lead to a false evaluation of status. While domestic labour undeniably involves hard physical work, long hours, and few monetary rewards, it is not esteemed as highly by either men or women as male wage labour. Among Central American immigrants, it is regarded as demeaning as well as burdensome for a husband to take over child care duties if his wife is the first to find a paying job. Some women will even refrain from seeking outside work until their husbands are employed. However, in Canada immigrant women are more likely to find jobs than are men.

In the Central American countries, general unemployment is very high, so that jobs for women are scarce, particularly well-paid and respected jobs. Even if the financial resources are available, women seldom pursue high school, technical, or university education, thus limiting their employment prospects even more. Instead, financial security is sought in marriage, which is seen to hold the promise of support by the husband for his wife and children. This valuation is so strong that a dependent wife is likely to tolerate her husband's mistress, albeit uneasily. The mistress is also seeking economic support, and by bearing a child with the man's name she makes a financial claim on him. This view of marriage reinforces a husband's belief that he can use physical force in arguments with his wife. Some women come to Canada seeking asylum for reasons of domestic abuse in their home country.

Nevertheless, women's role in the home and community has strengthening and enriching sides, and more often than not it is the women who hold the family together during the stresses of flight and relocation. Yet most women coming to North America enjoy a marked improvement in legal rights and social or work opportunities. This is certainly so for their daughters. This change in status can exacerbate marital and family tensions.

For many women, the biggest problem faced in Canada, aside from financial and immigration worries, is isolation. Language barriers, physical distance, reserved Canadian neighbours, and busy North American schedules put limits on Central American–style casual hospitality. Immigrant women learn to tolerate a degree of concern and anxiety which they would not unburden on their mothers even at home. Isolation can come in many forms. A typical sorrow confronting immigrant women arises when one or more children must be left behind in Central America. When parents leave their home countries, they do not always have sufficient resources to bring every child, either in money or in the sheer physical carrying power to walk to Mexico and swim the Rio Grande. They usually hope that money will be found quickly to bring the child north.

Men

Much attention has been paid to the concept of *machismo* in Latin American societies. Many Latin American men may describe themselves as "*macho*," but their understandings of the concept vary. Some see a *macho* man as courageous, acting with confidence as a leader in household and community, and keeping his problems to himself. Not all believe (though some may) that being *macho* involves dominating their families and resorting to regular physical and sexual violence to control their wives. It is important not to stereotype *machismo* as conforming to the aggressive image. Men's experiences of their gendered identities and roles in Latin American countries are diverse, and the changes that they face in Canadian society are complex, often affecting their health and well-being.

Many men have been raised to exhibit strength and courage, and to believe that sadness and depression are weak emotions, not to be expressed through crying or shared through talking to others, especially outsiders. For this reason, men may find it difficult to articulate their confusion and turmoil in Canada, and they may cling to rigid routines and the roles they previously held. "Life in a new country for Latin American men ... tends to be devastating to their sense of self," and in extreme frustration some men may begin to express themselves through violence towards others (Dunn 2000, 141). In these situations men may need encouragement in seeking help from outsiders, in relearning gender roles and new interpersonal behaviours.

Children

In Latin American countries children are universally welcomed, and a large family is often a measure of status, especially in rural areas. While the parents, especially the mother, are the primary sources of care, the extended family shares in these responsibilities. Young children often spend their playtime roaming the streets in groups, visiting neighbours, and playing games. Immigrants from urban areas will use bottle-feeding and disposable diapers for infants whenever possible as these are signs of technological progress and financial status. Child discipline is variable, though there may be more physical discipline among the urban middle and upper classes than among rural families.

The Elderly

At present there are few elderly Central Americans in Canada, although as younger refugees gain permanent resident status and begin to sponsor family members, this situation may change. Central America's life expectancies are generally lower than the Canadian average of seventy-nine years, but they have begun to increase.

There are no old people's homes in Central America. Rather, older members expect to live with or be cared for by younger generations in the family. Failure to provide care or shelter is a source of shame for the family. An older mother-in-law can be the focal point of a family, respected for the knowledge that a long life has given her. Learning English is particularly burdensome for these older people, and they often see no point in making the effort. This in turn can exacerbate their social isolation.

Names

The customary naming system in Central America differs significantly from that of North America in that when a woman marries she both retains her father's name and takes her husband's. For example, if Maria Sanchez marries

Juan Lopez, she becomes Maria Sanchez de Lopez. Her husband's name does not change. Their children will be, for example, Pedro Lopez Sanchez. Because the connecting "de" in a married woman's name means "belonging to" there are pockets of feminist resistance to its use.

Thus all elements in an immigrant family will have different last names, which can create bureaucratic confusion in Canada as well as hot tempers if questions are raised about the legitimacy of a marriage or child. Although some feel that the solution is for the family to take only the father's name, this can create problems for people returning to Central America since legal documents will not then be in acceptable order.

For a professional to call someone by his or her first name is seen as negative and patronizing. The same applies to calling someone by his or her family name (i.e., Sanchez), without adding Mr., Mrs., or Miss. Children are called by their first names and are addressed informally as "tu." Adults are formally addressed as "usted" to avoid appearing patronizing or presumptuous in using the informal "tu," which is used among friends.

Patterns of Communication

Compared to Canadians, Central American people relish physical warmth and closeness. This is as true of members of the same sex as of mixed couples.

People generally show deference and respect to those in positions of authority, such as physicians. For this reason they may feel uncomfortable about making immediate eye contact with strangers. Lowered eyes should not be interpreted as lack of interest or docility but rather as simple good manners.

Problems and sorrows often give rise to an apparent sense of fatalism. Misfortune is simply God's will and must be accepted, this being a reflection of socio-cultural realities in their countries of origin.

Shopping

Women are responsible for shopping for the daily needs of the household. For them, the differences between the lively Central American markets and the anonymous supermarkets of North America can be enormous. Initially, women may need guidance on comparison shopping, reading labels, bargains, and so on. Friends and family in the community will often rally to a woman's aid and help her find her way in the system. Husbands may be more responsible for decisions on major purchases, although wives will participate in the final choice of the individual product.

Time

The subject of many jokes, the Latin American sense of time is renowned for its flexibility. In practice in Canada, Central American respect for appointment times and deadlines varies among individuals. Many are very punctual, others less so. Explaining the importance of a health professional's timetable, and giving the assurance that the health professional will be on time, can help. It can also be useful to emphasize that the custom in Canada is to be punctual for appointments. Central American patients may be unaware that twenty-four hours' notice is required in order to cancel medical appointments.

Sleeping Practices

Depending on the social stratum of the family in the home country, family members may have slept in a single room or had separate bedrooms. In either case, once in Canada families quickly adjust to the idea that children sleep separately from their parents, although a baby is likely to share its parents' room. Many parents prefer their baby to share their bed and thus may need information about the dangers of this practice.

Recreation and Leisure

A significant difference in social life between Canada and Central America is the informal quality of visits and gatherings. While neighbours respect each other's privacy, doors are always open to the casual visitor who has time to spend chatting or sharing in a household task. A community will often have a few established meeting spots such as a park or bar where friends can be found during weekend afternoons or evenings. The custom of carefully arranging visits by phone ahead of time seems cool and stilted to many Central Americans.

Recreational activities depend largely on income levels, gender, and age, but group events are more likely to occur away from home. An extended family group may go to a restaurant; young people may go to a disco. Men particularly enjoy watching and playing soccer, and some Latin communities in Canada have established many teams. They may share a drink after a game, but otherwise alcohol has no particular social importance. The concept of drinking "to have a good time" is not prevalent. Women may come together and cook their favourite dishes when preparing for a family feast. Trips to a lake or the ocean are real treats, and hiking excursions into the mountains are holiday specialties.

Differences in languages and customs represent barriers between English-speaking Canadians and Central American immigrants, but when they do meet, the experience is generally positive for both sides.

Festivals and Holidays

Roman Catholic celebrations throughout the year are the biggest and most popular holidays. These include familiar events such as Christmas, but others, such as Lent, have much greater significance for Central Americans. During Lent weekends, carnivals, complete with games and cotton candy, are organized in church squares. Great efforts are made by congregations to enliven the churches with thousands of flowers, bountiful produce, and music. Another important festival occurs on 2 November but is not often observed in Canada. This is a more sombre occasion, in which dead family ancestors are honoured. People speak warmly of these different festivals and miss them as part of the familiar community life that they enjoyed in Central America.

Health Care Systems in Central America

The type and quality of care available in the region vary greatly with location and family income. Rural peasants and labourers have access to few Western-style medical personnel and facilities. The traditional views of health and illness are much more valid for them than for their urban counterparts. However, they are receptive to the spread of scientific medical practices, which they may see as a sign of sophistication. The traditional approach is largely based on a classification of hot and cold qualities. Certain sicknesses and conditions are considered hot, others cold. Food and medicines fall into the same categories. To maintain good health, the object is to establish temperature equilibrium. Using this logic the treatment of a hot condition (i.e., fever) with a "hot" medicine (some antibiotics) will be seen as counter-productive. Generally, people coming to Canada, with the exception of some Maya, will be familiar with using medicine, but because the hot and cold principles have been ingrained in every child, they are still occasionally apparent.

In urban areas, money is the biggest deciding factor in the type of health care available. For the wealthy, there are private physicians and hospitals that provide care on par with international standards. For the majority, however, local lay specialists and underfunded, overcrowded public hospitals provide the bulk of the medical care. Although hospital conditions are generally poor, and stories abound of emergency patients having to make do with shots of valium and of wounds being sewn up with a dressmaker's needle and thread, people still go to the hospitals for help.

Substance Abuse

Minors from Honduras may be vulnerable to substance abuse in Canada. Stories of individuals returning to their poverty-stricken home villages in Honduras with drug profits have spurred unrealistic ideas among other young men about the benefits of participating in the North American drug trade. Consequently young men who travel by themselves to Canada may have similar dreams of making fast cash to send back to their families, and will tend to be ignorant of the dangers that accompany the high-risk environment of the drug trade: the downward spiral of drug addiction, possible violence, trouble with the law in Canada, and increased contact with individuals who have infectious diseases, such as HIV, hepatitis, and syphilis.

Alcohol abuse has not been noticeable among Central Americans in Canada, although there are two Spanish chapters of Alcoholics Anonymous in Vancouver. Refugee claimants overall are highly motivated to prosper in Canada, and alcohol is seen as a troublesome distraction. It is sometimes used on social occasions such as after soccer games, but usually only by men. Tobacco is also not commonly used, partly because it is very expensive in Canada relative to Central America.

Prevalence of Disease

Since the immigration process screens out people with serious longstanding health problems, diseases are not common among Central Americans resident in western Canada. There is often radiological evidence of inactive cases of tuberculosis (primary complex), as people have been exposed to the mycobacterium via B.C.G. (Bacille Calmette Guérin) vaccination in infancy. An occasional case of syphilis is found, mostly at the S.E.L., early latent, stage but the incidence of other sexually transmitted diseases is about the same as for the general Canadian population, and may be lower for women.

Parasitic infections are common in people coming from this region and need attention. Giardiasis, amoebiasis, frichuris, and ascaris are the most prevalent. Evidence of torture may also be present, although the absence of physical evidence does not indicate that an individual has not experienced torture (see Chapter 8: Refugees in Canada). Professionals specializing in rehabilitating torture survivors emphasize that the emotional damage is far greater than the physical injury. While physical wounds may heal, the related psychological trauma may be extremely deep. For this reason it is not advisable to question a patient about scars or other indications of torture, unless the patient expresses a need to share this information. Once a relationship of trust has been established, and this can take years, the patient may voluntarily reveal his or her story. Until then it may be best to leave the subject untouched. Often the expression of past torture is manifested by psychosomatic illness, which may occur many years after the actual event.

Sexuality and HIV/AIDS

Sexuality and HIV/AIDS are not generally or openly discussed, especially with members of the opposite sex, including a male physician alone with a female patient. Parents may be unwilling to educate their children about these issues, and spouses may be reluctant to discuss prevention methods. Some heterosexual men may be resistant to women's efforts to use condoms to prevent HIV/AIDS and other sexually transmitted diseases (STDs).

Homosexuality in particular is taboo, although many Central Americans regard physical warmth between men as acceptable and desirable. Many people may be aware of the existence of homosexual men "in the city," but lesbianism remains very much closeted. Many heterosexual men link HIV/AIDS to homosexuality and therefore are reluctant to seek help for STDs for fear of being labelled homosexual. Some homosexual men and women may claim refugee status in Canada based upon experiences of persecution and "gay-bashing" in their home country.

The percentage of adults in Honduras with HIV/AIDS is 1.67, the largest of all Central American countries, several times the Canadian rate of 0.31 percent. In Central America itself, the rate of STDs may be very high relative to Canadian levels. Although STDs are rare in refugees entering Canada, there is evidence that some individuals from Honduras have entered Canada with syphilis. As stated in previous sections, most Hondurans in Canada arrive as young men or minors, and the absence of family can make these youth more vulnerable to becoming trapped in dire socioeconomic situations, and more likely to be exposed to infectious diseases such as HIV and hepatitis once they are here.

Mental Health

Pregnancy and childbirth aside, mental health disorders and related physical problems are the most frequent cause of Central American contact with the Canadian health system. The experience of being a refugee, from initial persecution to flight away from family and friends to the host country, is gruelling and draining. People have great hopes that when they reach Canada

Jorge Rodriguez, from El Salvador

Jorge Rodriguez was relieved to finally feel safe and be sitting in a doctor's office, prepared to talk about the ordeal that had brought him from El Salvador to Vancouver as an asylum seeker. Friends had recommended this Spanish-speaking doctor, saying that Jorge would be able to learn more about HIV and about group counselling services. However, Jorge felt guarded about sharing his story. He had been raised to keep his problems to himself; how could he tell this stranger that he was homosexual and had HIV? After everything he had been through, why should he believe that this doctor could somehow help him?

In 1997 Jorge fled El Salvador to seek refuge in Canada. In his homeland he had lived in a small province far away from the capital and its services. He worked as a successful engineer in an important international company. He had many friends, and at age thirty he had already accomplished many of his life's dreams. To outsiders he appeared to have the perfect life, and Jorge made sure that none of his family or friends knew that he was gay. He continued to fit in with his local male friends by occasionally dating women and telling stories about his exploits with them. He appeased his mother, who longed for more grandchildren, by claiming that he would settle down and have a family once he had become a director at his company. Meanwhile, under the pretext of going on business trips, Jorge made weekend visits to the metropolis where he could meet other homosexual men.

Keeping his sexuality a secret was a constant strain on Jorge, but there was widespread homophobia in the town where he lived. He lived in fear of what might happen if anyone were to discover the truth about him.

One day his boss announced that all employees had to undergo a blood test for HIV status. Jorge doubted that he had HIV, but as soon as he took the test he became filled with anxiety. After four agonizingly long days of waiting for the test results, Jorge was called into his boss's office and fired for being diagnosed with HIV. From that moment on, Jorge's world fell apart. He knew nothing about this disease, but it had cost him his job, his income, and all his medical benefits.

News quickly spread of Jorge's HIV status, along with rumours of his homosexuality. Former male friends began harassing him; even his family avoided him. He quickly moved away to a different town, where he applied for a job. He was almost offered one, but officials illegally passed on his diagnosis, and he was rejected. At the weekend a group of thugs came to his apartment to run him out of town. Fearing for his life, Jorge moved again.

After one year of continuous unemployment and harassment, Jorge had lost everything. The strain of these experiences aggravated the HIV symptoms he was beginning to experience, and his health rapidly declined. Without company medical coverage, he could not afford to buy the medications that would have helped to stabilize his health. With no family or friends to turn to, he stayed home and prayed almost constantly. His religious faith was all that kept him from committing suicide. Medical institutions refused to treat him with antiretroviral drugs, arguing that these were intended for families only. He suffered episodes of gay-bashing. Three years after learning about his HIV, Jorge packed his bags and headed for Canada with the idea of dying in a distant place where nobody knew him.

Jorge arrived in Canada with chronic depression and in very poor physical health, including injuries from severe beatings for which he had never sought medical help. As an asylum seeker, Jorge once again felt like a criminal. He had very little money, and ended up renting a room in a shabby hotel in Vancouver's Downtown Eastside. Thoughts of suicide intensified as he reflected on his past experiences, on his illness, and on the poverty and substance abuse that surrounded him. However, just when he was losing all hope, two other Latin American gay men befriended him. They had similar stories, and they directed him to several organizations that work with refugee claimants and with people with HIV/AIDS. He was relieved to finally receive some emotional support, and he began to make friends with refugees.

Now his friends had referred him to this doctor. He just hoped that the doctor would be the answer to his health problems. Jorge said very little as he observed the other man. Could he trust this doctor?

With permission of Storefront Orientation Services, Vancouver problems such as poverty, malnutrition, and persecution will disappear. Instead they are faced with the stressful immigration process and lengthy waits for landed immigrant status, work permits, jobs, and housing. Learning English is another major anxiety, especially for refugee claimants ineligible for sponsored language classes. These worries can lead to bitterness and anger.

As time passes, the roles of husband, wife, parent, and child begin to diverge from the models familiar in Central America. Many husbands are depressed in the early years in Canada as they see their traditional family position eroding.

For serious mental illness in Central America, people are institutionalized with the expectation that they will never recover or be discharged. Individuals from Central America may be reluctant or resistant to sharing their personal problems with close family or friends. Spouses do not habitually discuss intimate topics with each other, but may respond well when the suggestion is made to them. Here, as in Central America, drugs are readily prescribed to treat depression and anxiety. Counselling in Canada can be difficult because of the language barrier and the lack of Spanish-speaking practitioners. The extent of depression and its pervasive links with living conditions and life stresses also militate against effective counselling. As one woman noted, "It's difficult to counsel someone when everything can be a problem, even figuring out how to catch a bus to the Food Bank."

As people become settled, have their immigration status confirmed, and establish homes, jobs, and a place in the community, anxiety and depression usually fall away, as do the associated aches and pains.

Relationship between Patient and Professional

Canada's medical system is so different from that in Central America that an important part of a health professional's initial role is to advise patients on the resources available and the functioning of the system. People come expecting that health care here will be better, more technologically advanced, and more accessible. However, the practicalities of the system are unfamiliar and need explanation: things such as having a physician on call and a regular family doctor, well-baby clinics, community nurses, and so on. Some immigrants, most often male, from Latin America may perceive seeking help for health problems to be a sign of weakness; they keep their problems to themselves and do not wish to burden others (Dunn 2000). It is important to clearly encourage patients to ask questions and request help as a right. Some physicians have found that less of their time with a patient is spent on conducting diagnosis than on providing preventive education and information on the health care system.

Central American contributors described the following "ideal" model of interaction between physician and patient. The patient calls to see the doctor, who is either known or directly related to the patient's family. The physician takes a few minutes to discuss general unrelated topics, may walk around the room, guide the patient to a chair with a gentle arm around the shoulders, and so on. After the patient has been put at ease in this manner, the doctor takes a seat and listens very carefully to the patient's story. The physician is expected to take his client's concern seriously, label the problem for the patient, and prescribe suitable medication. It is also customary in some areas for a female relative to accompany a woman when she sees her male doctor. This is dictated by modesty and by the need to allay the husband's jealousy.

Regardless of education level or place of residence, most Central Americans appear to have some knowledge of prescription drugs and the conditions for which they should be appropriate. They will very often request from a physician a specific drug that they know to have been helpful in the past or offer a diagnosis to the attending physician such that it may take some convincing to have them understand why an antibiotic is not given. In these cases disappointment may be expressed when a medication is not prescribed. Prescribing medication is regarded as an indication to the patient that he or she is being taken seriously and treated well. Treatment of some kind – be it shots, tablets, or creams – is often the patient's criterion for success. Doctors who do not prescribe drugs are considered very poor. Doctors in Central America will freely prescribe antibiotics. For this reason it is often necessary for doctors in Canada to explain that antibiotics will not cure a cold or flu.

These expectations have several implications for Central American immigrants and their doctors in Canada. The idea that good care can be received from an anonymous doctor is initially foreign, and North American directness in medical interviews can aggravate the patient's uneasiness. The practices of limiting medication and performing comprehensive tests prior to treatment are welcomed by Canadians but tend to have the opposite effect on Central Americans. Some newcomers treated in this manner and unable to communicate effectively with their doctor believe that North American doctors "don't care" and "don't know their subject well enough to provide good treatment."

The idea that relaxation or exercise can help a problem may be poorly received. For example, an immigrant woman with a terrible headache went to Emergency for help. She was examined and told that nothing was physically wrong and that she should simply go home and rest until the headache passed. Feeling misunderstood and poorly treated, she went away resentful and in pain. Careful explanation, and the assurance that the patient is being taken seriously, can help to alleviate these tensions.

Practical details needing clear discussion will be useful for a general practitioner attending to a family's health needs over a period of years. For those Central Americans who received all their care from clinics, a long-term relationship with one doctor is novel. The purpose of regular check-ups and test procedures such as Pap tests, mammograms, and prostate checks is generally unfamiliar, as is the theory of preventive medicine. People are interested and concerned about their health, so that taking the time to explain things clearly will be highly beneficial. The concept of family medicine is in any case becoming somewhat harder to sustain with the growing availability of walk-in clinics. As one patient stated: "I go to the walk-in clinic for the easy things and I go to see my family doctor if it is more complicated."

Central Americans will want to see a doctor when they have a concern, even though some of their problems may appear minor to Canadian health professionals. For example, a slight rise in a child's fever at night can send parents quickly scurrying for help. The challenge for the physician is to avoid over-prescribing while still giving reassurance. Some physicians have found that as families adjust to life in Canada, the frequency of visits diminishes. The feeling is that people use physicians to confirm their well-being as much as to treat medical problems. As time passes the former need diminishes.

Though most women are satisfied with a male physician, some women patients may feel much more comfortable with a female doctor. When female doctors are not available, the presence of a nurse or other woman in the room during an internal examination can be a great help. However, this should not be automatically presumed. One Vancouver doctor discovered that his female patients grew perplexed when he asked his nurse to come in. The patients felt their private business was becoming too public.

While doctors in Canada and Central America hold a similar place in terms of training and prestige, nurses do not. There are very few professional schools for nurses in the region, and most receive their training on the job by working closely with a physician. Although nurses in Central America are able to do more of the mundane work usually performed by physicians here, such as sewing wounds, they are not as respected as Canadian nurses but rather seen as menial hospital workers. In places, notably Nicaragua, recent campaigns have aimed at boosting the status of nurses as health professionals and at enhancing their training to include community health work. For these reasons, nurses in Canada should be clearly introduced to newcomers as health care professionals. The abilities of nurses and the services that they provide to newcomers will confirm their status. Central Americans who have spent time in Canadian hospitals have generally been delighted with the skill and solicitude of nurses. As one woman noted, "The idea of being asked if I needed anything! This never happened to me at home in Guatemala." Public health nurses can be particularly helpful to immigrants in guiding them through the medical system and integrating them into the new community.

Hospitalization

Depending on a person's background, hospitalization in Central America can be associated with death rather than recovery. Though these fears may linger on in some immigrants, most trust the capabilities, high standards, and objectives of hospitals here and tend to become, in one doctor's opinion, model hospital patients. Privacy, clothing, and food present no problems, apart from certain postpartum food taboos concerning pork and other "cold" foods. Patients with fever may also resist bathing.

Central American families tend to visit convalescing relatives frequently and in large groups, but not to a disruptive degree. Consent forms are a novelty and need translation as well as explanation. As in other aspects of health care, language barriers present the biggest problem.

Postmortems are uniformly disliked unless absolutely necessary, the feeling being that the family member is already dead and should not be subjected to further trauma. Physicians will need exceptionally good arguments to overcome this sentiment.

Medications and Treatments

Although the technology and the theory behind much North American medical treatment will be new to many Central Americans, it is generally accepted and may be perceived as advanced. Points of contention arise when doctors do not prescribe medication for a patient, because this seems to signify that the physician is not taking the condition seriously. Some physicians work around this by giving simple vitamins or non-prescription drugs for symptomatic relief.

Some immigrants may attribute their pain or injury to bad luck, a curse, or to "the need to do penance for wrongdoing" (Cervantes and Lechuga 2004, 6). They may prefer to consult indigenous healers, particularly if they feel that physicians are dismissing their ailments. Common home remedies that people bring to Canada include herbal teas and the use of Vicks VapoRub for headaches, feverish babies, and a multitude of other discomforts. People from rural areas often use herbal packs for ailments such as fever, but many of the plants they need are not available in Canada. Eucalyptus is widely and variously used. Coins may be placed on a newborn's umbilical cord to prevent hernia. Rubbing (*sobar*) is a technique often used to try to alleviate sprains, strains, and arthritic-like symptoms. Religious faith and prayer may help individuals cope with pain.

Testing before treatment is also unfamiliar and may be interpreted as lack of concern. For example, a family grew angry with the attending physician when their son was hospitalized for severe pains in his legs. The extensive tests were seen as experimental procedures on a human guinea pig, while nothing appeared to be done to alleviate the pain. Language difficulties exacerbated the problem, but the story illustrates a common Central American fear. However, Central Americans are found to be as compliant as other Canadians when it comes to following a treatment schedule. As with others, there is a tendency to stop taking medication when symptoms disappear, thus necessitating clear prior instructions and explanations. Especially for new refugees, prescriptions may go unfilled because of a lack of money or the bureaucratic requirements involved in filing for medical insurance with the Department of Citizenship and Immigration. A Central American immigrant who is a Jehovah's Witness may refuse blood transfusions.

Common Canadian ideas about rehabilitation exercise will be unfamiliar to many Central Americans. They expect to spend the time in hospital inactively, convalescing. The encouragement of health professionals to get out of bed and exercise as soon as possible after surgery can be confusing and threatening. A Central American immigrant who had hand surgery to correct a long-term, slightly crippling condition could not believe the doctor who told him to start exercising and using the hand normally as soon as possible. When he disregarded suggestions, his hand became stiff and painful, thereby reinforcing the patient's initial lack of faith in the surgeon. However, when rehabilitation practices are explained as being a part of the healing process, people have generally been very responsive and expect to recover fully and resume normal activities. Some men may have been raised to bear their pain with dignity (*aguantor*) (Cervantes and Lechuga 2004, 8). Such men may need coaxing to convey the extent of their pain, though subtle efforts to communicate may be hindered by language barriers.

The Disabled

The quality of life for persons with either mental or physical challenges in Central America depends greatly on the financial resources and social position of their family. In most countries, there are no public social services for the disabled, and their care is the responsibility of the family, although the patient will be loved and protected. Disabled people will not often appear in public, partly for fear of ridicule and insult and partly because there are no facilities or jobs for them. The exception to this for some poor families is that a disabled person may be sent out to beg, which may make all the difference to the family's financial survival.

In recent years a program was initiated in Nicaragua for people in wheelchairs to play basketball. People expressed initial incredulity and then delighted surprise when the project turned out to be fun, exciting, and popular. In short, like other people in Canada, Central Americans may initially doubt the abilities of disabled people.

Family Planning

For Central Americans, talking about sexuality and related subjects does not come easily, although many women are concerned enough about contraception to initiate the discussion with their physicians. For problems of sexual dysfunction, such as premature ejaculation, men are much more likely than women to approach a doctor, although even here numbers are very small.

Knowledge about fertility can vary greatly along class, age, and gender lines, with large segments of the population being very ignorant of the biology of reproduction. Although Central American families tend to be larger than Canadian families, wives are very interested in controlling their fertility. Birth control may be seen as a "woman's problem," and methods which require male participation, such as condoms, are unlikely to be well received. The pill is widely accepted, the intra-uterine device (IUD) is tolerated, but diaphragms are unpopular. Withdrawal is probably the most commonly used practical method of birth control. Central American families have also been found to express a preference for the contraceptive injection.

In the event of unwanted pregnancy, about 50 percent of women favour abortion, once they know it is a legal procedure in Canada and despite their strongly Roman Catholic backgrounds. Abortion is illegal throughout Central America, although many unlawful abortions are performed under often terrible circumstances. Frequently these illegal terminations lead to sepsis with resulting infertility and even death. It is not unusual to find women who have undergone illegal abortions among the immigrants to Canada. However, it is important to note that Spanish uses the same word for miscarriage and abortion.

Pregnancy

Class and geography determine the kind of prenatal care a woman experiences in Central America. For rural women, pregnancy and childbirth will be overseen by a local midwife, and mothers and other older women in the community will provide the necessary support, knowledge, and household help. For working-class and poor urban women, the situation is similar except that they usually deliver in a hospital or polyclinic, though they may have had no formal prenatal medical care. Rich urban women will use the best physician and hospital services available.

Prenatal classes are unheard of in Central America, although those classes offered in Spanish in Canada have been well attended. Husbands need firm encouragement to go, but once they see the presence of other male participants they may make good-spirited efforts to take part. Since birth procedures in Canada are so unfamiliar, clear information on the working of the system as well as tours of the hospital would be an invaluable resource to Central American couples.

Childbirth

Women from urban areas in Central Latin American countries would usually rather have a baby in hospital than at home with a midwife. However, hospitals may be so crowded that there may be no available recovery beds. In rural areas, and especially in indigenous communities, traditional approaches to childbirth are preferred, using experienced community midwives to assist with birth and to provide the mother with care and emotional support.

Central American immigrant women's experience of childbirth in Canada has been very positive, despite the unfamiliarity of customs. Language presents the greatest problem, and often husbands have to translate. Fathers are not normally permitted into hospital delivery rooms in Central America, but with appropriate encouragement many attend in Canada. However, some women feel uncomfortable at the prospect and prefer to bring a female friend or relative. Health care workers should respect this choice. Oftentimes many members of the family are in the hospital premises while the delivery is taking place, and it is not unusual for two or three members of the family to be present in the birthing room.

Newborn babies often have their waists tied with a belly band, or they have a coin placed on the umbilicus to prevent a hernia. These practices may seem unnecessary to Western doctors or nurses, but they bring peace of mind to the new parents. Infant sons will not be circumcised. Baby girls often have their ears pierced after two or three months, and if doctors refuse to do the piercing, parents will do it themselves or find someone else.

Most women, except perhaps Mayans, are familiar with Caesarean sections and generally accept whatever procedures the physician deems necessary to deliver a healthy baby. At the same time, they may tolerate considerable pain before asking for an anesthetic.

Individuals who practise traditional health prevention consider childbirth and the postpartum period as very "cold" times, and sometimes new mothers in Canadian hospitals will be shocked to be served ham, a notoriously "cold" food.

Postpartum Period

The degree to which women follow traditional practices will dictate how much the postpartum period diverges from mainstream Canadian customs. Rural women new to North America are the most likely to observe the traditional forty-day postpartum period during which they ideally remain indoors, away from drafts, and with their head, ears, and feet covered. They are expected to not watch television or listen to the radio, to eat proper "warming" foods such as tortillas, and to avoid "cold" foods such as pork. Bathing is considered risky because of its potential for chilling the new mother. She will also wear a special girdle to prevent the uterus from becoming dislocated or, in more recent times, to aid its return to its original size. It must be remembered that these practices represent one end of the spectrum. Most women will retain what they consider to be the most valuable parts of the tradition, while others dispense with tradition altogether.

A major issue facing new mothers in Canada is the strong pressure exerted by medical staff in favour of breastfeeding. Infant formula food companies have mounted very successful advertising campaigns in Central America which have convinced women of the superiority of bottle-feeding. In Central America the bigger the baby the better, and mothers believe that babies grow faster on the formulas. Having the tables turned so emphatically is confusing and causes distrust, so that the women do not know whom to believe. Lots of encouragement and explanation will help.

There is no real preference for either male or female children. Sick infants may provoke great concern. Sometimes deformity in a baby will be attributed to wrongdoing by the mother during pregnancy, such as attempted abortion, excessive emotion, or an unsatisfied food craving.

Childhood Health and Illness

Poverty is the root cause of many of the diseases common to Central American children living in Canada. Lack of money can lead to crowded living conditions and diets deficient in fresh fruits, vegetables, and protein. Malnutrition in turn encourages the spread of scabies, colds, fevers, bronchitis, and eczema. Parents use over-the-counter products to treat their children at home but will readily bring them to see a doctor. This may not be done by new refugee claimants, who have no medical coverage apart from the complicated bureaucratic emergency procedures provided by the Department of Citizenship and Immigration. Vicks VapoRub is used extensively to treat sickness in children (and adults), and a feverish baby may be completely covered with Vicks to help it fight the infection. Since bathing is thought to chill people, sick children will generally go unbathed. Swallowing a scrap of paper is believed to cause constipation in children, and parents may want to obtain a laxative.

Overall, people are receptive to vaccination. Many will be familiar with it from public health campaigns in the urban barrios of Central America, although they may not have been vaccinated themselves.

Children, like adults, sometimes suffer the consequences of having lived in countries filled with violence. Sleep disorders such as insomnia may be a problem, and children who have witnessed violence may have recurrent nightmares.

Chronic Diseases

Parasites and worms are chronic problems in Central America, although they can be treated and eliminated in Canada. An occasional case of active tuberculosis is found, and X-rays show evidence of many more inactive cases. Malnourishment can be an ongoing problem, exacerbated by the poor condition of some arriving refugee claimants and their lack of money during the first months here.

Death and Dying

Because Central American countries do not generally have social programs, people look after dying members of the family themselves. If a condition is stable, the person will be taken home from the hospital to die. In urban areas, after a death occurs the body is taken to a funeral chapel, where it is prepared for burial. A wake for family, close friends, and sometimes a priest is held, usually in the presence of the open casket, and people generally stay up all night with the body. For both religious and secular people, this event is very important, as it is the last time the family will be together with the deceased. Burial is the norm, cremation being a foreign idea. Catholics and Protestants will follow their customary rituals.

The mourning period traditionally requires that close family members wear black for a year. If a child dies, white clothes will be worn for a shorter time, although both practices have become less common in recent years. A stillborn baby of religious parents will be baptized and given a burial service. Autopsies are disliked, as it seems unnecessary to cut open a person who is already dead. Some of these customs may continue to be followed in Canada.

Nutrition: Food and Drink

Central American people enjoy the traditional foods of the region, such as tortillas, bean dishes, and rice seasoned with peppers and strong spices. The financial status of the family determines how much meat is eaten, with poorer working-class people perhaps having meat only for Sunday dinner. Newcomers to Canada find local meat prices very high.

Breakfast is generally a substantial meal shared by the whole family, and consists of eggs, beans, and tortillas. Lunch will be eaten by family members in different locations, and may include rice, beans, or plantain (banana) as its major ingredient. Supper is a lighter family meal, perhaps of mixed vegetables. Dairy products are popular, although there is some lactose intolerance in this group. On coming to Canada, people continue to make their own tortillas at home, often buying supplies from East Indian shops where prices are the most competitive. Teenagers in North America often eat more processed and fast foods than in Central America. Overall, dietary quality seems high, but financial constraints make quantity a problem. Poverty also encourages diets high in carbohydrates, with resultant weight gain and the expression of Type II diabetes in adults.

Dental Practices

Except for the very small minority of wealthy immigrants, the dental status of refugee claimants is uniformly poor. Cavities, periodontal disease, and missing teeth are very common. Poverty and the absence of public health education mean that dental hygiene is unknown to most Central Americans. The custom has been to pull a painful tooth rather than undertake restorative work. Once in Canada, people are receptive to preventive techniques, although cost considerations will push visits to the dentist far down the list of priorities.

Bathing

People coming from poor urban barrios may have had access to water only from a single tap situated a few blocks away. Once in Canada most people bathe regularly because of the abundance of available water.

Sometimes menstruating women will not want to bathe or wash their hair for fear of stopping the flow of menstrual blood. More common is the belief that people with fevers should not get wet.

Current Patterns of Use of Health and Social Services

The refugee and immigration process determines the availability and standard of medical services that can be utilized by Central Americans new to Canada. Before refugee status is granted, claimants have extremely limited access to health insurance; Interim Federal Health (IFH) is mostly for emergencies and hospitalization, and using these services often requires lengthy paperwork. Refugees will be very conscious of their vulnerability and will wait a long time before seeking help. They may fear that mental or physical illness will adversely affect their applications for refugee status or subsequent permanent residence. Alternatively, they seek free services from places such as the Pine Free Clinic in Vancouver. Refugees who have been accepted and who qualify for provincial health insurance often make frequent initial visits to the doctor and for apparently minor problems. But as they adjust to the community and their lives become less stressful, the frequency of visits declines. People will also use emergency services as necessary. Once they accept the notion of a long-term family physician, they may try to find Spanish-speaking doctors, who in 2004 are in very short supply. Alternatively, they use a volunteer translator to accompany them.

Social programs have a mixed reception. Welfare can be demoralizing and can increase stress levels.

Counselling Central Americans

Many individuals, especially from Guatemala, El Salvador, and Colombia, have endured political and psychological violence, so the need for adequate counselling facilities may seem self-evident. However, convincing individuals and families to participate in counselling may prove challenging. First, the lack of available Spanish-speaking professional counsellors creates an immediate hurdle; providing services with an interpreter is awkward and impersonal, yet it can be extremely stressful for individuals to try to express themselves in English or French, especially while discussing events that are already distressing for them.

Like most people, Central Americans may be guarded about engaging in "talk therapy" unless they form a trusting and personal relationship with their counsellor. In particular, for men to discuss private matters with strangers is considered to be a weakness; cultural *machismo* may dictate that courage and strength are displayed by resolving one's own problems and not burdening others.

Individual counselling may serve to exacerbate family conflict. Extended Central American families may be extremely close. In dealing with family conflicts, Western health professionals may consider the interference of extended family members to be burdensome and the dynamics to seem co-dependent. However, Central American cultural assumptions about family relationships may perceive conflicts as inevitable and as reflective of attempts to fulfil family responsibilities towards one another. "The client might verbalize the conflict by saying: 'I am not in agreement with what my grandmother wants me to do but *ella puede* (she can); *tiene derecho* (has the right).' What this actually means to the client is that he has to deal with how the grandmother feels about an issue since she can interfere and she cares. The therapist has to assist the client in dealing with the significant other in a fashion that will enable him to appropriately handle the conflict without breaking away from that person" (Sandoval and De La Roza 1986, 180).

Central American individuals and families may become more engaged in counselling or family services when they see that these sessions have resulted in concrete changes to their living conditions. It may be helpful to offer referrals to other agencies that can assist with finding employment, the refugee claimant process, accommodation, English as a Second Language classes, church groups, and so on. Moreover, encouraging individuals to participate in sports or church groups may create much needed networks of social support that help relieve isolation. Individuals may also need reassurance that they are not "crazy," that their feelings and mental health problems are normal reactions to what they have been through. Encouraging individuals to participate in family or group counselling may be more effective in facilitating the healing process. "Since the family has proven to be an effective system for buffering some effects of trauma, the reconstitution of the biological family or creation of a foster family (integrated with known and familiar persons) must be one of the main therapeutic goals, especially when working with children" (Garcia and Rodriguez 1989, 80).

Political Violence and Torture

Physicians examining refugee claimants frequently come across evidence of torture and brutality. The natural temptation is to ask the patient, albeit with compassion, for explanations. But this may be a grave error that will only occasion distress in victims of this type of violence. The pain goes far deeper than physical wounds, and a lengthy period, perhaps two or three years, is needed before professional and patient develop the necessary degree of mutual trust.

The legacy of civil war and politically sponsored abduction, murder, and torture will also often show up in people's sleep patterns. Children are haunted by nightmares, anxiety, depression, and phobias; adults are plagued by sleeplessness, depression, substance abuse, aggression, family violence, relational problems, and somatic illness (Garcia and Rodriguez 1989, 77). Families mourn those who have been killed, imprisoned, or caused to "disappear." Although not everyone has been a victim, everybody knows a friend or family member who has suffered. For the Canadian health professional, it is very important to take account of this background – but not before the patient raises the subject. (For more information on survivors of torture and post-traumatic stress syndrome, see Chapter 8: Refugees in Canada.)

Methods of torture used in El Salvador and Guatemala include covering the victim's head in a rubber mask, repetitive submersions of the victim in water, selective beating of parts of the body, electrical shocks to especially sensitive areas of the body, forced witnessing of torture or executions of others, including relatives (Garcia and Rodriguez 1989, 74). Individuals may also have seen mutilated bodies, including those of pregnant women, left out in the open by the army.

In addition to experiencing these horrors of war, many refugees have been beaten, raped, or robbed during their journeys to Canada. Some may have been arrested by officials in other Latin countries and forced to pay money for their freedom.

Delivering Culturally Sensitive Health Care

The old adage about putting yourself in the other person's shoes is perhaps the best advice for providing compassionate and appropriate health care to refugees and immigrants from Central America. Uncovering the details of a patient's story will help in building this understanding. Indications of the situation left behind can be inferred from country of origin, social background, current immigration status, and length of intermediate stay in the United States. Likely current problems are suggested by language skills, familiarity with North American customs, and employment.

Refugees are in a very stressful position and need social as well as medical support. On the other hand, it is essential to guard against being patronizing. Poverty and limited English do not preclude pride and mental alertness. As one physician put it, "People are more fragile because of what they have been through. They really don't want to be bothersome, they don't want to make waves. So a doctor will have to take time and be gentle, but the rewards will be great." Another Vancouver physician has prepared a mimeographed sheet in Spanish that explains how the medical system works, what a call schedule is, and what to do in case of emergency. Some physicians have found that giving a patient written information, in point form (for example, how to take the medicine, when to return to physician, doctor's phone number), is helpful. For people with limited skills in English, instructions should be very clear and direct, such as "see your family doctor tomorrow" or "come back in one week." Hospital forms will need translation. People should be told clearly that they have a right to ask for help and care. And health professionals should not mistake apparent passivity for acceptance. The patient may simply not understand the English expressions being used.

Further Reading

Acker, Alison. 1986. *Children of the Volcano.* Toronto: Between the Lines Press.

Amnesty International Canada. 2004. *Colombia: Human Rights under Attack.* http://www.amnesty.ca/Colombia.

Cabezas, Orar. 1985. *Fire from the Mountain: The Making of a Sandinista.* New York, NY: Crown.

Calvert, Peter. 1985. *Guatemala: A Nation in Turmoil.* Boulder, CO: Westview Press.

Cervantes, Joseph, and David Lechuga. 2004. "The meaning of pain: A key to working with Spanish-speaking patients with work-related injuries." *Professional Psychology: Research and Practice* 35, 1: 27-35.

Cohn, Jorgen, Kirsten Holzer, Lone Koch, and Birgit Severin. 1981. "Torture of children: An investigation of Chilean immigrant children in Denmark, preliminary report." *Child Abuse and Neglect* 5: 201-3.

Conchita, M. Espino. 1991. "Trauma and adaptation: The case of Central American children." In F. Ahearn and J. Athey, eds., *Refugee Children: Theory, Research and Services,* 126-34. Baltimore: John Hopkins University Press.

Cosminsky, S. 1982. "Childbirth and change: A Guatemalan study." In Carol MacCormack, ed., *Ethnography of Fertility and Birth, 205-30.* New York, NY: Academic Press.

Dunn, Samuel. 2000. "Keeping the pain: Health, belonging and resilience among Guatemalan immigrant men." Master's thesis, Social Anthropology, York University, Toronto, ON.

Economist. 2004. "Holistic Healing. A better approach to civil-war recovery." 373 (16-22 October): 34-36.

Encarta. 2004. "Guatemala" and "Maya civilization." Microsoft Encarta Online Encyclopedia.

Garcia, M., and P. Rodriguez. 1989. "Psychological effects of political repression in Argentina and El Salvador." In D. Koslow and E. Salett, eds., *Crossing Cultures in Mental Health,* 64-83. Washington, DC: Society for International Education, Training and Research.

Ferris, Elizabeth G. 1985. "Regional Responses to Central American refugees: Policy making in Nicaragua, Honduras, and Mexico." In E. Ferris, ed., *Refugees and World Politics,* 187-211. New York, NY: Praeger.

Leslie, Leigh A. 1992. "The role of informal support networks in the adjustment of Central American immigrant families." *Journal of Community Psychology* 20: 243-56.

Maduro, Renaldo. 1983. "Curanderismo and Latino views of disease and curing." *Western Journal of Medicine* 139: 64-70.

Menchu, Rigoberta. 1984. *I, Rigoberta Menchu: An Indian Woman in Guatemala.* London: Verso.

Mennonite Committee Council. 2004. *Kidnappings and Detentions in Colombia.* http://www.mcc.org/areaserv/latinamerica/colombia/detention/index.html.

Randall, Margaret. 1981. *Sandino's Daughters.* Vancouver, BC: New Star Books.

Sandoval, M., and M. De La Roza. 1986. "A cultural perspective for serving the Hispanic client." In H. Lefley and P. Pederson, eds., *Cross-Cultural Training for Mental Health Professionals,* 151-79. Springfield, IL: Charles C. Thomas Publisher.

UN Security Council. 1993. *From Madness to Hope: The 12-Year War in El Salvador: Report of the Commission on the Truth for El Salvador,* S/25500, 5-8. New York: Un Security Council, Annex.

Contributors to the first edition

Augusto Arana, Immigrant Services Society, Vancouver
Roxana Aune, MOSAIC, Vancouver
Gill Bentzen, Immigrant Services Society, Vancouver
Bernardo Berdichewsky, Capilano College, North Vancouver
Althea Brown, Vancouver Health Department, Burrard Unit
Yaya de Andrade, VAST, Vancouver
Esther Frid, Family Services, Vancouver
Miriam Maurer, MOSAIC, Vancouver
Carolina Palacios, Vancouver
Peter Quelch, Richmond
Sheila Shannon, MOSAIC, Vancouver
Lucia Silva-Zarate, Inland Refugee Society, Vancouver

Contributors to the second edition

Cheryl Anderson, Physician, Ravensong Community Health Centre, Vancouver
Alexandra Charlton, Director, Storefront Settlement Services, Vancouver
Bayron Cruz, Bridge Health Clinic, Vancouver
Yaya de Andrade, Psychiatrist, Vancouver
Eduardo Emmandio, Simon Fraser University, Vancouver
Luis Garrigo, Settlement worker, Storefront Orientation Services, Vancouver
Noe! Hermida, Immigrant Services Society of British Columbia, Vancouver
Cecilia Mascayano, Mennonite Centre Committee for Refugees and Newcomers, Vancouver
Zoila Ramirez
Mary Regester, Nursing, University of British Columbia
Alihandro Ruiz

2
People of Chinese Descent

Ka-Ming Kevin Yue

Several waves of migration have brought people of Chinese descent to Canada from various parts of the world over the last 150 years, the vast majority from mainland China, Hong Kong, and Taiwan. The largest wave came from Hong Kong from 1985 to 1994. In 1998 mainland China overtook Hong Kong and became the major source of immigrants of Chinese background. In fact, in 2000 mainland China sent more immigrants to Canada than did any other country. Chinese have arrived from other countries as well, including Singapore, Thailand, Malaysia, the Philippines, Vietnam, Cambodia, and Laos, and from Africa, South America, and the West Indies.

Chinese have been in Canada for up to five generations – since before Confederation. Some were pioneers and built the railways that consolidated the nation, with whose history their names are interwoven. Chinese Canadians have achieved great success as mayors, members of the Legislative Assembly of British Columbia, members of Parliament, and the current governor general of Canada is a Chinese Canadian. Yet others, such as refugee claimants from China, are viewed by some as unwelcome.

Though people of Chinese descent share many physical characteristics, they are culturally heterogeneous. A recent immigrant from rural China is vastly different from a person born in Canada whose family has been in Canada for three generations. The Chinese refugees who were forced out of Vietnam and spent long periods in refugee camps have had quite different experiences from people born in Hong Kong who come to Canada as "business class" immigrants.

The culture of Chinese immigrants varies according to place of origin, socioeconomic status, level of education, and experience with and adaptation to Western culture. People who come from mainland China, Hong Kong, and Taiwan have many cultural, religious, and socioeconomic differences. Research and clinical experience tell us that people who are affluent and from urban areas are usually more familiar with Canadian medical practices, having had access to high-quality Western health care before coming to Canada. They may also have used a variety of healing practices taken from Chinese medicine. The less well-off, those from rural areas, and those who do not speak English may know less about Western medicine and generally have difficulty navigating the Canadian health care system.

It would therefore be inappropriate for health professionals to deal with all people of Chinese descent in the same way. An understanding of each patient's background and his or her familiarity with the Western health care practices is an important starting point of any interaction.

Geography and History

China

China is the third-largest country in the world in area (after Russia and Canada) and has the world's largest population. In 2003 the population was estimated to be about 1.3 billion, more than forty times the Canadian population. China's vast geography encompasses deserts, mountains, and farmland. Its climate ranges from long, cold winters in Tibet and northern Manchuria, to subtropical warmth and rain in the coastal areas of the southeast, to arid desert conditions in the west.

Most of China's population resides in the eastern third of the country, where the major cities and fertile plains are located. About 80 percent of the population lives in rural villages. Agriculture is the backbone of China's economy, although industry is rapidly expanding. China now has the second-highest Gross Domestic Product (GDP) worldwide. With its abundance of human and natural resources, China attracts investments from Hong Kong and from all Western countries. Not only do many major companies have production plants in China, but China's large population is also one of the world's largest markets.

About 94 percent of the population of China is Han, the largest ethnic group. The Han people share a common history, culture, and written language, but their dialects vary from region to region. The rest of the population is composed of about fifty minority groups, most of which live in the border regions of the far north and west.

"China" is a translation of "the Middle Kingdom." The country has a rich culture that developed during the course of many successive empires. Dating back 3,500 years, Chinese history is one of the oldest in the world. In 221 BC a strong, centralized Chinese empire was established, and subsequent dynasties lasted in one form or other for a period of two thousand years. During the 1800s, the empire finally started to weaken, and it was overthrown by revolutionaries in 1911. In 1912, China became a republic ruled by the Nationalist party. China fought against Japan from 1938 to 1946 in the Second World War. The Chinese Communist Party, started in 1921, defeated the Nationalists in 1949 and founded the present government, the People's Republic of China. Beijing became the capital city, and Mandarin became the official dialect.

Under Communist rule, all important industries, trade, and finance were placed under state ownership and control. Land once owned and farmed by individual families was turned over to state ownership and management. People dissatisfied with Communist domination fled to neighbouring and Western countries.

After years of political hardship and turmoil, the government not only dramatically increased industrial production but also expanded and improved education and medical care. The latter is now completely socialized. Professional government workers are provided with free medical insurance, and insurance fees for other workers, mostly farmers, are deducted from their wages.

The recognition of the People's Republic of China by Western countries and China's desire to promote technological advance by opening its doors to the Western world have led to further changes in the lives of the Chinese. Moreover, the Chinese government's recent emphasis on private ownership signifies further economic changes to come.

Hong Kong

Situated on the south coast of China, Hong Kong is about the size of Greater Vancouver. Its 410 square miles include Hong Kong Island, the Kowloon peninsula, which is attached to mainland China, and more than 235 islets. Hong Kong has a subtropical climate with hot, humid summers and dry winters.

Originally, Hong Kong was part of China and consisted of a few small fishing and farming villages. After the Opium War of 1839, Hong Kong was ceded to Britain, which added control of the Kowloon peninsula in 1860. In 1898, China leased more adjacent land, the New Territories, to Britain for ninety-nine years. In 1997, China reclaimed all of Hong Kong through negotiations with Britain.

Almost all (98 percent) of the residents of Hong Kong are Chinese. In the past, large numbers of people have migrated from China to seek employment and, more recently, to escape Communist rule. The two official languages in Hong Kong are Chinese and English. Cantonese is the most commonly used Chinese dialect, though Mandarin has become more important since Hong Kong returned to China in 1997.

Hong Kong is one of the most densely populated places in the world. Because of its strategic location and its status as a free port, it is a bustling centre of economic activity, with one of the strongest and most varied economies in Asia. The vital importance of international trade, finance, and tourism means that most residents work for manufacturing firms or have jobs in commerce. Fewer than 3 percent make their living by farming or fishing.

In the past three decades, especially as the handover from Britain to China set for 1997 came closer, large numbers of skilled, educated, and wealthy people from Hong Kong have immigrated to countries such as Canada, the United States, and Australia. Then the North American recession in the late 1990s saw expatriates returning in large numbers to work in Hong Kong. Some continue to hold dual citizenships in Western countries for protection against political instability.

Hong Kong is now a Special Administrative Zone. Its economy is changing from manufacturing to commerce. Since mainland China has cheap labour and Hong Kong has managerial expertise, Hong Kong has become an exporter of business managers to the mainland.

Taiwan

Taiwan is a mountainous island in the South China Sea situated about ninety miles off the Chinese coast. It has a subtropical climate with hot, humid summers and mild winters.

Most Taiwanese are Chinese whose ancestors originated in the Fujian and Guangdong Provinces of mainland China. Although the people speak various Chinese dialects depending on their regional birthplaces, almost all speak Mandarin, the official language. Most Taiwanese are involved in manufacturing and foreign trade, and about one-third of the population are farmers.

The Chinese of Taiwan began to come to the island from mainland China even before AD 600, but large-scale settlement did not begin until about 1600. In 1895, Japan gained control of Taiwan as a result of the First Sino-Japanese War and developed and expanded Taiwan's agriculture, industry, and transportation networks. After the Japanese were defeated in the Second World War, China regained Taiwan.

In 1949, when the Chinese Communists took control of mainland China, the defeated Nationalist government under Chiang Kai-shek settled in Taiwan. Both the Communist and the Taiwanese Nationalist governments consider Taiwan a province of China, but each claims to be the legal ruler of all of China. In the 1970s, a number of nations, including the United States, cut diplomatic relations with Taiwan and established ties with Communist China.

The 2000 election of Chen Shui-bian of the pro-independent Democratic Progressive Party brought an end to more than fifty years of Nationalist rule in Taiwan. In response, China stated that it would be keeping a close eye on Chen and would never allow Taiwan independence.

Migration to Canada

Like other ethnic groups, most people of Chinese descent have come to Canada hoping to improve their quality of life. They felt that Canada would offer better job opportunities for themselves and better educational facilities for their children. Some came to join relatives already settled here. Others came for political and religious freedom.

Early migrants, 1858-1923

Canada's first Chinese arrived in British Columbia in 1858 from California. They were mostly men from the Guangdong Province in Southern China. They were merchants and labourers who had escaped the famines and rebellions of home to search for gold and fortune. They filled jobs shunned by Anglo-Europeans and worked in mining, laundries, restaurants, and fish canneries and as domestic servants. They came to make money to send home or to earn enough money to return home to retire.

Between 1881 and 1884, more than 15,000 men were "imported" from China to serve as construction workers on the Canadian Pacific Railway. Many lost their lives doing the most treacherous work in railway building.

Chinese Exclusion Act, 1923-62

In 1923, with the passing of the Chinese Exclusion Act, the entry of Chinese into Canada virtually ceased. Immigration began again in a small way after the Second World War when Canada allowed close relatives of Chinese residents to enter the country.

Renewal of Chinese Migration, 1962

The repeal of the discriminatory clauses of Canadian immigration laws in 1962 and the development of the "point system" encouraged a large number of Chinese to immigrate to Canada, especially after the Hong Kong riots in 1967.

New Immigration Act, 1978

In 1978, a new Immigration Act came into effect in Canada and marked a turning point in Chinese immigration; the point system was revised to emphasize occupational experience and demand. With this new policy, Chinese immigrants, especially those with skills and potential for employment in Canada, were encouraged to settle. As a result, between 1978 and 1981, Asians of all countries accounted for 44 percent of all immigrants to Canada. Chinese from Hong Kong and Taiwan with relatives resident in Canada, skilled workers, and professionals began to arrive.

Following the Geneva Conference of 1979, organized by the United Nations secretary general to deal with the refugee question, Canada accepted

60,049 Indo-Chinese refugees between 1979 and 1980, about 30 percent (18,012) of whom were linguistically Chinese (Li 1998, 94-95). These were refugees from Southeast Asia who had been displaced from Vietnam, Laos, and Cambodia (Kampuchea).

Prior to China's takeover of Hong Kong in 1997 and her threats to repossess Taiwan, more affluent people from these two places, those with investment capital and the capacity to create employment, moved to Canada. Then, in the late 1990s the global economic downturn resulted in decreased immigration from Hong Kong and Taiwan. A significant number of expatriates consolidated their portfolios, sold their homes and assets in North America, and returned to Asia.

Recent Migration, 1988 Onward

China's relative poverty, overpopulation, political system, and restrictive policies, such as the one-child rule and anti-Christian and anti-union policies, have provided persistent motivation for people from China to migrate to Canada. By 1998 mainland China supplied more immigrants to Canada than any other country – almost 20,000 – and that number had doubled by 2001. Concomitant with this major shift, the number of immigrants from both Hong Kong and Taiwan plummeted. Hong Kong, from which there were more immigrants than any other country as late as 1997, dropped to seventeenth place by 2000; in the same period, Taiwan shifted from fourth to fourteenth place. In 2001 the largest group of mainland Chinese settled in Metropolitan Toronto, followed by Vancouver, with its mild climate and relative proximity to Asia, and Montreal.

Immigrants from mainland China were mostly of the independent category – highly educated and skilled – but in Canada they became underemployed or unemployed, usually because of the language barrier and lack of Canadian experience. They came with high expectations, hoping they would be able to find the same level of employment as they were used to. They believed that passing the immigration interview was sufficient. However, they found they needed further training in Canada to become qualified for the labour force. People from Hong Kong usually have good social support networks of either friends or relatives in Canada; those from mainland China may not have similar supports on arrival in Canada.

Refugees

Refugees from varied backgrounds have been coming from mainland China to North America since after the Second World War, and especially after 1949, when China became a Communist country. Following the Cultural Revolution in China in the 1960s, people were prohibited from leaving the country. Leaving China even to visit relatives in Hong Kong or the United States was considered a betrayal, but in the 1970s some people went illegally to the United States. Most Chinese were more willing to go to the United States than to Canada. A relatively large number of refugees came to Canada from Southeast Asia as resettled, or convention, refugees in the 1970s, escaping from the repercussions of the Vietnam War.

Most refugees from mainland China came to Canada after the June 1989 Tiananmen Square massacre. Some came on student, business, or visitor visas and later made a refugee claim here. Many have come from Fujian Province (the boat people). Other refugees are members of the Falun Gong, an organized movement for health and well-being, also known as the Falun Dafa. A very small number came because of religious persecution, mostly Christians, or political persecution.

Health professionals should be aware that many refugees are suspicious of the authorities because of their experiences with governments in China. They are usually afraid to talk to health professionals, whom they believe will pass on the information to the government, and are hesitant to share private information.

Socioeconomic Status

Socioeconomic status among immigrants varies from well-to-do families who bring their lifelong savings to invest in Canada to low-income refugees who have to work long hours to support their families. Educational backgrounds also range from university-educated professionals to people with no education who are entirely illiterate. Refugees from mainland China are mostly factory workers, whereas many young immigrants are well-educated professionals in the independent category. Many immigrants coming from Hong Kong and Taiwan are in the "business class" category and they are usually affluent.

In recent decades, some Chinese Canadians have achieved great economic and political success. Yet some immigrants experience downward mobility in employment or even unemployment through lack of English or different skill demands in Canada. Foreign professionals' credentials are often not recognized in Canada. A mathematics professor from mainland China may work as a janitor. Some people go back to school for further training. Others go into small businesses unrelated to their education. Language training programs – English as a Second Language (ESL) – may not be feasible or readily accessible. The level of training provided may not be high enough to prepare them for the Canadian labour market.

Experience with Canadians

The early Chinese immigrants were mainly labourers, who faced extreme hardship and racial discrimination. Chinese labourers were used exclusively to set the charges to blast through the mountains for the railway. They were housed and fed separately from the Anglo-European workers. Their descendants fought for Canada in the Second World War even though they were not allowed to vote. It was only in the last few decades of the twentieth century that people of Chinese descent became more widely accepted as part of Canada's multicultural society.

In general, immigrants operate in survival mode. In Canada their first priority is to achieve economic sustenance. They focus on pragmatic matters – work, housing, and education for their young.

The later immigrants, who are urbanites, better educated, and well-off, have far more resources and connections than earlier immigrants. But since they come from highly competitive societies, Canadians and the established Chinese Canadians may at times find them overly competitive. The newer immigrants tend to live among their own social networks, maintain connections with their places of origin, and travel back and forth often. Out of familiarity and safety they tend to stick together, and their integration into the larger community will take several generations.

More recent immigrants from mainland China are independent class immigrants. They are young professionals who had good jobs at home, though in Canada they may not find the jobs they expected and may need to upgrade their English and training. Some would like to live in communities where they can be exposed to the larger Canadian society, to prepare them for the Canadian labour market. They have no family in Canada, have little connection with China, and are more committed to staying in Canada.

Religious and Philosophical Beliefs

The Chinese have been influenced by a number of religions and philosophies. While most individuals do not adhere strictly to one religion, ideas from these religions and philosophies have blended in harmony over the centuries. Thus most Chinese in Canada hold strong convictions that are deep sources of spiritual support in times of crisis, such as illness. Health professionals will find that these beliefs can be important to people even after they and their families have lived in Canada for a long time. The following religions and philosophies can be strong influences on the Chinese coming to Canada from Hong Kong, mainland China, and Taiwan.

Confucianism

Confucianism, the most influential philosophy in China, was the state doctrine and basis of education for over two thousand years. It strives for a harmonious society based on the utmost moral discipline of citizens. Its rules prescribe the social structure, one's role, and one's relationships with others.

Confucius defined codes of conduct for ruler and subject, father and son (filial piety), husband and wife, older and younger brothers, and between friends. The central theme is submission to authority.

Being a gentleman, preservation of equilibrium and moderation, obedience to parents, and loyalty to family and state are valued. Education and hard work are the main means of achieving a higher station in class status. The study of Confucianism, culminating in a nationwide exam, was one means by which a peasant could become a government official.

Buddhism

Originating in India 2,500 years ago, Buddhism focuses on suffering, with spiritual and physical self-discipline to attain enlightenment. It teaches avoidance of killing, of taking what is not given, of misconduct, falsehood, and intoxicants. Charity, atonement, and prayer can relieve pain and lead to eternal happiness after death.

Buddhism stresses a holistic world view that is based on the belief that all life is interdependent. Not only is all of human society interdependent, but human society is interdependent with the physical realm as well. The Buddhist world view also includes a belief in karma, the later consequences of what one does. The effects of karma extend not only throughout one's life but also beyond, because life is not limited to a single individual existence. The idea of past lives impinging on one's current life sometimes opens the door to a sense of fatalism: "It is my fate; there is nothing I can do about it."

The notion of karma is an important one for health professionals to understand because it affects attitudes to health and disease. In Buddhism there is a relationship between health and morality. To live well, which means to practise moral and religious values such as compassion, tolerance, and forgiveness, is to live a healthy life. Patients who have these beliefs may well interpret disease as due to lack of moral or mental discipline.

Health is holistic; it is the expression of harmony within oneself, in one's social relationships – family, work – and in the environment in which one lives. Disease is the expression of disturbed harmony in our lives. Healing, in Buddhism, is not the mere treatment of physical disease or of measurable symptoms but rather the realignment of mind and body to overcome disease. The goal is to bring back harmony within the self, within relationships, and with the natural environment. Buddhists may find it congruent with their beliefs to adopt a vegetarian diet, traditional Chinese herbal medicine, Tai-chi, and chi-kung exercises.

Buddhist temples in Canada have gradually become more than places of worship. Vegetarian meals, regular prayer, meditation, and ceremonies on special days are offered. Most worshippers are older recent immigrants. Some Buddhist organizations participate in philanthropic endeavours. Some temples provide ESL classes, Tai-chi, and computer classes, and seniors' and children's activities.

Daoism (Taoism)

Daoism is a Chinese philosophy which is second to Confucianism in influence on Chinese culture. Daoism was founded by Lao Tzu in the sixth century BC. His teachings were passed down orally before they were compiled in the third century BC in a book titled the *Classic of the Way and Its Power*.

Dao means "way." It is understood that the Dao is the underlying pattern of the universe, which can neither be described in words nor conceived in thoughts. The goal of Daoism is to bring all elements of existence – heaven, earth, and man – into harmony. To be in accordance with the Dao, the individual must empty himself of doctrines and knowledge, act with simplicity and humility, and above all seek nature. The main belief in Daoism is that nature has laws and will take care of itself. This philosophy slowly evolved into a religion that promised, among other things, to be capable of exorcising the spirits and pacifying the dead.

Christianity

Christianity, spearheaded by the Jesuits, established a foothold in China in the sixteenth century. The Jesuits learned the Chinese language, studied Confucianism, adopted Chinese customs, and brought knowledge in mathematics, astronomy, and navigation to China. At the end of the nineteenth century, when European powers tried to establish trading posts by force and colonize China, Christianity was seen as colonialism in disguise and was then rejected by the state. Later, the Communist government in China stressed loyalty to the state and suppressed all religions, Christianity included.

Christian churches operate many schools, orphanages, hospitals, and other charitable organizations in Hong Kong and Taiwan. Most private schools in Hong Kong are run by churches.

In Canada, Chinese Christian churches provide important support networks and services for their immigrant and local-born members, including child care, schooling, youth programs, and visitation for the aged and the sick.

Cosmology

Yin and yang are two diametrically opposed forces that are the foundation of the universe, including the human body and its health. Yin represents negative energy, femaleness, darkness, coldness, and emptiness. Yang represents positive energy, maleness, light, warmth, and fullness.

Qi (Chi) is the cosmic force of vitality and righteousness that exists in the universe and the human body and is closely related to blood. Illness and surgery drain vitality, while rest and Qi Gong exercises restore it.

The concept of yin and yang, central to classical Chinese medicine, is influential in the Chinese community and important in understanding Western and Chinese therapies. For example, Chinese medicines are often seen as preserving the balance of the self, whereas Western medicines may be seen as bringing immediate symptomatic relief but not necessarily balance.

Astrology and Feng Shui

Originating with farmers, the Chinese calendar offers daily guidance as to what is safe and what should be avoided, thus in part enabling one to control one's fate.

Feng Shui originated with the choosing of a burial site so that the soul can settle peacefully and go on to protect the living. It has evolved to choosing the location and layout of one's home or business.

Chinese pronunciation for the word "four" approximates that for the word "death" and four is therefore considered an unlucky number. The words for "three" and "eight" approximate "life" and "prosperity," respectively; thus, three and eight are lucky numbers.

Festivals and Religious Holidays

Events and holidays are celebrated by families and communities. Family gatherings for meals are central to celebrations. Major Chinese festivals include Chinese New Year, the Mid-Autumn Festival, and the Dragon Boat Festival. Chinese in Canada usually celebrate both Chinese and Canadian festivals and holidays.

Language

Early immigrants from China spoke mainly the Toisan dialect of Cantonese. More recent arrivals from Southern China and Hong Kong Chinese speak Cantonese; those from other parts of China speak Mandarin; and most Chinese from Taiwan speak Mandarin or the Fujian dialect of Cantonese.

The more urban or educated immigrants may speak Mandarin as well as their own dialect. Those from rural and less educated backgrounds may understand only their own dialect. Unless they know each other's dialect,

Mandarin and Cantonese speakers will not understand each other – though they read the same newspaper.

Many people from China do not speak English, although professionals from northern China are likely to speak it. Those from Hong Kong and Taiwan have often learned English in school.

In Canada, attendance at English classes may be difficult for those who have little access to transportation or who work extended hours. It is also particularly difficult for restaurant workers who work in the evenings. Some first-generation immigrants have not acquired English even after several decades. They survive in the local Chinese community and rely on young family members and friends as interpreters. When family members are not available, friends, neighbours, church members, or service organization volunteers help as interpreters.

Family Structure

Traditional Chinese Families

As in many agricultural societies, in the past the family in rural China was often large, headed by the eldest male, with extended family members living in the same dwelling. Large families were encouraged as a source of labour; sons were favoured for their greater strength and their ability to carry on the family name. Birth order implied power and prestige, and, when a powerful man had several wives, being a child of a senior wife carried greater power, responsibility, and prestige. Unmarried children were expected to live at home.

Traditionally, the elderly were highly respected, and the young were obliged to take care of them. Grandparents were expected to look after grandchildren and educate them, and were never relieved of parental duties. An elderly mother, for example, might remind her adult son to dress warmly, to drink the soup that she had prepared, and to avoid injuring himself at work or in sports. The eldest son was expected to assume responsibility and to make decisions if the parents were no longer able to do so. Adult children were expected to care for and serve elderly parents and not send them to institutions in old age.

Chinese Families in Canada

Urban families in Hong Kong, mainland China, and Taiwan, and immigrant families from urban areas today, do not usually fit this profile. Institutionalization of elderly parents may be a necessity for those who have to work. When families immigrate, both parents usually work and may not be able to meet an aging parent's expectations and needs. Grandparents may become the household babysitter and be expected to look after household chores as well. Those unable to communicate with neighbours may feel isolated and abandoned in their homes during the day when their sons or daughters are at work. In addition, there might be intergenerational conflicts. Grandparents may hold traditional ideas and speak only Chinese. Children and especially grandchildren may adopt Western culture and speak English. The language of the grandparents may soon be forgotten. In a few families, grandparents, parents, and children can hardly communicate.

In the immigrant Chinese family, as in other Canadian families, there may be a division of roles – husbands managing finances and child discipline, wives taking care of the household and everyday family needs. Like many other women in Canadian society, Chinese women in the workforce usually have to balance paid work outside the home with housework and child care, feeling inadequate as they try to juggle multiple roles. In some instances, the woman becomes the family breadwinner. Even though her husband may be highly educated, his credentials may not be recognized in Canada, and it is often easier for women to find low-paying jobs.

In addition, women are usually responsible for day-to-day health care decisions. However, major decision making in the family will likely involve all family members, including extended family. Therefore, health professionals should find out the preferences of the families they are working with when important health care decisions are to be made. In some families, the eldest son may still be expected to make major decisions or control the flow of information to the family and patient, so health professionals need to be closely attuned to family dynamics.

Communicating with Outsiders

Parents having poor command of English may depend on young school-aged, English-speaking children to communicate with outsiders, including health professionals. A child may be expected to provide the history and interpret investigative questions and treatment instructions. Sensitive information may be withheld and technical information incorrectly translated because the child lacks vocabulary. Both health professional and patient may end up with inaccurate or inadequate information, to the detriment of treatment outcomes.

Relationships

With immigration, family members may be separated because of work, education, and immigration regulations. Labouring immigrants often work hard to send money back home to family members left behind.

In the recent past, families among the entrepreneurial class in Hong Kong sent wives and children to Canada for the children's education while husbands stayed in Asia to maintain their business. These fathers planned to move to Canada when they retired. In the meantime they regularly commuted between the two countries, and these families came to be called "astronaut families." A second, more recent, family situation arose with the global recession in the late 1990s. At that time some husbands lost their jobs in Canada or sold off their Canadian businesses and returned to Asia to seek better employment or tend to their Asian holdings. In these situations weakened family ties sometimes put all parties at risk. Wives left in Canada may suffer from neglect, while children may lack adequate supervision and emotional support. A few returned husbands established new relationships and raised second families in Asia.

Child-Rearing

Traditional Child-Rearing in Chinese Cultures

In rural China, male children were desired for their physical strength in agriculture and to inherit the family property. If a wife were "unable" to bear a male child, the husband might take a second wife in an effort to gain a male heir. Male children may be given more power and offered more opportunities for education. In recent decades in mainland China, a policy of one child per family has been enforced in order to curb population growth. This allowed fewer opportunities for producing a male child. Parents circumvented this policy by escaping to the countryside or by paying large fines.

Confucianism heavily influences child-rearing even today. A leading Confucian principle, filial piety, requires the child to be absolutely obedient to the parents. The parents are devoted to the well-being of the child and expect to dictate the child's education, career choice, and marriage. The child who fails to achieve expectations brings disgrace on the family. Education and work are highly valued and are seen as the only means of attaining success. Spending time on schooling and employment is considered much more important than pursuit of leisure activities. These expectations create tensions between parents and children in Canada.

Child-Rearing in Canada

In the traditional Chinese family, the very young child is cared for at home by the mother or grandmother. Now use of daycares is common when mothers work outside the home. In the past, the rich hired "wet nurses" to breastfeed their babies. Babies are now more often formula-fed than breastfed. Frequent feeding to pacify or promote sleep can cause "baby bottle tooth decay." This may develop when mothers too frequently offer breast milk, baby formula, cow's milk, and soft drinks. Rice becomes a staple food very early in the infant's diet. Toilet-training is initiated at an early age. Babies are bathed often, and parents tend to overdress their children to prevent them from catching cold.

Some Chinese parents still want to raise their children in the traditional Confucian ways and find it a challenge to raise children in Canada, where children have more autonomy and freedom. This is the origin of many conflicts. The father is expected to be the solemn disciplinarian, holding back on open gestures of affection. At times he may become distant and harsh. The mother, the intermediary between father and child, develops a much closer relationship with the child. She subtly assumes the role of major decision maker, even though the father retains his official status as head of the household. While parents may be lenient with young children, strict discipline is imposed when the child gets older and is assumed to understand that actions have consequences.

Migration to Canada brings many tensions between traditional values and present realities. The balance of power may shift from parents towards children. For parents who lack a command of English, the oldest child who speaks English may be given a great deal of family responsibility.

Marriage Patterns

Chinese families in Canada who have lived here for years or for generations might not conform to traditional practices. For example, it is now rare for a Chinese marriage to be arranged by parents. But some customs persist today in Canada and in the countries of origin, with expectations of the families of both groom and bride.

In Canada, the marriage partner is usually chosen by the individual. However, arranged marriages occur, sometimes in order to immigrate to Canada. A matchmaker may be called upon to match couples based on social status and their ancestors' place of origin. Some men go back to China to find a wife, and the future wife may agree to come because she sees the West as better than China, perhaps not realizing that because she has little or no English she will face acute isolation in Canada. Some women come because of the one-child policy in China. Many couples become pregnant immediately after arriving in Canada. Others arrive pregnant and make a refugee claim.

Divorce is rare. Some wives may remain subservient to their husbands even when their relationships have deteriorated. As in all families, relationships vary widely.

Interracial marriage in Canada is becoming more common but tends to be discouraged by the elderly. The expectation is to marry within the "race," and it is not unusual to be threatened with excommunication if parents do not agree with their child's choice of spouse.

The Elderly

Some Chinese seniors were born in Canada. Although they grew up in an era where life was difficult for their minority group, they are relatively accustomed to Western ways and the health care system in Canada.

Chinese seniors in Canada migrated in several groups. A small and shrinking number of railway builders and labourers, now in their advanced years, migrated to Canada in the early 1900s. These men came to make money to send home or to earn enough money to return home to retire. Most were unable or unwilling to return to China. Legislation passed between 1885 and 1923 prevented the families of these men from joining them. As a result they formed clan associations to provide mutual support and care. They live now in bachelor rooming houses in Chinatowns, deprived of children and family support.

A second group migrated in their youth, worked, and retired here. They maintain some traditional Chinese values but have been influenced by the experience of living many years in Canada.

A final group immigrated recently in their old age, along with their children or came later in family reunification. They hold a relatively higher degree of traditional Chinese values, incorporating Chinese herbal medicine and acupuncture into their medical care. They may be isolated because of lack of English and means of transportation. A weekly trip with their children to Chinatown may be their only chance for socialization. While the elderly expect attention and care from their adult children, the latter are often busy with their work and expect the grandparents to perform household and child care duties. Facing a combination of generational, language, and cultural barriers, this group of elders is vulnerable to neglect or abuse.

Elderly Chinese maintain varying degrees of Chinese culture, more so than do the young. In general, seniors from politically unstable homelands are satisfied with the stability of Canada and its medical and social programs. Many live with their families; others live separately with close access to family. Most require family help to access resources when they become ill.

Cultural Values and Behaviour

Names

A Chinese name usually consists of a one-word surname followed by a two-word given name. Some families from South Africa had their names reversed by immigration authorities. A woman may keep her own surname or use her own and her husband's surnames in hyphenated form. The traditional Chinese may give a child a second name when schooling commences

Mrs. Kit Fan, from China

Mrs. Kit Fan, now eighty-seven, immigrated ten years ago from a small town in Fujian Province to live with her son and his family in Richmond. When her son brought her to see the doctor, she had eaten very little for one month and had lost five kilograms. She told the doctor she had had an appendectomy in China and had also been troubled with a duodenal ulcer. The physician ordered several tests, and on a second visit a week or so later, she had lost more weight and was slightly jaundiced. Her sixty-year-old daughter told the doctor privately that the "appendectomy" in 1979 in China was actually surgery for colon cancer. Her family had asked the Chinese surgeon not to tell her, believing she would suffer even more if she knew.

Further tests found a tumour in the common bile duct. Because of her age, the physician did no surgery but instead gave treatment to relieve the stricture and make her more comfortable. She was not in pain. The doctor talked with the family about Mrs. Fan's prognosis, and the probable progression and management of her symptoms. Mrs. Fan's son gradually informed her of her condition. The palliative care team visited her family in their home to discuss her terminal care, and her family decided that they wanted her to be hospitalized near death because everyone worked long hours and could not stay home with her.

Four months after Mrs. Fan first saw the doctor, she was hospitalized with increased jaundice, edema, low fever, and chills. At first she was reluctant to go into the hospital, but her attitude changed when she found it to be quite comfortable. Some of the staff spoke Chinese, and she could ask questions and chat a bit. When the social worker mentioned to Mrs. Fan's son that she might be discharged, the family went into a panic because caring for her at home was impossible.

As Chinese New Year approached, Mrs. Fan asked the doctor if she could go home for dinner with her family on New Year's Eve. Instead, her entire extended family came to eat with her at the hospital. Her grandson brought his laptop computer to help her send New Year's greetings via the Internet to all her out-of-town relatives. A few days later Mrs. Fan passed away peacefully with her immediate family at her bedside.

and a third name when marriage occurs. In Canada, most children have an additional English name.

Personal Relationships

Confucianism still influences cultural values and behaviour. Even among those acculturated to Western ways, deep meanings, based on philosophies that have influenced generations for centuries, may underpin everyday life. Some values may be held in high regard, such as respect for authority, abiding by the law, and heeding the wishes of the elderly. As well, certain patterns of behaviour may be evident. For example, people may greet one another by bowing their heads and smiling. Avoidance of eye contact may be a sign of respect, rather than a lack of engagement, and looking downwards is meant to project humility. Nodding and smiling connote civility and should not be interpreted as signalling understanding and agreement. Except for a handshake, body contact, such as kissing and hugging, is uncommon and usually avoided with strangers. To the Westerner, the polite and formal Chinese may appear reserved and unassertive, whereas the Chinese may perceive the informal manners of the Westerner as rudeness.

To the Chinese, confrontation is usually to be avoided. One may attempt to reply in an indirect way and try to handle a situation diplomatically. Both sides should be left with a way out of a situation, in order to "save face." The Westerner may perceive this as submissiveness and not being forthright.

High Value on Basic Family Needs

Chinese are generally viewed as pragmatic people who give priority to satisfying practical family needs, particularly sufficient food, housing, and clothing. It may then be hard for parents to understand why in Canada further demands are made on them, for example, to meet a child's emotional needs or hold meetings with the teacher. Completing a task to the best of one's ability is expected. Traditional parents may stress shortcomings rather than achievements. Career and academic achievements are emphasized, while extraneous activities such as sports and arts may be discouraged. Social status is measured in terms of level of education, as well as age and wealth.

Hospitality

An invitation is usually required to visit someone's home, and hospitality is very important. Typically, the Chinese like to be surrounded by many relatives and friends, the more people the better. Some common pastimes include having a Dim Sum lunch, Tai-chi exercises, or games of Mah Jong.

Traditional Concepts of Health and Illness

Concepts of health and illness in China began with classical Chinese medicine, which later evolved into Chinese folk medicine. Elements of these concepts affect modern Chinese.

Classical Chinese medicine was recorded in an ancient text, *Huang Ti Nei Ching (The Yellow Emperor's Classic of Internal Medicine),* written between 1698 and 1598 BC. "Man" is part of and inseparable from the universe, which exists in harmonious balance. The universe consists of five elements: wood, fire, earth, metal, and water. Yin and yang are universal complementary opposing forces. Yin represents the female, negative energy, darkness, coldness, and emptiness. Yang represents the male, positive energy, light, warmth, and fullness.

Illness arises when yin and yang are in imbalance. Wind, cold, heat, dryness, and internal fire can trigger an imbalance. To avoid disease, one should avoid an environment where a particular factor is abundant. For example, exposure to wind and rain can trigger an internal excess of wind and wetness and may give rise to rheumatism. Giving birth is a "cold" event since the warm newborn and blood are passed out. The new mother should therefore avoid bathing and cold drinks, which are also viewed as "cold."

Illness is a manifestation of internal imbalance, diagnosed by measuring the pulse and studying the complexion, eyes, and tongue. Very little history is taken; in fact, a good traditional Chinese doctor is supposed to be able to diagnose without asking any questions. Diagnosis and explanation are simple and brief. Confirmatory laboratory testing is not performed, as in the past this did not exist. Treatment is prescribed immediately.

Herbal treatment is the main treatment modality of Chinese medicine. One authoritative book, *Ben Cao Gang Mu,* was written in the Ming Dynasty (AD 1368-1644) and listed 1,892 herbal ingredients. Each dose of herbs is prescribed to restore balance. In Chinese medicine this knowledge is passed down from masters to apprentices.

Organs are connected by channels called Meridians, which transport life energy called Qi. The Meridians also connect the interior of the body to the skin at specific points called Meridian points. Stimulation of these points by the acupuncture needle restores the flow of Qi to enable the organs to heal themselves. Treatments include acupressure and moxibustion, the burning of small quantities of herbs at these Meridian points.

Bonesetters originated from Kung Fu masters who treated soft tissue and bony conditions. They employ massage, poultices, and herbs in their treatment.

In folk medicine, the focus is placed on a balance between cold and hot. Illness can be caused by transgressions in the past or present, even ones committed by an ancestor, by evil spirits, poisons, bad luck, and even by nature itself. Religious figures, fortune tellers, and Feng Shui experts may be consulted.

Food is central to health. Medicinal and preventive functions are performed by sometimes drinking special soups prepared with herbal ingredients and avoiding certain foods at other times. Drinking warm or room-temperature fluids helps maintain balance in health, especially when one is ill.

Health professionals need to be aware that Chinese immigrants and people who have lived here for years, even if wealthy and speaking fluent English, may use traditional therapies because they are "natural." For that matter, the use of Chinese medicine, particularly acupuncture and herbal remedies, is becoming widespread among people who are not Chinese.

Attitude to Illness

In Confucian, inner strength is a virtue that is highly valued and may have implications for responses to illness. For example, many women were brought up to endure pain and suffering through self-discipline and mental strength. Sometimes, it might therefore be difficult to tell whether physiological pain is present. A Chinese patient may have a high pain tolerance and may hesitate to accept painkillers. "It is not clear whether they actually have a high physiological threshold for pain or they are less willing to express pain due to their upbringing, beliefs, or values" (Fung 1998, 73).

Some illnesses are attributed to transgressions and sins committed by the patient or the family. This can cause the patient and the family to hide the illness, especially infectious disease, cancer, and mental illness.

Health Care Facilities in China, Hong Kong, and Taiwan

How immigrants interact with the health care system in Canada is affected by their past experience. Their expectations may be of a system that allows use of multiple practitioners, simultaneous use of Chinese and Western medicine, seeing a specialist without referral, and paying to obtain a service immediately rather than being put on a waiting list.

Mainland China

In mainland China, everyone can access the medical system for a nominal fee. Medical insurance is offered to public servants, factory workers, and farmers in communes. Most are first seen in local clinics but may be referred to district hospitals, city hospitals, and then finally to university hospitals if more specialized treatment is necessary. Thus each patient is accustomed to seeing many doctors. In recent years a small number of private facilities that serve the affluent and accept private payment have appeared.

Most doctors in mainland China have some training in both Western and Chinese medicine, and most facilities employ both together. Western medicine is offered along with Chinese medicine, including herbal medicine, acupuncture, and bonesetting. When patients seek care directly from hospitals, they may encounter frontline specialists rather than general practitioners.

Hong Kong

There are several systems of care in Hong Kong. Most people access government clinics operated by the Hospital Authority, where fees are nominal, waits may be long, and referrals can be made to specialists. There is a smaller sector of semi-private care funded by employers through private insurance plans, where patients are attended by doctors on contract. Then there is a completely private sector where the affluent, having social contacts and able to pay high fees, access the specialists with the best reputations – although for the treatment of chronic disease, such as cancer, even the wealthy may choose to go to public hospitals. Most large hospitals are government-funded. These include state-of-the-art university hospitals. Government hospitals have first-, second-, and third-class rooms available depending on what the patient can afford.

Yet another system of care is provided by unlicensed doctors trained in Western medicine and practitioners of the traditional modalities of Chinese medicine. This broad and informal system appeals to the poor because fees are generally low despite the lack of government support.

Taiwan

The system of medicine in Taiwan includes government-sponsored health services, private physicians and hospitals, and physicians who practise traditional Chinese medicine. Taiwan now has a mandatory comprehensive National Health Insurance Plan, with the cost of health care being shared by the government, the employer, and the worker. The government provides health services, including educational programs, to the mountainous regions and offshore islands. The medical facilities in Taiwan are usually very good, and people migrating to Canada should not have difficulty adapting to the health care system in this country. Both Western and Chinese medicine are practised side by side.

Most Chinese have had varying degrees of experience with both Western and Chinese medicine. But many are puzzled by the Canadian health care system. Not only are they surprised at long waiting lists but also many think they should be able to get better service if they pay more. Affluent immigrants, used to a private health care system, often expect to receive the best services in Canada by paying for them.

Attitudes towards Western and Chinese Medicine

In traditional Chinese medicine, illness is seen as the imbalance of forces within the body. The restoration of balance by "natural" herbs is preferred over the artificial chemicals in Western medicine. Herbs are believed to maintain balance and prevent the imbalance that causes illness.

Western modalities like blood tests, biopsies, and surgery are seen as invasive. Many believe acute illnesses, particularly those requiring surgery, are best treated by Western medicine. Chinese medicine is usually used to treat chronic conditions. When serious complications or relapses occur, Western medicine may be sought as stronger and more immediate. Blood or organ donations are not common. Among immigrants who have retained ties to China, some will venture back to China to seek treatment when they develop a hopelessly terminal illness.

Prevalence of Diseases

Some medical doctors have found that certain diseases such as diabetes, hepatitis, tuberculosis, intestinal parasites, renal failure, and renal stones are more prevalent in the Chinese. Sexually transmitted diseases and HIV/AIDS are increasingly prevalent in mainland China. Some types of cancers are also common: nasopharyngeal, esophageal, gastric, and liver cancers. Many men smoke, thus contributing to cancer. Many Chinese are intolerant of lactose and experience gastrointestinal problems with milk or milk products.

Mental Health

Health professionals in Canada may encounter Chinese patients with low awareness, understanding, and acceptance of mental illness. Mental illness evokes considerable shame and guilt and leads to attempts at minimizing by denial or normalization.

Medical papers published in China showed unexpectedly low prevalence of all mental illnesses. Neuroses are under-reported, while psychoses, which are much more feared, are typically ignored or not reported at all. Schizophrenia, for example, has a worldwide lifetime prevalence rate of approximately 1 percent, but the rate reported in China is almost one hundred times lower.

Traditionally, emotions are linked to different organs. For example, anger is associated with the liver, and joy and depression with the heart. Mental illness is usually attributed to external factors, such as evil spirits, transgression, or cold wind. The problem is usually presented in the form of somatic

Jason Wong, from Hong Kong

Jason, eighteen, emigrated from Hong Kong to Calgary when he was nine. He recently finished high school in the city and took a job in a relative's restaurant in a small town seventy-five miles away. About a month after he began work, he came home to see his parents and high school friends.

That weekend at midnight Jason's family doctor was paged by Jason's uncle asking him to "get Jason out of the hospital." Jason had just been committed to the psychiatric ward, referred there by the Mental Health team. The physician arrived to learn from the ward nurse that Jason's family had earlier threatened to physically remove him from the ward and had backed down only when confronted by security guards. The ward nurse added, "They don't speak English, but luckily Jason can translate." The attending psychiatrist reported that, in addition to exhibiting psychotic symptoms, Jason had said, "I will kill myself if I am going crazy."

The doctor knew something of Jason's family because his uncle and grandmother were regular patients and he had successfully treated the uncle for depression. Jason had seen the doctor a few times for minor ailments and seemed to have a tendency towards hypochondria. The physician had met with Jason's mother once, but she had not raised any concerns about her son.

Later, piecing together what had led to Jason's hospital admission, the family physician discovered that Jason had a "learning disability." A year earlier his special education teacher, who knew him well, had taken him to see someone at the Mental Health team. At that time his family said that they had not seen any change in his behaviour, mood, or social interactions, but Jason told the team that his brain had been damaged by antibiotics. Believing that a drug addict had gotten into his car and put a needle inside him, Jason had gone to an emergency room to demand an X-ray. The Mental Health team gave him medication for schizophrenia, but after two visits Jason failed to return to the clinic. It was about a year later that Jason was admitted to the hospital.

complaints. It is acceptable to seek relief for somatic symptoms but not to discuss emotions. For example, an elderly woman may say that her heart hurts and may go to the coronary care unit for help when she is actually suffering from depression.

Some conditions may be normalized or mislabelled. Developmental disorders in children may be labelled as laziness or disobedience, depression as boredom, anxiety as neurasthenia, addiction as weakness.

The family plays multifaceted roles. In the traditional family, the submissive role of the wife may mask depression; the passive role of the child may mask depression or prodromal schizophrenia. Since mental illness may be attributed to misdeeds of the patient or the family, it brings a great deal of shame, and the patient and family may be reluctant to seek help. There is also fear that mental illness may be inherited. Discussion of family dynamics may be viewed as disloyalty.

Health professionals must find ways to ensure that the patient has access to good care. Patience is needed to win the trust of patient and family, who need to be reassured that the patient is not crazy or possessed and that mental illnesses are common and are now found to be treatable brain dysfunctions. Reassurances about strict confidentiality may provide some comfort. An alliance with the family's decision maker may be needed to allow commencement of therapy.

The use of medication to alleviate negative symptoms and improve the functioning of the patient is most acceptable. Patient and family need to learn that medications require time to take effect and must be maintained following instructions. Chinese people tend to need smaller doses than Anglo-Europeans and to be more sensitive to side-effects.

Acceptance of psychological counselling is poor, although pragmatic "talking therapies" such as lifestyle modification, cognitive-behavioural therapy, and stress management may be acceptable. Some people are less amenable to psychological counselling. Payment for private consultation with psychologists and counsellors may be an obstacle.

Relationship between Patient and Professional

A patient and a health professional who are both of Chinese descent may be from different places of origin, different socioeconomic classes, and different cultures. They may not share the same health beliefs. Chinese health professionals who work in Canada are likely to be educated either in Canada or in Taiwan or Hong Kong and re-qualified in Canada. It is important for Chinese health professionals in Canada to be aware of their own cultural and class bias and not to assume that their Chinese patients follow practices and beliefs similar to their own. There is great diversity, and Chinese health professionals should ask questions that will help them understand a particular patient's perspective.

From the patient's perspective, the dress, age, and affiliation of the health care professional and the busyness of the medical practice may imply expertise. Endorsement from someone trusted is important.

Traditional Chinese patients are submissive to authoritarian figures. They respect the physician, who back home is usually from the educated class. Out of respect, patients may avoid eye contact and answer always in the affirmative or with a nod, even when they disagree or don't understand. They are taught to avoid confrontation and not to question a doctor's recommendation. To the Western health professional, such a patient may appear to be aloof or uninterested.

Traditional Chinese patients expect to be instructed what to do with little discussion; they may be afraid to "bother their doctor." Too much discussion might even be seen as indecisiveness on the part of the health professional. Chinese patients in Canada therefore may find it helpful to learn about their right to make choices and to be self-determining in the Canadian health care system. However, health professionals need to bear in mind that some might interpret a non-authoritarian approach as uncaring and suggestive of incompetence on the part of the health care provider. Moreover, a recent immigrant encountering a treatment differing from the expected traditional one may suspect the Canadian doctor of incompetence.

Patients from Hong Kong or urban areas in China and Taiwan may be accustomed to seeking health care from multiple health care professionals, at times simultaneously from Western and traditional Chinese practitioners. Affluent patients are used to getting prompt attention and may have expectations of preferred treatment. To a Western health professional such a patient may seem demanding, untrusting, disloyal, and aggressive. It helps to understand that such attitudes arise from unmet expectations.

The concept of preventive medicine may be unfamiliar to those who seek help only when they feel ill. People may be unfamiliar with the concept of annual check-ups, such as for cervical and breast cancer, and the regular monitoring of health for asymptomatic diseases such as hypertension and diabetes.

The language barrier remains a considerable obstacle for many, especially older people who have recently immigrated to Canada or less educated people. Patients who speak only a Chinese dialect are usually limited to the small number of health care workers who speak their language. Family members, young children, or Chinese-speaking hospital workers are sometimes asked to interpret, at times inappropriately. Interpreters who are relatives can sometimes filter or alter information and may pose confidentiality risks.

Chinese women may prefer female professionals, especially for obstetric and gynecological care. If they must have a male physician, the doctor or nurse should invite the woman to bring along her husband or a friend, or should provide a chaperone. Similarly, Chinese men may be uncomfortable with female physicians and male nurses.

Some patients may prefer older, more experienced health professionals. They may also expect immediate results from medical treatment. It is important that the real limits of the treatment are explained to avoid misunderstanding and disappointment.

An immigrant who speaks only Chinese and who encounters a Chinese-speaking health care professional may feel the need to have a closer relationship, expecting the professional to be a friend and be ready to help in non-medical matters.

Some Chinese may not be familiar with the need to make appointments with health professionals, and sometimes appointments may be missed through work obligations. Health professionals should investigate apparent tardiness and poor manners.

For those Chinese who are used to a hierarchy of practitioners in their home country, the Western health care system with its team approach may be confusing. The patient may not understand the roles of various team members. This can affect attitudes to nurses, for example, because general nursing is not highly regarded as a profession in China. However, the patient will respect discernible specific responsibilities and expertise, as in the case of community health nurses or professionals who are entrusted with specific tasks, such as prenatal classes or teaching home management of diabetes.

Hospitalization

The hospital can present both language and cultural barriers. Language is the most significant barrier in health care, creating problems when doctors, nurses, and paramedical personnel do not speak the patient's language, when instructions and signs are only in English and French, and when appropriate interpreters are missing.

Cultural expectations can conflict with hospital policies. When a person is hospitalized, family members may prefer to visit as a group and may expect to help in nursing the hospitalized person, especially an elderly patient. Some family members may have employment with unconventional hours and cannot fit in with the standard hospital visiting or discharge hours. This is a common source of friction in hospitals. Hospital food may be completely different from food at home. Soups, sometimes with herbs, are traditionally valued in helping the sick in their recovery, but the ingredients may interact with treatment given in hospital. It is therefore important to remember to ask about such things, but to do so respectfully and open-mindedly.

Since elderly Chinese often associate hospitalization with death, they may be reluctant to be hospitalized. And indeed, family members may rush the sick to the hospital, not only to receive better treatment there but also because death at home is considered to bring bad luck to the family.

Medication and Treatment

Self-medication is a common practice. A patient may take both Western and Chinese medicine simultaneously or consecutively to avoid interaction.

Western medicines, perceived to be "stronger," are expected to bring immediate results. For this reason, antibiotics prescribed for a certain course of time may be prematurely discontinued if results are not immediately forthcoming. Prolonged use of medication for chronic illness, especially asymptomatic illnesses, may not be readily accepted.

"All things in moderation" is a commonly held belief among the Chinese. Thus Chinese patients may feel that taking medicine over an extended period of time will weaken their bodies. As well, they may think that Western medicine is too potent and may reduce dosages to a level they believe suitable. All these factors can be perceived as non-compliance, but it is crucial for health professionals to give patients explanations and clear specific instructions about medications.

Some people regard injection as more potent than pills, and pills in turn are considered more potent than drops, creams, and ointments. Blood tests and biopsies are considered invasive. Surgery is most invasive. Invasive procedures may be refused out of fear.

Traditional Chinese medicine may be perceived to be naturally compatible for people whose ancestors invented and used it for thousands of years. Herbal remedies are perceived to "get to the cause" and thus to correct the underlying imbalance, whereas Western medications are understood to treat only the symptoms and are accordingly judged by the degree of symptomatic relief they bring. Some Chinese patients may believe that a particular medicine must be compatible with their particular body – a unique fit. The wealthy may seek the newest and most expensive treatment.

It is not uncommon for a patient to attribute cure to the skill of the doctor rather than to the medicine. A poor outcome, therefore, results in a perceived need to change doctors.

Rehabilitation

Rehabilitation services for a physical ailment may be avoided. The concept of moderation and restoration of Qi implies that exercise and active physiotherapy may be strenuous and therefore harmful. Rest and passive non-painful modalities such as massage are preferred.

The family of a physically or mentally disabled patient may prefer to accept the condition rather than use rehabilitation services, believing that the disease results from past or present family transgressions. They may refuse help from outsiders because of shame and a bad reflection on the family. As a result, the handicapped person may be sheltered, not diagnosed, not properly cared for, and kept from the outside world. This holds true as well for the handicapped child and the demented elderly.

Sexuality and Family Planning

There is virtually no sex education in a traditional Chinese family. Talking about sex is considered improper and embarrassing. Consequently, there is little or no knowledge of contraception or sexually transmitted disease, including AIDS. Although sex education may be mentioned in biology classes in junior high school, most adolescents gather at times incorrect information from their peers or the media. Proper terminology may be lacking for sexual practice or body parts.

While traditional Chinese prefer large families, mainland China has a policy of one child per family which has been more or less enforced for decades. The male child is more valued, partly for Confucian reasons and to preserve the family tree. This has led to social issues, such as widespread abandonment of female babies, escape from urban to rural areas where the policy is less strictly enforced, and emigration from China.

The policy of one child per family has also encouraged contraception. These include the use of more permanent methods such as the intra-uterine device and tubal ligation. While the mainland Chinese state promotes these methods, tubal ligation is not popular with many individuals because of its invasiveness. Vasectomy is doubly unpopular because of its invasiveness and the perception that it robs the man of his virility. On the other hand, therapeutic abortion is common. The rhythm method, withdrawal method, and birth control injections are also used. Birth control pills and barrier methods such as condoms are seldom used.

Several factors have led to the recent drastic increase in sexually transmitted diseases (STDs). When mainland China established the "open door policy" in 1986, a relaxation in strict social controls led to changing morals and a re-emergence of prostitution. Moreover, since the late 1980s, 100 million people, largely the young rural poor, have migrated to the urban eastern seaboard in search of work, creating a population most susceptible to STDs. Fostered by the low use of barrier methods to contraception, STDs are now the third-most-common infectious disease in China after dysentery and hepatitis.

Residents in some poor rural areas of mainland China, such as Yunnan, have been paid to donate blood. The use of unsterilized needles led to transmission of AIDS and hepatitis, and the problem was complicated by a tradition of denial among the officials. There is little or no treatment for AIDS, of which the government now estimates there are one million cases nationwide.

STDs and AIDS are considered sinful and immoral, leading to further denial and lack of recognition. Homosexuality, though occasionally mentioned in literature, is considered immoral and sinful as well, although in large cities by the end of the millennium some gathering places for homosexuals became public. The more urban and educated Chinese have relatively more knowledge of contraception and STDs and more tolerance of alternative sexual orientations.

In Hong Kong, Taiwan, and Canada, the pattern of contraception use among Chinese approximates that of the general Canadian population, except that Chinese seldom use cervical caps or diaphragms because women are uncomfortable inserting such objects inside their bodies.

The sexual behaviour of immigrant youth or young second-generation immigrants needs to be addressed by health care providers. They are at high risk of STDs and unplanned pregnancies through a combination of lack of education at home, more permissive liberal attitudes in Canada, relative lack of parental control of teenagers, and the teenagers' need to break away and fit into the larger society. The same is true for consumption of illicit substances.

Pregnancy and Prenatal Care

Prenatal care in rural mainland China is sometimes not sought until very late in pregnancy, because of a lack of health care personnel. Midwives are common in China and Southeast Asia. Doctors are involved in complicated cases. A female attendant may be preferred. In rural areas home births are usual, but in urban centres all births are hospital births. Pregnancy care and delivery in Taiwan and Hong Kong are similar to those of Canada.

In Canada, couples may not be able to attend prenatal classes because of work commitments or language barriers, although prenatal classes in Cantonese and Mandarin are available in some parts of Canada, such as Vancouver. There may be over-reliance on older female relatives during pregnancy.

Some women follow certain cultural practices to safeguard the fetus. For example, women may avoid foods that are classified as excessively "hot," such as lamb, or excessively "cold," such as watermelon and banana, or "poisonous," such as shellfish or turkey. Food with a slippery texture may also be avoided for fear the fetus may slip out. Physical exertion, such as vacuuming or moving furniture, may also be avoided during pregnancy. Even well-educated women may follow these practices under the influence of their mothers or mothers-in-law.

Childbirth

Childbirth can be a difficult time for newcomers to Canada with little English. The expectant mother may be unable to communicate with hospital staff about her needs. She may be misinformed about procedures such as the epidural, which is believed to cause permanent back problems. Caesarean section may be perceived to be easier on the mother's health than vaginal birth.

In Taiwan, Hong Kong, and mainland China, a woman can request a Caesarean section and pay for her choice. Chinese women may not understand why they have no choice in Canada. They may not want to go through the pain of delivery, or they may wish to have the baby on a specific day due to particular beliefs.

During the perinatal period, the expectant woman's mother, mother-in-law, aunts, and sisters may expect to provide assistance, and the health care professional has to gain their trust. A traditional husband may feel uncomfortable about participating in the birthing process and baby care. However, the absence of an extended family in Canada may oblige the husband to help care for the newborn.

Postpartum Period

After discharge from hospital, the mother may expect help from a female relative, and wealthy families may have a nanny. This does not indicate a lack of interest in the child. Health professionals should make sure that all the family members who will be involved are included in newborn care teaching.

The postpartum period is perceived as a vulnerable, "cold" period. The woman is expected to "sit for one month" (or "stay home for one month") and to avoid cold foods such as fruits, vegetables, or cold water. She has to eat more "hot" foods such as ginger vinegar soup and certain herbs. Ice packs to the breast or perineum may not be readily accepted, as the woman must avoid cold exposure including hair washing, bathing, or going out of the house. Heavy lifting is to be avoided to safeguard the uterus. Failure to comply with these practices is believed to result in infections and rheumatism. At the infant's one-month birthday, it is tradition to have a grand banquet, sometimes on the scale of a wedding, to celebrate the mother's and child's successful passing through the "vulnerable" period. Couples may abstain from sex for one hundred days after childbirth.

Nutrition and Food

Food has very important social meaning since the family gathers together at mealtimes. Feasts take place on special occasions, such as births, birthdays, weddings, and funerals. At these times, adherence to a prescribed diet can be a challenge.

The relationship between diet and health has long been interwoven with the traditional Chinese concepts of wellness and illness, much earlier than a similar awareness in Western medicine. A good diet restores, creates, and preserves health. It can prevent and treat illness.

The balancing of yin and yang is presented by the balancing of "cold" and "hot" foods. Individuals are thought to differ in their ability to tolerate hot and cold foods. Different foods are considered to contain varying degrees of heat or cold, quite apart from their actual temperature. Hot foods give strength and blood but in excess cause fever and related illness. Cold foods bring rest and relief but in excess produce weakness and chills.

Hot foods include strong alcohol, meats, spicy and fatty foods, and foods prepared by long cooking or at high heat. Cold foods include herbal teas, bland vegetables, most fruits, beer, and foods prepared cold.

Soup is a common home remedy, is consumed almost daily, and is valued as much as medicinal therapy. One often drinks the soup broth, but leave the vegetables or meat ingredients unconsumed. Immigrants accustomed to an unsanitary water supply may refuse to drink unboiled water, and such a person may refuse to take pills with tap water.

Steamed rice is the major staple. Rice cooked into a broth and noodles made from flour or rice are other sources of starch. Meat is eaten in small quantities, usually cut into bite-size pieces and stir-fried with vegetables. Polyunsaturated oils, especially peanut oil and sesame oil, are used in cooking. Buddhists may be vegetarians on account of their belief that one should not cause suffering by killing. Soybean is the other main source of protein. Cow's milk and its derivatives are not traditional foods, and many Chinese have an intolerance of lactose. Before refrigeration and canning were commonplace, food was preserved by drying. As a result, dried foods such as vegetables and seafood are still consumed even when equivalent fresh ingredients are available.

The traditional diet is low in fat, calories, and sugar. Obesity is relatively rare. The wealthy and the Westernized tend to eat more rich foods high in calories, such as fat, meat, and sweets. Consequently, in Hong Kong and North America, obesity, diabetes, and cardiovascular disease are becoming more common in Chinese families, along with breast and bowel cancer. Obesity is viewed as a sign of good nutrition and prosperity. Even though many Chinese are aware that MSG and a high fat content are not good for health, adherence to a prescribed diet can be a challenge.

Northern Chinese do not have year-round access to some fruits and vegetables and rely on preserved foods. They have increased incidence of esophageal and gastric cancers. Southern Chinese have more barbecued meats and salt-preserved fish. They have an increased incidence of nasopharyngeal cancer.

Many Chinese have a relatively slow metabolism of alcohol, but drinking problems are uncommon.

Bathing

In the past, with poor water sanitation in the homeland, bathing and hair washing were to be avoided during illness, during menstruation, in the postoperative period, and in the postpartum "sitting for one month" period. However, sponge baths were permissible. Infants may be bathed frequently, because cleanliness is highly valued, especially among southern Chinese.

Aging

Chinese people value longevity greatly, and it is a status symbol implying a sinless, healthy life. Old age is considered a time to enjoy the fruits of a lifetime of hard work and one's children and grandchildren.

Confucianism valued caring for elderly parents. Traditional responsibility for care of the elderly rests with the children, in particular with the eldest son and his wife. Next in line are the unmarried children. Daughters usually end up doing much of the work. Seniors who did not marry or have children are considered unfortunate.

Age is perceived to bring wisdom and warrants status and respect. Most Chinese political and religious leaders have been elderly.

Nursing homes are loathed. Moving into a nursing home represents loss of prestige for the elderly and shame for their children. However, there are now long-term care facilities operated by Chinese organizations, and these are well used. In Canada, placement in these nursing homes is slowly increasing. In many families all adults work, and many are unable or unwilling to quit work to look after the physically frail or demented elders. Well-to-do families may hire a full time caregiver to look after the elderly family member when dependency or reliance on family members increases.

Death and Dying

Among Chinese, any discussion about death and dying is sensitive. Timing of the discussion and who is to be involved must be carefully considered. The older generation believes death can be postponed if it is not mentioned or discussed. Families are often reluctant to tell the elderly dying patient the diagnosis and prognosis. Consequently, estate planning is seldom done, hospice and palliative care are seldom sought, and anticipatory grieving seldom takes place. It is helpful for the health provider to clarify whether the patient already knows about the prognosis or, if not, wishes to know. Some patients may want to delegate the receiving of information and decision making to another family member.

Though death is viewed as natural and inevitable, families often prefer that health professionals not reveal the prognosis to the dying. Filial piety requires the children to ensure the last days are free of worry and pain. Decisions to establish level of care, to not resuscitate, or to withdraw life support are difficult. The decision is often made collectively by the family, and the health care professional may need to address all involved. Death at home brings misfortune.

When illness is incurable and terminal, many will seek traditional Chinese therapies. At times this can be expensive, interfere with prescribed medications, and contribute to unrealistic denial. Health care providers should remain open to this and be ready to negotiate.

Because of the importance of food, families may be overly enthusiastic in feeding the terminal patients when they have loss of appetite and nausea from the illness or treatment. Chinese families, at times more so than the patients themselves, may insist on pursuing interventions such as intravenous hydration and tube-feeding to prolong life even if these do not add to the quality of life.

Upon death, the body should not be disturbed, so that the spirit can leave in peace. Angry spirits can bring misfortune to the living. A postmortem is almost always refused, being perceived as most invasive and disrespectful to the dead. Organ donation and cremation are also not acceptable. Buddhists want the body to remain unmoved for several hours. The health team should learn about such things ahead of time.

Burial rituals are dictated by the person's particular religion. Family and friends attend the funeral, which often ends with a simple dinner. Traditionally, pregnant women, even if they are close family, are often not allowed to attend a funeral for fear that it would harm the pregnancy. In the past, males wore black armbands and females wore white woollen flowers in their hair. Clothing with bright colors is avoided. Relatives of the deceased may not visit others or attend celebrations during a mourning period. To do so would bring misfortune to the host. Relatives mourn for forty-nine days following the death of a loved one, and a memorial service is held every seventh day for this period of time.

Delivering Culturally Competent Health Care

Chinese culture has been in existence for 3,500 years. The subject of innumerable books and scholarly writings, it is intricate and complex. This chapter barely touches on those aspects that relate to health and illness.

The Chinese have been in Canada since the nineteenth century, if not earlier, and because of immigration patterns are an extremely heterogeneous group. An individual's cultural beliefs and attitudes can fall at any point along a continuum between the traditional and the fully Westernized. Influencing factors include place of origin, gender, socioeconomic status, education, exposure to Western culture, and length of time in Canada. Even among highly Westernized individuals, such as Canadian-born Chinese, some Chinese traditions and culture are deeply ingrained and integrated into their family structure.

With such diversity in the culture, generalizations and stereotypes are misleading. Each person is a unique individual with a distinct background and values. Time is well spent in determining each individual's background, present life circumstances, and beliefs in a non-judgmental and respectful manner. In order to optimize the delivery of culturally appropriate health care, health care professionals need to be willing to negotiate a mutually acceptable plan of care that addresses the individual, including his or her cultural beliefs.

It is essential to communicate in a language that the patient and family can understand. Involvement of the family is important, and is usually an integral part of providing effective and acceptable care. However, when interpretation is required, a professional interpreter, rather than a family member, should be utilized. Health care providers who speak the language and have experience with Chinese people may be sought as consultants.

Further Reading

Bowker, John, ed. 2002. *Cambridge Illustrated History of Religions.* Cambridge: Cambridge University Press.

Chan, A. 1985. *Gold Mountain: The Chinese in the New World.* Vancouver, BC: New Star.

Fung, Kwok-Keung. 1998. *Understanding Chinese Cultures: A Handbook for Health Care and Rehabilitation Professionals.* Toronto: Yee Hong Centre for Geriatric Care.

Fung, Yu-Lan. 1948. *A Short History of Chinese Philosophy.* New York: The Free Press.

Hong Kong Apothecary: A Visual History of Chinese Medicine Packaging. 2003. Vancouver, BC: Raincoast Books.

Kleinman, A. 1980. *Patients and Healers in the Context of Culture.* Berkeley, CA: University of California Press.

Li, Han. 2004. *The Water Lily Pond: A Village Girl's Journey in Maoist China.* Waterloo, ON: Wilfrid Laurier University Press.

Li, Peter S. 1998. *Chinese in Canada.* Toronto, ON: Oxford University Press.

Ratanakul, P. 1999. "Buddhism, health, disease, and Thai culture." In H. Coward and P. Ratanakul, eds., *A Cross-Cultural Dialogue in Health Care Ethics,* 17-33. Waterloo, ON: Wilfrid Laurier University Press.

Sethi, Sarla, David C. Este, and Maya B. Charlebois. 2001. "Factors influencing child-rearing practices of recently migrated East Indian and Chinese women with children from infancy to age six." *Hong Kong Nursing Journal* 37: 14-20.

Stewart, M., J. Anderson, M. Beiser, A. Neufeld, and D. Spitzer. 2003. "Multicultural Meanings of Social Support for Immigrants and Refugees (Edmonton, Vancouver, and Montreal)." Research study funded by the Social Sciences and Humanities Research Council of Canada, Ottawa.

Wong, Jan. 1999. *Jan Wong's China: Reports from a Not-so-Foreign Correspondent.* Toronto, ON: Doubleday Canada.

Woo, Sophia, and Raymond Lee. 2001. "Spirituality and mental health in Chinese culture." *Visions: BC's Mental Health Journal* 12: 23-24.

Contributors to the first edition

Sharon Boyce, SUCCESS, Vancouver

Raymond Chang, Strathcona Community Care Team, Vancouver

Rita Kwan, SUCCESS, Vancouver

David Lee, Ministry of Social Services and Housing, Vancouver

Shirley Leung, SUCCESS, Vancouver

K.C. Li, Strathcona Community Care Team, Vancouver

Centina Low, SUCCESS, Vancouver

Elaine Lui, Health Sciences Centre Hospital, University of British Columbia

Margaret Ma, Vancouver Health Department

Contributors to the second edition

Francis Chan, Program Director, SUCCESS, Vancouver

Lorraine Cheung, Cultural Studies and Health Research Unit, School of Nursing, University of British Columbia

Alice Choi, SUCCESS, Vancouver

Wallace Chung, Retired surgeon, University of British Columbia, and former chairman, Chinese Cultural Centre

Jane Crossen, Cultural Studies and Health Research Unit, School of Nursing, University of British Columbia

Truus Kotwal, Physiotherapist, Holy Family Hospital, Burnaby

Magdalene C. Lai, Community Health Nurse, Vancouver Coastal Health Authority; Co-author of chapter on Chinese in first edition of this book

Donna Lee, Registered Nurse, Vancouver Hospital

Kwok Chu Li, Clinical Professor of Psychiatry (Emeritus), University of British Columbia

Agnes Luk, Counsellor, Healthiest Babies Possible, Evergreen Community Health Centre, Vancouver

Sui Mei, Settlement worker, Storefront Orientation Society, Vancouver
Hiram Mok, Psychiatrist, Cross-Cultural Clinic, Vancouver Hospital
Peijian Shen, Instructor of Traditional Massage, Langara College, Vancouver
Allan Wong, Psychiatrist, Vancouver Hospital
Angela Wong, Psychiatrist, Cross-Cultural Clinic, Vancouver Hospital
Tracy Wong, Instructor, Faculty of Dentistry, University of British Columbia
Sophia Woo, Multicultural Mental Health Liaison Worker, Vancouver/Richmond Health Board
Douglas Yiu, Family Physician, Vancouver

3

People of Cambodian and Laotian Descent

Chansokhy Anhaouy, Elizabeth Richardson, and Nancy Waxler-Morrison

Although people from Cambodia and Laos are discussed together in this chapter, they are linguistically and culturally distinct from one another and usually form socially separate communities in Canada. They nevertheless share certain historical and cultural features, including the fact that the overwhelming majority in both communities came to Canada as refugees in 1979 and thereafter.

Cambodia and Laos, neighbouring countries in Southeast Asia, share certain historical and cultural characteristics. Both experienced the early influence of Indian culture and follow the Theravada Buddhist religious tradition. They formed part of French Indochina, remained French colonies until independence in 1953, and have therefore inherited a legacy of French language and culture. During the colonial period, large numbers of Chinese migrated to Indochina as merchants and eventually gained control of rice trading. The Chinese remained a distinct ethnic minority in both countries and were generally resented by the majority because of their dominant economic position. Also during the colonial period, Vietnamese were brought in by the French to staff the government bureaucracy, a policy that strengthened the historical antipathy of Cambodians and Laotians towards the Vietnamese.

The refugee experience is another factor common to Cambodian and Laotian immigrants, one that they share with the Vietnamese. Departure from their home countries was largely forced on them by political upheavals beyond their control, so their migration was neither voluntary nor planned but hurried and often dramatic. For the Cambodians in particular, escape followed several traumatic years under the Khmer Rouge when the social fabric of family and society was destroyed. During the flight from their countries many suffered extreme hardship. In many cases escape was followed by long periods of uncertainty in crowded refugee camps. Acceptance by Canadian immigration authorities and arrival in Canada, though solving many problems, added others, such as culture shock, language difficulties, financial worries, discrimination, and unemployment. At the same time as they were attempting to settle in and adjust to Canada, they also had to come to terms with the recognition that the loss of their home would be permanent.

By 2003 almost all of the original refugees from Cambodia and Laos had become Canadian citizens, though a few remained landed immigrants. Some have sponsored family members to join them in Canada.

Cambodia

Cambodia is a tropical kingdom situated in the southwestern part of the Indochinese peninsula and bounded by Thailand, Laos, and Vietnam, with a southwest seacoast on the Gulf of Siam. The climate is hot and humid, with monsoon rains in the summer.

Of Cambodia's 13.8 million people, three-quarters live in rural areas, where they grow rice and other food crops; urban dwellers work in business, services, and manufacturing, mainly of garments. The Cambodian economy has not completely recovered from earlier conflict and continues to rely heavily on foreign aid. One-third of Cambodians live below the poverty line, and average life expectancy is low, fifty-four years for men and fifty-nine years for women.

The population of Cambodia consists of three main ethnic groups, the largest being the Khmer, representing roughly 85 percent. Vietnamese constitute 5 percent of the population and Chinese about 3 percent, and there are other smaller minority groups. Traditionally, the majority of ethnic Khmer were farmers working primarily in rice cultivation, the Chinese minority were urban dwellers involved in business enterprises, and the Vietnamese were generally fishermen or small businessmen.

History and Reasons for Migration

Gaining independence from France in 1953, Cambodia became a constitutional monarchy under Prince Norodom Sihanouk. In 1970, Sihanouk was overthrown by a military coup and replaced by a pro-American, anti-Communist regime headed by General Lon Nol. Fighting ensued between government forces and the Communist Khmer Rouge, a radical guerrilla movement. In 1975 the Khmer Rouge were victorious and established a government under Pol Pot.

The situation in Cambodia in the four years that followed has been described as genocide, in which an estimated 1.7 million people died from hunger, disease, and execution. Upon seizing power in 1975, Pol Pot's Khmer Rouge regime embarked on a policy of de-urbanization. Cities were forcibly evacuated, and urban dwellers were expected to join the peasantry in agricultural production. Parents and children, male and female, were separated and forced to work at building dams, farming, and so forth. The regime abolished all religions as well as markets and money. Education was limited to political dogma. Persecution and execution were the fate of Cambodians who were educated, had been exposed to Western culture, were associated with the previous regime, or resisted the new one. Thousands of others died as a result of starvation and disease. Food was rationed and inadequate, and medical care was limited to traditional medicine. To attempt escape was a crime punishable by death. Nonetheless, a few did manage to flee to Thailand or Vietnam, some walking for as long as two months, day and night, and suffering en route from malnutrition and disease.

In late 1978, Vietnam invaded Cambodia, defeated the Khmer Rouge, and set up a puppet government. These events set off a huge wave of refugee departures as, for the next thirteen years, the ousted Khmer Rouge cadres waged a guerrilla war against a coalition government. During this time most freedoms were restored, although under very difficult conditions. In 1991 a United Nations–sponsored peace agreement led to free elections in 1993 and the restoration of the monarchy with Sihanouk as king. Relative political stability was established soon after, and efforts were made to rebuild the economy.

Waves of Migration from Cambodia to Canada

Before the major influx of refugees began in 1979, only about two hundred Cambodians lived in Canada. Most had come to Canada for education in French-language universities and had remained as professionals; some were joined by family members. The majority lived in Quebec.

From 1979 to 1983, after the overthrow of the Khmer Rouge, there was greater opportunity to escape, and tens of thousands of Cambodians fled across the border into Thailand to the refugee camps set up by the United Nations. These were people of all backgrounds – professionals, workers, fishermen, businessmen – but the majority were farmers and labourers drawn from the countryside. Few spoke English or French, many had not completed elementary school, and many were young families or single men. Camp conditions were very poor, and decisions by sponsoring countries were delayed.

In the first few years after 1979, about 7,000 Cambodians were accepted by Canada, of whom approximately three-quarters were Khmer and one-quarter were Chinese and others. All were classified as "convention refugees" and therefore became landed immigrants upon arrival in Canada. Most were sponsored by government and a few by private groups, especially churches; both government and private sponsors helped with such things as housing, jobs, and school enrolment for one year. By 2002 most of these Cambodian refugees had become Canadian citizens. While initially many settled near their sponsors, later they moved on, mainly to metropolitan areas, particularly Montreal, Toronto, and Vancouver. The more educated people tended to settle in Montreal where their knowledge of French was useful.

From 1983 until the 1990s, the Cambodian government imposed many barriers to leaving the country. However, the Canadian government had begun to encourage family reunification in 1982, and some were able to take advantage of that program. It is estimated that of the 6,330 Cambodians living in Canada in the 1980s, 20 percent had come as sponsored relatives. Many were siblings, some were children, a few were parents, but there were very few elderly people.

More recently, some unmarried Cambodian men in Canada have chosen to find wives in Cambodia rather than to marry "modern" Cambodian girls who grew up in Canada. Often these are men who can sponsor a wife, for which the criterion under the Immigration Act is having a job rather than a certain income level. The number of immigrants from Cambodia has dropped progressively from about 700 per year in 1990 to about 200 per year in 2002.

Laos

Laos (the "s" is silent) is a small, landlocked country composed of densely wooded mountains and fertile river valleys with a tropical monsoon climate. Laos shares borders with Vietnam, Cambodia, Thailand, and, in the north, with Burma (Myanmar) and China. In 2002 Laos had 5.5 million people, 80 percent of whom lived in rural areas where they grew rice, corn, tobacco, coffee, and cotton. Only around the capital, Vientiane, has some industry developed. In the largely rural north, 53 percent of the population is poor, in contrast with a poverty rate of 22 percent in and around Vientiane, which is in the south. Large numbers of families depend upon remittances from relatives abroad for their main source of income. As in Cambodia, life expectancy is low: fifty-three years for men and fifty-six years for women.

About half the population is ethnic Lao, who are farmers or educated urban lowlanders. Of the several minority groups, one of the largest is the Hmong, a generally illiterate mountain people who have retained a distinctive language and cultural tradition. A Chinese minority were traditionally city dwellers involved in business enterprises.

History and Reasons for Migration

Until the French takeover of Indochina in the late 1880s, Laos was a kingdom largely controlled by Thailand. Following independence from the French in 1953, fighting broke out between the Royal Lao government and the pro-Communist Pathet Lao. A period of almost continuous warfare ensued, with the French and later the United States supporting the Royal Lao government, and the Vietnamese Communists backing the Pathet Lao. During this period of civil war, families were uprooted and driven from their homes.

In 1975, following Communist victories in Cambodia and Vietnam, the Pathet Lao seized control in Laos and has continued to form the government since then. After 1979 large numbers of Laotians fled to refugee camps in Thailand. Contributing to the exodus were economic collapse, the new government's policy of reprisals against those who supported the former regime, and the general hardening of Communist government policies. Initially, refugees were from the upper and middle classes – professionals, students, merchants, and administrative and technical employees of the former regime. As the economic situation deteriorated and resistance to the new government increased, Laotians from rural areas joined the exodus. Another major refugee group from Laos was the Hmong, the rural hill people mentioned above, most of whom found asylum in the United States.

In order to escape from Laos and get to Thailand, refugees had to cross the Mekong River by swimming or by paying for transportation in boats, and sometimes those who were caught were shot. As with the Cambodians, most of the Laotian refugees underwent extreme physical and emotional hardship while escaping and during their ensuing lengthy internment in Thai camps.

Waves of Migration from Laos to Canada

Before 1979 there were about 200 Laotians in Canada. Like the Cambodians in similar numbers, most Laotians were students who had come to Quebec for university education in French and had chosen to remain. A few were professionals.

From 1979 to 1983 came the major wave of migrants, when about 7,700 Laotians were accepted by Canada as "convention refugees" who became landed immigrants upon arrival. Many were young families and single men and the majority were ethnic Laos. In this wave approximately 20 percent were of Chinese background; a very small number were Hmong. In contrast to the Cambodians, Laotians were often sponsored by churches, with the Mennonite Church being particularly active.

When the Canadian government offered the possibility of family reunification, many Laotians did not have sufficient income to meet the financial levels required for family sponsorship. However, some family members did arrive, so that by 1990 there were 14,000 persons of ethnic Lao origin in the country. From 1990 to 2000, immigration from Laos dwindled to less than 100 persons per year.

Groups Discussed in This Chapter

This chapter discusses the majority groups: the Khmer of Cambodia and the Lao of Laos. Substantial numbers of ethnic Chinese from Cambodia and from Laos arrived in Canada in the large wave of migrants that began in 1979. But they have gravitated to the larger Chinese community and so are discussed in Chapter 2 on people of Chinese descent. The Hmong from Laos went mainly to the United States; the few who came to Canada live mainly in the Kitchener-Waterloo area (for more information about the Hmong, see Fadiman 1997).

Early Settlement Problems in Canada

The initial experiences of refugees from Cambodia and Laos differed widely, in part because of the diversity in socioeconomic and political backgrounds within each group. Some were well educated and urban, while others were from rural areas, with little formal schooling or exposure to Western values.

The Khmer

Many urban, educated, middle-class Khmer were either executed by the Pol Pot regime or fled when it came to power or after the Vietnamese invasion. Consequently by 1979 when migration to Canada began in earnest, the majority of Cambodian refugees were drawn from the countryside. Most were farmers and labourers, and many had not completed elementary school. Because they were mainly sponsored by government, they settled initially near the relevant Canadian government offices.

Though some Khmer had learned English in the refugee camps, knowledge of English in the Khmer community was generally very poor and relevant job training absent; as a result the jobs the Khmer could obtain were unskilled and poorly paid. Many families were forced to supplement part-time or marginal incomes with financial assistance from the government. It was noted at the time that the Khmer "have been the least well served by public and private attempts at refugee assistance and have had to carry on primarily on their own. This has led to difficulties in finding employment, underuse of social and health services, social isolation, and a lack of public and government awareness of Khmer [Cambodian] problems and concerns" (Indra 1985, 456).

Initially the Khmer were unable to sponsor family members because the Canadian government did not recognize the Vietnamese-backed regime. Only family members who were able to escape to refugee camps outside the country could be sponsored. Thus many Khmer had no relatives in Canada, and they commonly experienced isolation and homesickness.

The Lao

The Laotian community was composed primarily of young families, with very few elderly people. Because the majority were sponsored privately and people settled near their sponsors, the community tended to be widely scattered.

Downward occupational mobility was common among Laotian refugees because of their poor English and inability to find employment in occupations for which they had been trained. Needing to support their families, they also lacked time and money for retraining. The overwhelming majority did not find the type of employment they were used to. Former teachers, army officers, administrative personnel, and technicians were employed as farm workers, factory workers, and janitorial staff, positions they would never have considered at home because of their education, training, and social status.

When the Khmer and Lao arrived in Canada, money and employment were crucial issues for them. Generally, their savings, if any, were used up during their escape and in the refugee camps, and many felt obliged to send money to assist relatives still in Southeast Asia, an obligation that continues to this day. Underemployment led to frustration, humiliation, and depression and was especially difficult for members of these cultures because class and status distinctions are taken very seriously. Many Khmer and Lao had periods of unemployment due to layoffs from marginal jobs, and the experience caused feelings of shame and incompetence as well as tension in familial and social relationships.

Language

The predominant language in Laos is Lao, a language related to Thai. In Cambodia, the Khmer speak their own language, also called Khmer.

Since French was the language of government, business, and education during the colonial period in Indochina, some older or educated Khmer and Lao immigrants spoke or were familiar with French. Those with some French have had an easier time learning the language. Few had experience with English.

In 1991 in Canada, neither English nor French was spoken by 22 percent of Khmer and 14 percent of Lao, perhaps reflecting the somewhat lower levels of education among the Khmer. By 2004 the large majority had learned these languages through ESL classes or daily experience.

Young Khmer and Lao who have been educated in Canada have fluent English or French but often do not know Khmer or Lao since there are few formal schools for these languages. This creates a communication gap between young and old at home, where older family members are more

Mrs. Sochua, from Cambodia

Mrs. Sochua, now fifty-five, has been in the hospital for a week with pneumonia. She came to Canada with her daughter and son in 1981 after three years in a Thai refugee camp. The family lives mainly on her son's occasional work as a labourer and sometimes on social assistance.

Every day, eight or ten anxious friends crowd around Mrs. Sochua's bed during visiting hours, speaking in Khmer; a few try to ask questions of the nurses in broken English. The nurses have difficulty understanding the questions and find the crowd of people somewhat intimidating. They find it difficult to focus on Mrs. Sochua's condition and respond to her needs when she is surrounded by so many people they can't talk to.

One day a Cambodian girl just out of high school accompanied the visitors. She overheard one nurse say to another, "These people have been in Canada for such a long time and they still can't speak English! I don't see why we should put ourselves out to cater to them. Why can't they just learn English and get on with it! They take up so much of our time." Everyone went away feeling very upset: the girl, the visitors to whom she relayed what she had heard, and the nurses themselves.

comfortable speaking their traditional language. Young people sometimes look down upon their elders who do not speak the Canadian languages.

Religion

Lao and Khmer cultures are similar largely because of the influence of Theravada Buddhism, one of the main streams of Buddhist thought, which is adhered to by 90 percent of the population of both countries. A notion central to Buddhism is that desire for pleasure and possessions causes suffering, which, however, can be avoided through non-attachment to things. In other words, man can avoid undue pain and suffering through moderation in all aspects of behaviour, including the expression of strong emotions. Another basic and interconnected belief is reincarnation and the theory of karma, that is, that one's present life is the consequence of one's deeds in a previous one. Through correct and meritorious behaviour, man can improve the condition of his next life. Buddhism tends to be family-centred, and rituals are frequently practised in the home.

Before the advent of Buddhism in Cambodia and Laos, there existed an animistic cult marked by the worship of spirits that lived in people and in nature. The Lao, for example, believed in thirty-two spirits inhabiting the human body. At the time of death, these spirits were believed to separate and then combine with others to be reborn in a new body. However, the spirits of those who died in childbirth, accidents, or other violent causes were considered evil and were prevented from being reborn. More precisely, these spirits were doomed to roam the earth, tormenting the lives of others by, for example, causing physical or mental illness. Such animistic beliefs continue to be held in varying degrees, particularly by those from rural backgrounds, and coexist with Buddhist tenets.

Both the Khmer and Lao communities have made efforts to establish their own Buddhist temples in Canada, plans made more difficult because many monks and priests in Cambodia and Laos died in the pre-1979 conflict. As a result, by 1993 the few Khmer and Lao temples established in Canada often did not have monks. In 2004, for example, the closest Khmer temple for residents of southern British Columbia was in Washington State. Many BC Khmer and Lao worship at the Thai temple in Vancouver, where there are no ancillary social or supportive activities for their groups.

Small numbers of Khmer and Lao have converted to Christianity as a result of close relationships with their Christian sponsors. Within the Lao community there is a tendency towards social distance between Christians and Buddhists.

Family Structure

Traditionally in Cambodian and Laotian society, the family is the key social and economic unit. The extended family forms a network of support and assistance, both financial and emotional. The role of women is subordinate, although compared to some other parts of Asia their status is quite high. They are responsible for child-rearing, for performing most household duties, and often for managing family finances. They are expected by men to be virtuous, gentle, modest, and obedient. The husband as head of the household has authority and is the decision maker and breadwinner. Typically, in Southeast Asia, women are not employed outside the home, although before immigrating many women were forced to support families when husbands and male relatives died in the war or were conscripted for military service.

Once in Canada, Khmer and Lao women were forced by economic necessity to do outside work. This change upset the traditional family balance in which the woman was financially dependent on her husband, and it sometimes undermined the self-esteem of men whose traditional role was that of the family breadwinner.

The genocidal policy of the Khmer Rouge in Cambodia instilled great fear in the Khmer survivors and has resulted in continued dysfunction in family relationships many years later in Canada. The Khmer Rouge abolished traditionally strong family ties and encouraged family members to spy and report on one another; children were taught to distrust parents. This fear continues to be felt in Canada today, where adult children may still distrust older parents.

In urban areas of Cambodia and Laos, a household usually consists of a married couple and their unmarried children. In rural Laos, households tend to be extended, while in rural Cambodia they are nuclear. When first in Canada and income levels were low, families often shared housing with other adult relatives in order to enjoy a higher standard of living. Since the mid-1990s, Khmer extended families have sometimes pooled their resources to buy a house together.

In Cambodia and Laos, family problems are considered personal and private. Solutions are sought within the family, or sometimes with the assistance of close friends. However, in most cases, the doors are firmly closed to involvement by outsiders, including professionals. Even after many years in Canada some Khmer and Lao are uncomfortable with the fact that in Canada government figures such as social workers and school counsellors use their authority to mediate or force solutions upon family members rather than allowing this role to be taken by a close associate such as an elder or valued friend of the family.

Marriage

In Laos and Cambodia, marriages are typically arranged in the sense that the parents of both partners are closely involved. In some cases the wishes of the young couple are taken into consideration. The man's family is generally interested in the girl's character, social reputation, and ability to perform household tasks. The girl's family is concerned about the prospective husband's character, family background, and social status. In Cambodia dating is rare; courting takes the form of group activities, such as parties, and is seen as leading to marriage. Premarital chastity for women is highly valued, and an unwed girl who becomes pregnant brings shame to her family. In rural areas she may be considered an evil person who will attract bad fortune. Divorce is rare and disapproved of strongly.

Following a wedding in Cambodia, the young couple lives with or near the groom's family. The bride is expected to serve the husband's family and this makes her vulnerable to abuse. In Laos, the couple generally starts married life with the bride's family, sometimes moving later to the husband's family home, or out on their own.

Over the years of residence in Canada, many Khmer and Lao parents recognized their children were being socialized as Canadians, and they attempted to find some middle ground between their own cultural values and those of their children. Today, dating is becoming more common. Some parents arrange marriages; in other families children choose their own partners. Young married couples usually live independently from the outset but often reside close to their families. Divorce is becoming more common as well. Some intermarriage is occurring, sometimes between Khmer and Lao, sometimes with mainstream Canadians.

In 2004 it is slowly becoming the norm for working Khmer men in Canada to return to Cambodia to find a wife. These men are searching for "traditional" women, not the "modern" Khmer girls who have grown up in Canada. Most of these traditional brides are young, and they have no relatives of their own in Canada.

Child-Rearing

Children in Cambodia and Laos are taught to respect and obey parents and other adults. There is a hierarchical order among siblings whereby the younger ones are expected to defer to and respect the older ones, who in turn are often required to care for their juniors. This is particularly true in the case of the eldest male child, who in his teenage years has almost parental authority and responsibility for his younger siblings.

Infants are seldom left to cry, are carried more, and tend to walk later than Canadian children. Generally bottle-feeding continues longer, sometimes up to three or four years of age. Some Khmer believe that prolonged bottle-feeding will strengthen the baby, while others simply do it out of convenience. Toilet-training, which is learned through observation rather than deliberate conditioning, comes later. For the most part there is a more relaxed attitude towards the stages of childhood and thus towards developmental delays in walking or speech. Parental indifference to a delay in learning to talk sometimes leads to problems when the child first enters school. From infancy, children take their place at social events; only at very formal events are they excluded.

Discipline is usually not physical, especially for young children, tending instead towards persistent verbal admonition. Children are expected to learn correct behaviour by observing and imitating adults. However, among the Khmer in Canada physical punishment does occur, and some parents do not understand that such punishment may be judged to be "child abuse" which can lead social services to step in and remove children from the home. In Khmer culture it is normal for adults to touch children in a way that might be construed to be sexual. It is also normal for children to sleep in the same bed as their parents. Often children are allowed to play naked, both inside and outside the house. However, in some regards Khmer children are more strictly controlled than Canadian children. Open disagreement with parents is unusual. Swearing at or looking down upon parents is shameful and insulting, and towards grandparents such behaviour is unheard of.

Khmer parents may give gifts, usually money, to their children as an incentive to behave and cooperate. They may use gifts to entice their children to attend school every day. The gift is given before the child cooperates and is therefore not a reward for good behaviour. In fact the desired result may not occur.

Cambodian and Laotian cultures are very protective of girls, who tend to be brought up more strictly than boys because their reputations must be beyond reproach if a suitable marriage partner is to be found. They are taught a helping role within the family, are given a greater share of household tasks, and are, traditionally, not expected to achieve the same level of education as boys. Over the years in Canada parents have accepted the idea that education is important for both boys and girls. As well, Laotian parents have allowed girls to have more freedom to date and to participate in school activities.

Children's and Adolescents' Experiences in Canadian Schools

In Cambodia and Laos, traditionally, the role of the teacher was highly authoritarian. Teachers were respected by parents and children, so parents turned their children over to the teacher during school hours and did not question or participate in school affairs. Khmer and Lao who arrived in Canada with young children or who established families after migrating brought the same expectations here. Many young Khmer had disrupted and incomplete educations in Cambodia as a result of Pol Pot's destructive policies, and came to Canada with very little educational experience of any kind.

In the early years of immigration to Canada, school children were caught between two cultures, between the traditional values of their parents and the pressures to conform to peer values and behaviour. Children sometimes expected more freedom and were less willing to defer to the authority of parents. Some experienced confusion, loneliness, and alienation in a school environment which differed so much from their home countries. In Canada the role of the teacher is more relaxed and familiar. Behavioural expectations are different. For example, some children were extremely embarrassed at having to undress in school locker rooms, so many avoided activities such as gym or swimming.

Khmer families with teenagers who were born in Cambodia or in refugee camps had an especially difficult time in Canada. Children had been indoctrinated to inform on parents; they were separated from parents and lived for long periods in collective work camps. These adolescents tended to have difficulty coping with other students and with school work, and the majority dropped out of school in Canada before grades 8 or 9.

Even today, children's schooling continues to be affected by Khmer experiences in Cambodia and the continuing struggle of poorly educated and trained parents to overcome poverty and become established. Many Khmer parents do not know how, or do not have the time, to support their child's schooling, and most continue to see teachers as authorities to whom they cannot talk. Parents do not participate in school affairs. Furthermore, when their parents are constantly stressed, children face special challenges, and they express their frustration and confusion by getting into trouble at school.

Most Khmer adolescents still do not finish high school, leaving them eligible only for low-level, often part-time, employment. Many of these young people are financially unable to establish their own households and continue to live with parents. Of the small proportion who do complete high school, very few go on to higher education. Most Khmer students do not have the emotional and financial support necessary to sustain their interest and enthusiasm for college or university. Many young Khmer lose their Khmer identity and simply become "poor Canadians" faced with all the challenges of poverty.

Laotian children have had somewhat similar experiences in Canadian schools. Many parents do not have time to go visit the school. Many continue to fear authorities, to avoid confrontation, and to be intimidated by language problems. However, parents tend to trust their teachers and their children and do not mind not participating in their children's education. In Laotian families still struggling to establish themselves economically, Laotian boys sometimes drop out of high school in order to work and contribute their income to the family. Girls tend to be more successful in school than boys.

The Elderly

The elderly have great authority and receive considerable respect in traditional Laotian and Cambodian societies, particularly the men, who are called on to advise and make important decisions for family members.

Elderly parents typically live with their families, never alone, and adult children feel a strong responsibility to care for them. In these extended families, grandparents give practical help with household tasks and often with the care of grandchildren.

Names

In the Laotian naming system, as in Canada, the personal name comes first, followed by the family name. Traditionally the family name is not very important, and people are generally addressed and referred to by their personal names. Nicknames are common. When a Lao woman marries, she takes her husband's family name. Most Lao family names are polysyllabic, for example, Koulavongsa or Sysavoth.

Among the Khmer, by contrast, and unlike Canadian names, the family name comes first, followed by the given name. As with the Lao, given names are used more frequently than family names. So for example, if a man's family name is Vong and his given name is Sararith, he will be addressed as Mr. Vong Sararith or more commonly, Mr. Sararith. Similarly, if his wife's personal name is Maly, she will be called Mrs. Maly or Mrs. Vong Maly – though at marriage most Khmer women keep their own last names. Therefore, addressing a female spouse as Mrs. [husband's last name] would not be appropriate. A child is often given a nickname shortly after birth, a custom originally intended to confuse the evil spirits that might want to cause harm.

Family identity and last names are highly valued in Khmer society. This is expressed by respect for others' last names. Insults to the family name may incite physical retaliation.

Cultural Values and Behaviour

Time

In Southeast Asia, time is generally more elastic than in Canada and the pace of life more relaxed. Punctuality tends to be considered unimportant. The important thing is simply to be present. However, people adjust quickly to Canadian expectations, and keeping appointment times is usually a problem only for some newcomers.

Greetings

The traditional greeting involves pressing the palms of one's hands together at chest level accompanied by a slight bow. This gesture is also used to express thanks. While some Khmer and Lao men have adopted the Western custom of shaking hands, women may not feel comfortable with this practice. Traditionally, the head of the family is greeted first. Khmer are not accustomed to saying "excuse me" when passing others. In Cambodia it is traditional for children to show respect when they pass an adult by bowing the head and going quietly by, but this custom is rarely practised in Canada.

Hospitality and Gifts

Hospitality is a strong tradition in Khmer and Lao cultures. The concept of the "Dutch treat" is foreign, and the host is expected to pay for his guests, say, at a restaurant. Casual visits do not require an invitation, and there is much entertaining of family and friends at home.

Khmer and Lao may initially respond to invitations with a refusal, so as not to appear over-eager or impolite. Typically, the offer or invitation is then made several times, after which it is considered appropriate to accept.

Gift-giving is less common than among Canadians and is usually not associated with special occasions, except weddings. Acceptance by a woman of a man's gift signifies encouragement of romantic intentions and may not be considered entirely proper. People may be reluctant to accept favours where they feel unable to reciprocate. Occasionally, thanks may be expressed by giving an extravagant gift.

Expression of Emotion and Courtesy

Physical expressions of affection between members of the opposite sex, including married couples, are considered improper when performed in public or even in front of friends. Body parts are seen to exist in a hierarchy, the most supreme and respected part being the head, with other parts diminishing in importance towards the feet. Touching the head or shoulder of another person in casual contact, particularly if he or she is older, is viewed as extremely disrespectful. When communicating, an avoidance of eye contact is an expression of respect.

In accordance with Buddhist beliefs, the traditional attitude towards life stresses harmony and interdependence; direct confrontation is avoided, and the expression of anger or displeasure is considered rude. Conflicts and disagreements are approached indirectly, and a person may simply withdraw when offending appears unavoidable. Thus an overt "yes" does not always signify true agreement but may simply indicate a desire to maintain politeness and harmony. For example, if someone does not wish to see a health professional, he or she may agree to an appointment and then fail to keep it. Similarly, a smile does not necessarily express approval, pleasure, or acceptance; it may be intended only to prevent social discomfort or to conceal anger, embarrassment, or grief.

In both Laos and Canada, Lao show respect to all older people, even those who are strangers, by addressing them as "aunt" or "uncle."

Clothing

In Canada, Cambodians and Laotians wear Western-style clothing, and remove their shoes when entering a home. Some Cambodians and Laotians dislike using second-hand articles, especially clothing. This attitude may stem from fears that the previous owner died, or was a carrier of a communicable disease or of general bad luck which might then transfer to the new owner.

Special Customs

Laotians traditionally celebrate a special custom called *baci* (pronounced "bassi") whereby individuals receive blessings and wishes of good health and prosperity. During the ceremony, cotton strings are tied around the wrists of the persons being honoured and are subsequently worn for three days. Often a community potluck dinner follows the ceremony. Baci is celebrated on many occasions, such as the birth of a baby, marriage, recovery from illness, graduation from high school or university, or to mark any other happy event. It continues to be practised by Laotians living in Canada.

Recreation and Leisure

In Cambodia and Laos, sports, especially soccer, are a popular pastime, and recreation is generally family-centred. In Canada, families from these countries tend not to spend money on entertainment such as movies or restaurants, but rather enjoy their free time at home or visiting with friends and relatives at home or in public parks. For some men gambling and drinking alcohol are pastimes in Canada. The Khmer have big gatherings on weekends in their homes which may include a potluck dinner and karaoke. Activities outside the home include a day at the park, fishing, and clam digging. Khmer and Lao sometimes socialize together as well as with others from Southeast Asia.

Festivals and Holidays

Pimay, the Laotian New Year, is the only traditional holiday that continues to be practised by Lao living in Canada. According to the Buddhist calendar, it falls near mid-April and marks the end of Laos's dry season and a return to growth and prosperity. In Canada, it is celebrated by the ceremony of baci, followed by a party with food and dancing.

Khmer in Canada observe several religious celebrations during the year, with a Buddhist monk officiating when possible. As in the Laotian tradition, the New Year is determined by the Buddhist calendar and is celebrated in mid-April, when the community gathers together for a party. Other religious celebrations during the year involve large parties, as many as four hundred people, financed by community fundraising.

Relationships with Canadians

Khmer and Lao from rural areas are used to friendly, relaxed relationships with neighbours. Doors and windows are left open and neighbours' voices carry easily from one house to the next. Early in their life in Canada, immigrants frequently experienced a major difference in Canadian neighbourhood life, finding that Canadians are quiet and keep to themselves. Many felt lonely and isolated as a result.

Health Care Systems in Cambodia and Laos

In Cambodia there is no medical insurance system, and patients are required to pay cash for treatment. Hospitals exist only in major urban centres, and rural areas have few health services, including dental care. People from these areas rarely travel to the cities for treatment because of the expense involved.

In Laos, while residents of urban areas have access to clinics and hospitals, only company and factory workers have medical insurance, often paid for in part by the employer. In rural areas, even the most remote ones, non-government organizations and aid agencies have recently established primary health clinics where no health services existed before.

In both Cambodian and Laotian medical centres and offices, patients must wait their turn to see a doctor or nurse because there is no appointment system. Some wait a whole day and some must return to the queue the next day as well. Pharmacists, called "Doctor," often recommend and sell medicines as well as traditional remedies; a sick person's relative may describe the symptoms and purchase medicines to take home to the patient.

Prevalent Diseases

In 2000 major health problems in Cambodia and Laos included tuberculosis, malaria, trachoma, diphtheria, typhoid, cholera, dysentery, hepatitis, intestinal parasites, malnutrition, dengue fever, filaria, encephalitis, AIDS and other sexually transmitted diseases, as well as drug addiction. Moreover, leprosy sometimes occurs in outlying rural areas. Infant mortality rates are high: ninety-six and eighty-seven per 1,000 live births for Cambodia and Laos, respectively. In Laos maternal and neonatal mortality and morbidity remain high.

In the late 1970s when Khmer and Lao arrived in Thai refugee camps, many were ill, and the conditions in the crowded camps, combined with insufficient medical attention, made recovery difficult. When the first wave of refugees came to Canada, they were sometimes found to have tuberculosis, intestinal parasites, anemia, hepatitis B, and dental caries. At that time, in a study of the health status of Indochinese refugees, recently arrived Khmer were found to be in poorer health than other groups, probably because of the extreme deprivation they had suffered during the prior decade, including lack of food, shelter, and medical care.

Currently, Cambodia has the highest prevalence of HIV/AIDS of any of the Southeast Asian countries. While both Cambodia and Laos have major funding for prevention programs, there is concern for the spread of the disease by large numbers of transient persons seeking work across country borders. Condom use in Laos is very low, sex with prostitutes is a common leisure activity for men, and thus HIV/AIDS may be passed on to their wives. There are commonly accepted myths about the disease. Many believe that young boys and girls are not susceptible, especially young people from rural areas.

Traditional Health Care Beliefs and Practices

In Cambodia, health care was abolished during the Pol Pot regime. Instead, both urban and rural Khmer used medicine provided by traditional doctors, *loke kru,* to care for themselves, or they were simply left to die. Medicines made of herbs, leaves, and roots, as well as marijuana, were commonly used. In general, traditional healers are greatly revered and trusted, especially in rural society, and they are missed by many Khmer in Canada.

In Canada, self-medication and treatment may tend to be more common among Khmer and Lao than in many other Canadian residents. Few homes are without Tiger Balm, a mentholated ointment, which is used to treat a variety of conditions including colds, upset stomach, bruises, and insect bites. It is believed that some people may be allergic to the ointment. Medicines made from fresh herbs are used widely in home countries, but not in Canada, as the ingredients are not easily obtainable. Drinking tonics, such as ginseng, and avoiding excess are common ways of maintaining health.

Many Cambodians and Laotians, like Vietnamese, use a traditional practice known as coin rubbing in which an area of the body is rubbed with a metal object, usually a coin or spoon, until the skin becomes red. The area may be massaged first with a mentholated ointment, such as Vicks VapoRub or Tiger Balm, or with baby oil. This practice is commonly used to treat headaches, colds, fever, stomach aches, dizziness, and fatigue. Different areas of the body are rubbed depending on the symptom or problem. Coin rubbing is a common home remedy that continues to be used widely in Canada, especially when symptoms first appear and before a doctor is consulted. If the problem persists or is particularly troublesome, medical attention is usually sought. Another traditional treatment practised in Canada is the pinching of the skin between the eyebrows until it becomes red. This is used as a remedy for headaches and dizziness. Both coin rubbing and pinching cause bruising of the treated areas and when used on children can be mistaken for evidence of child abuse.

In Canada, many people will often try traditional medicines and treatments at home before they seek help from a health professional. If symptoms do not improve, medical attention is generally sought. Traditional treatments and medicines, such as herbal infusions, may be continued in conjunction with prescribed medical treatment without the physician being informed.

Doctor-Patient Relationships

Typically, in Khmer and Lao cultures, the role of the health professional is authoritarian while that of the patient is passive and dependent. The professional is expected to ascertain quickly what is wrong, and the cure, or disappearance of symptoms, is expected to be fairly rapid. Doctors are highly respected and trusted members of society.

At a medical consultation a patient expects to receive some medication or treatment. It is unacceptable for the doctor or health professional to suggest that there is nothing seriously wrong and that the condition will heal by itself. Most Khmer and Lao would be left feeling that the physician is uncaring and unhelpful. Similarly, many people find medical tests meaningless before treatment is prescribed because the tests are not seen as part of the therapeutic process. Health professionals in Cambodia and Laos typically view the psychological support afforded to their patients as an important part of their healing role. The provision of some type of medication or treatment is regarded as integral to this support. Placebos are widely used by practitioners in Southeast Asia.

Lack of fluency in English is a major problem for many older adult Khmer and Lao in obtaining satisfactory care from health professionals in Canada. Unlike for some other immigrant groups, there are no professionals who speak their native languages in most areas of the country. For some it becomes necessary to rely on interpreters or on broken English, a less than satisfactory arrangement. Those people who can communicate in Vietnamese, Chinese, or French are sometimes able to consult practitioners who speak these languages. Most prefer any Asian doctor over a Western one.

Women, particularly older ones, prefer female physicians, especially for obstetrics and gynecology. However, in Canada, most have male doctors and may thus be reluctant to discuss complaints and undergo regular checkups. A Khmer woman quoted her elderly mother as saying, "I'd rather die than be examined by a doctor who is a man." However, many Khmer women prefer a male doctor for serious procedures like surgery.

Many Lao and Khmer in Canada see a doctor only when they feel seriously ill. This is especially true of men. This reluctance to seek early medical attention may stem from language difficulties and discomfort at the cultural differences that divide patient and professional. Many Lao and Khmer continue to be wary of all authorities, a fear learned during the terrible destruction of their own societies. But in Canada, many also fear the unknown: "What will the doctor do to me?" Older people in particular will not go to a physician unless there is a very severe problem. As well, Khmer and Lao with low-level jobs may want to avoid the loss of income they incur when attending medical appointments.

Mr. Sararith, from Cambodia

Mr. Sararith, sixty-one, was admitted to hospital in Nanaimo for hernia surgery. He, his wife, and their youngest child came to Canada in 1983 after two years in a Thai refugee camp. They accepted refuge in Canada knowing almost nothing more than "it's cold there." Mr. Sararith had been a fisherman in Cambodia before the terrible chaos and genocide began. He had begun working with his father as soon as he was strong enough to pull the nets. He took only three years of school. His wife never went to school and could not read their own language, Khmer.

Once in Canada they were relieved to be finally safe, but they knew no other Cambodian immigrants, having only a few names of fellow Cambodians from the camps who "lived in Canada, somewhere." Both Mr. and Mrs. Sararith were intimidated by ESL classes and finally stopped attending. He managed to find seasonal work on the fish boats with the help of another Cambodian he had met, but mainly they depended on welfare.

When Mr. Sararith was well enough to be discharged, the nurse caring for him came to the room to explain to the couple what Mr. Sararith could expect to do at home and what help he would need from his wife. She talked about what he could eat, how to bathe; she cautioned him against lifting; she told him to book a follow-up appointment with his doctor. Mr. Sararith did not understand the technical terms, and his wife understood almost nothing. All the information went by very fast, while they nodded and smiled. But Mrs. Sararith became very worried.

About five days after he had been at home, late at night, Mr. Sararith began to have swelling and severe pain in his abdomen. These were symptoms that he had not had before. Neither of them knew what to do. Should they telephone someone? But Mr. Sararith could not get to the phone. Who to phone? Should they go to the hospital? But it was almost impossible for him to walk up the steps to a taxi. Their upstairs neighbours might be able to tell them what to do, but it was the middle of the night and they did not want to disturb them. They finally decided to wait, to see if he would get better.

Mental Health

Mental illness is stigmatized by Khmer and Lao cultures. An individual who has mental health problems brings disgrace and shame to his or her family and is considered to be "crazy." Being labelled as mentally ill is devastating to the individual and to his or her family. As a consequence, mental illness tends to be feared and denied. Not infrequently, people suffering from mental health problems are sheltered and hidden by family members until the family can no longer cope. At that point they may seek professional help. Mental illness may be attributed by those with rural backgrounds to evil spirits or by some Buddhists to karma, that is, to the consequences of bad deeds committed in previous lives.

In Southeast Asian culture, where stoicism is a virtue and emotional weakness is unacceptable, "somatic complaints represent a cultural means of expressing psychological and emotional distress" (San Duy Nguyen 1984, 88). Khmer and Lao with mental health problems are likely to display a variety of physical symptoms, such as headaches, insomnia, aches and pains, fatigue, and dizziness. Because complaints are somatic, people tend to seek help from medical practitioners rather than mental health professionals, and they generally expect to receive medication. Health professionals may need to ask indirect questions to obtain information about the patient's symptoms. By 2004 mental health workers had become more common in Cambodia. This may contribute to a slightly more receptive attitude towards mental illness among the Khmer.

Most mental health problems among Khmer and Lao in their early years in Canada were linked to severe loss, the difficulty of cultural adjustment, and uncertainty about the future. These refugees had typically gone through many traumatic experiences in rapid succession with little time to adjust. Often it was only after they began to settle into their new environment that the full impact of the losses and experiences was felt. Some suffered "survivor guilt"; they felt that they had no right to be alive or to live well when other family members and compatriots had died. Added to the stresses rooted in the past were those of the present: culture shock, language difficulties, social isolation, financial problems, and unemployment or underemployment. It was not surprising that, in their early years in Canada, depression was one of the most common mental health problems found in Southeast Asian refugees.

Especially for the Khmer, many of the early stresses continue today. The survivors of genocide never forget their experience, and some continue to suffer from symptoms of post-traumatic stress. Problems of employment and education add to the burden. Mental illness continues to be stigmatized. Those suffering from it are sheltered at home and will be taken to a hospital emergency room only when the family feels that the person is seriously ill, that is, "crazy."

Treatment and Medication

It is commonly held among Khmer and Lao in Canada that medicine may lead to side-effects such as dizziness and even death. Further, Khmer distinguish between North American medicine and the French medicine that they received in their home country. One Khmer living in Canada reported, "Some people died in Cambodia after the Red Cross sent medicine from America," the implication being that the American medicine was not strong enough. People sometimes increase the strength and frequency of the prescribed dosage. For example, a person who is told to take an antibiotic capsule four times a day might take two capsules each time, or take them five times a day. Further, many Khmer may stop taking a course of antibiotics as soon as they feel better; the remaining pills may be given to a relative or friend.

Among the Khmer there is a widely held belief in the effectiveness of injections over other forms of treatment. People who hold this view are likely to feel discouraged about the prospects for cure if only pills are prescribed. Many Khmer and Lao are especially fearful of anesthetics and believe they will never recover from them. Associated with this fear is the great fear of any kind of surgery, minor or major. Surgery for gallstones is felt to be especially dangerous. If a Khmer wants to insult someone he says, "You don't have a gall bladder!" It is important that the need for surgical procedures, both major and minor, be carefully and clearly explained.

Many fear X-rays because they believe a lifespan is reduced by one year with each exposure to an X-ray. Some fear blood tests, thinking that the loss of blood causes dizziness and fatigue. People in a weakened state, such as following surgery, may feel that a blood test is actually life-threatening and may therefore need considerable reassurance before they consent. Many older Lao will not go for a blood test unless it is absolutely necessary.

A Khmer or Lao patient may appear to agree to a prescribed treatment and then not comply, or may behave in a manner that effectively undermines it. Lack of compliance may be due to disappearance of symptoms or to the influence of family or friends. It is important to realize that others besides the patient and the immediate family may be involved in decisions about treatment. Extended family members and friends and even important community leaders may all offer advice and guidance.

Beliefs about Specific Diseases

In Cambodia many Khmer are very afraid of cancer. They sometimes confuse hepatitis with cancer because of the jaundice they have in common. The disease that a Canadian physician might diagnose as cancer may, from a Khmer point of view, be called an "infection" that is best treated with traditional medicine. In Canada, most know about breast and lung cancer, but other forms of cancer are frightening and need explanation.

In general, the Khmer and Lao communities in Canada know little about AIDS, sexually transmitted diseases, or diabetes. Efforts are now being made within the Khmer community to educate elders about these diseases. Young people learn about these diseases in school, but in the Khmer community it is important for this information to be validated by the elders.

Hospitalization

In Cambodia and Laos, family involvement with a hospitalized patient is extremely important. Generally speaking, the entire family is expected to visit daily. In Cambodia, a relative usually stays in the same room with the patient and helps with care. In both countries, visitors bring food and are encouraged to do so. In many cases, meals are brought in as substitutes for hospital food.

In Cambodia, the physician usually visits a hospitalized patient twice daily, and the Khmer in Canada may interpret the relative infrequency of contact with their doctor as lack of concern.

Rural immigrants who have not had ready access to hospitals may view them as places where one goes to die, since that is in fact what often happens in Cambodia. For this reason, they are likely to fear and avoid hospitalization in Canada.

Most Khmer and Lao are familiar with the idea of being asked for consent for procedures, but in their home countries the consent was verbal, not written, because of their complete faith and trust in doctors. In Canada today, while younger Khmer and Lao do not have language difficulties, older people may need an interpreter to explain the details in each case.

Lack of fluent English is a major problem for some older Khmer and Lao hospitalized in Canada. The inability to communicate with hospital staff makes the experience frightening and lonely, and many miss the traditional close support of family members. Using children to interpret has huge pitfalls. Many children lack sensitivity as well as the necessary vocabulary; often young people have one language strongly but the other language is weak. Differences in food create a further difficulty; most Southeast Asians eat rice three times daily and generally do not eat bread, potatoes, cheese, butter, or milk. Hospital gowns, however, are accepted as they are used in home countries.

Family Planning

In 1999 family size in both Cambodia and Laos, at an average of four or five children, was larger than in neighbouring Vietnam and Thailand. Many women have never taken ongoing, daily responsibility for birth control. Only one-quarter of women used modern methods of birth control and more commonly in urban than rural areas. Men do not use condoms. In Laos today, abortion using over-the-counter medicine is becoming a common choice. Some women will choose tubal ligation once families are complete. In general there is no special preference for the sex of offspring; boys and girls are equally welcome.

In Canada, most Lao and Khmer couples prefer smaller families, with two or three children being the norm. There is a prevailing feeling that child-rearing is more expensive here and that a smaller family gives children a better chance of gaining a good education. In the case of an unwanted pregnancy in Canada, a Lao or Khmer couple may decide on abortion.

Pregnancy and Prenatal Care

Khmer and Lao prenatal customs vary with ethnicity, region, rural and urban domicile, and level of education. Some Khmer women believe, for example, that hard physical work during pregnancy will result in easier delivery. Some hold that beer consumption during pregnancy will give the baby a beautiful, clear skin. Another notion is that an easy delivery will be assured if the mother imbibes a traditional white wine containing medicinal herbs when she is seven or eight months pregnant. There is a traditional Lao belief that a pregnant woman should not attend a funeral or visit anyone who has had a recent death in the family. Because practices vary, it is essential that health professionals find out from individual women what they believe to be important in their prenatal care.

When a woman becomes pregnant in Cambodia and Laos, she first tells her husband and then her immediate family. It is happy news, and pregnancy is considered a normal, healthy period in a woman's life. Until very recently only those living in urban areas received regular medical attention. In Canada, some, but not all, Lao and Khmer women are interested in attending prenatal classes. Their husbands generally do not attend because men do not discuss "women's problems" in public, nor do they discuss such things with their wives.

Illegitimate pregnancy is stigmatized in Cambodia and Laos, where it sometimes leads the woman to commit suicide using over-the-counter medicine. When it occurs in Canada, families may arrange an abortion. However, illegitimacy is somewhat more acceptable in Canada, so an unmarried Lao or Khmer mother may receive some support from her family, but attempts will be made to "save face" and keep the pregnancy hidden.

Childbirth

In Cambodia and Laos, the birth of a child is an occasion for celebration and ceremony. In rural areas, childbirth is generally at home. The mother and newborn are attended by a midwife who usually stays for three or four days following the birth. In urban centres, childbirth is generally in a hospital, and a female member of a woman's family may stay with her during the period of hospitalization.

Traditionally the father does not participate in the birth, and in Canada few Khmer and Lao men choose to be present in the delivery room. Initially, in Canada, women who had already given birth in their home countries often felt uncomfortable delivering in a Canadian hospital because of the contrasts. In Laos, for example, as soon as a woman delivers, she must drink hot water; she should definitely not consume anything cold. There is a general fear of invasive procedures such as Caesarean section and episiotomy, and the need for such measures should be carefully explained. Circumcision is not typical. Younger women who have grown up in Canada and know the system do not have much difficulty.

Postpartum Period

According to both Khmer and Lao traditional beliefs, it is extremely important for women to keep warm after childbirth, and many find Canadian hospitals too cold. After giving birth in rural areas of Cambodia, the woman rests on a special bamboo bed under which a charcoal fire is kept burning for up to a week. Windows may be closed, and a woman usually covers her head. Khmer also traditionally believe that women must not take showers or cut their hair for the first month postpartum; a woman washes in a mixture of warm water and a special wine that is believed to have medicinal properties. Laotian women traditionally take hot baths and drink warm fluids for twenty-one days to a month following birth. Hot food is very popular for postpartum mothers, and ginger and peppers are added to their food. They also consume herbal white wine. Many traditional beliefs and customs continue to be practised in Canada and need to be recognized.

Traditional food restrictions may also obtain during the perinatal period. A traditional Laotian belief requires that a new mother should avoid soup and spicy food and should eat only dry food. During the postpartum period some Khmer women may avoid beef, chicken, and raw vegetables. Because of the diversity of dietary beliefs and practices, it is necessary for the health professional to determine what the individual patient holds to be important in her health care.

For the first month postpartum in Cambodia and Laos, women are expected to stay at home and rest in bed while family members help with household tasks. In Canada, women stay home for as long as possible, but if they have jobs they return to work when their unemployment benefits expire. Couples usually abstain from sexual relations for three months. In their home countries, women generally breastfeed for up to a year and sometimes two years in rural areas. In Canada, many choose to bottle-feed either because they have to return to work or because they feel it is more acceptable.

Childhood Health and Illness

In rural Cambodia and Laos, children are usually treated for minor illnesses at home with traditional medicines and remedies, usually as prescribed by grandparents. For the Khmer, Tiger Balm or an equivalent ointment is routine treatment for infants and young children to prevent stomach aches and to relieve gas. The ointment is rubbed on the child's stomach two to three times a day, especially after bathing and before bedtime. In Canada, because medical care is inexpensive and accessible, Cambodian and Laotian families are generally prompt in seeking medical attention for sick children.

Food and Nutrition

The traditional staple of the Laotian diet is a glutinous variety of rice which is steamed, while the Khmer eat standard rice. In addition, fish, poultry, beef, pork, vegetables, and fruit are common items. Lactose intolerance, that is, the inability to digest milk or milk products, is common in both Khmer and Lao; thus milk does not feature in the traditional diet. In Canada people are usually able to find necessary spices and other ingredients in Chinese food stores. While most Khmer and Lao in Canada eat with forks and spoons, some still prefer to eat with their fingers. Over the years here many have taken to junk food, but there is not yet a substantial problem with obesity.

Food preferences or taboos may be practised during periods of illness. Khmer believe, for example, that stomach ache sufferers should not eat fresh vegetables or oily food or drink orange juice or anything acidic. Some Cambodians maintain that any type of skin disease requires avoidance of beef, chicken, bamboo shoots, and eggplant. There are people who prefer not to eat at all when they are sick.

Food was scarce and nutrition very poor during the Pol Pot regime in Cambodia. Many suffered from malnutrition and were forced to eat whatever was available, including lizards and snakes. Many Khmer in Canada link their stomach problems to this experience.

Alcohol and Tobacco

In their home countries, alcohol, most commonly traditional rice wine, is consumed by men. This rice wine, which may contain 40 percent alcohol, is much stronger than typical Western white table wine. Use of alcohol by women, especially young unmarried women, is generally considered improper. Alcoholism is extremely rare. In Canada, Lao and Khmer men drink socially at parties or with visitors in the home. Women, although they drink less than men, are more likely to accept alcohol here. In Canada, excessive alcohol use by Khmer men was fairly common early in their stay; it was believed that drinking showed they were "strong." More recently, Khmer men seem to have become aware of the dangers of alcoholism and are drinking less and consuming alcohol only with food.

While many Cambodian and Laotian men smoke cigarettes, few women do so.

Dental Practices

In Cambodia and Laos, dental care exists only in urban centres. Personal dental hygiene is generally good, and teeth are cleaned daily. In rural areas, salt or lemon is frequently used in place of toothpaste. Most older people chew tobacco mixed with other ingredients. The malnutrition experienced by the Khmer and Lao and the poor conditions in refugee camps meant that many people lost their teeth and many had gum and teeth problems upon their arrival in Canada.

Because the majority of Khmer and Lao in Canada have low-level jobs with no dental insurance, most cannot afford private dental care and thus use it only for severe emergencies. School children are more likely to receive dental care through the school system. Older Lao fear all kinds of health care and thus do not want their teeth extracted; they would prefer to have a diseased tooth fall out on its own. As well, many do not understand gum disease and why it should be treated.

Care of the Elderly

Elderly people in Cambodia and Laos are important members of the family and are generally highly respected by the young. There are no nursing homes or care facilities as families are expected to, and want to, care for the elderly. In Canada these families continue to honour their traditional responsibility. They believe that nursing-home care is improper, and a daughter would rather quit her job to care for an aged parent than allow him or her to be placed in a nursing home. To do otherwise would invite censure from the community. In 2000 the numbers of Lao and Khmer over age sixty-five were still very small, about 5 to 7 percent of the population of these groups, so few families have had to find ways to care for old people. When such care was needed, one working Lao couple arranged for their older children to go home from school at lunchtime to see that their elderly grandfather had his lunch. There are probably no elderly Lao who have no family; any such would be cared for by the Laotian community.

Death and Dying

For Khmer and Lao who are Theravada Buddhists, the funeral is by cremation. Those who are Christian converts follow the particular church's practice.

In Cambodia and Laos, according to the Theravada Buddhist belief, the deceased's body is washed and placed in a casket in the home. A wake is held for three days and nights during which family and friends visit, food and drink are provided, and the atmosphere is generally festive. On the third day, the body is taken to a temple where cremation takes place. On every anniversary of the death, family and friends participate in a memorial ceremony.

A person who knows that he or she is dying may request the family to gather so that last wishes may be expressed and belongings bequeathed to family members. Traditionally, Khmer and Lao prefer to die at home if at all possible. In home countries, a hospitalized patient who is terminally ill is often discharged so that he or she can return home to die, and elders and priests are invited to pray in the home.

In Canada patients want to die at home, and they are usually taken home by family members. Cremation is commonly preferred, although burial is also used. Families generally do not understand and will not agree to an autopsy.

Attitudes towards Public Health and Social Services

When the large wave of immigrants arrived from Cambodia and Laos in the late 1970s, few of them understood the purpose of public health and social services, let alone how to use them. There were no such services functioning in their home countries. By 2004 some social services have been introduced into Cambodia and Laos. In Canada, home visits by social workers may be accepted, but many people are unlikely to understand the relationship or know how to respond, since involvement by strangers in personal matters is a foreign notion.

Young women are generally anxious to receive information and help from public health nurses about nutrition and infant care because most do not have older female family members in Canada to educate and assist them. Many women do not know the purpose of mammograms or Pap tests and thus do not go for them, although young and educated women are more likely to do so.

Providing Culturally Sensitive Health Care

In relating to Khmer and Lao immigrants, formality and politeness are essential as a basic cultural expectation in clinical encounters. A slower pace and a quiet, unhurried manner are likely to reassure patients and will be more successful in establishing rapport and trust.

It is very important to remember the traumas that Khmer and Lao experienced before and during their escape from their home countries. Families were broken, education and health services were unavailable, human rights were ignored, food was in very short supply, many people died. The past must be remembered in order to understand why many Lao families, and particularly many Khmer families, continue to struggle to establish themselves in Canada even twenty years or more after their arrival.

Above all, it is necessary to recognize that Khmer and Lao are not homogeneous groups. Considerable diversity exists, based on ethnicity, rural or urban background, level of education, and degree of exposure to Western health care. It is only through approaching patients as individuals that health care can be truly sensitive and appropriate to cultural and personal needs.

Further Reading

"Asia survey, Hong Kong." 1973-88. *Far Eastern Economic Review*.

"Cambodia and Laos." 2002. *Asia 2002 Yearbook*. Hong Kong: Far Eastern Economic Review.

Catanzaro, Antonio, and Robert John Moser. 1982. "Health status of refugees from Vietnam, Laos, and Cambodia." *Journal of the American Medical Association* 247: 1303-8.

Chan, Kwok B., and Doreen Marie Indra, eds. 1987. *Uprooting, Loss, and Adaptation: The Resettlement of Indochinese Refugees in Canada*. Ottawa, ON: Canadian Public Health Association.

City of Vancouver Task Force. 1980. *Background Paper on the Laotian, Cambodian, and Hmong Refugees*.

Dorais, Louis-Jacques. 2000. *The Cambodians, Laotians and Vietnamese in Canada*. Ottawa, ON: Canadian Historical Association.

Fadiman, Anne. 1997. *The Spirit Catches You and You Fall Down: A Hmong Child, Her American Doctors, and the Collision of Two Cultures*. New York, NY: Farrar, Strauss and Giroux.

Garry, Robert. 1980. "Cambodia." In Elliot Tepper, ed., *Southeast Asian Exodus: From Tradition to Resettlement*. Ottawa, ON: Canadian Asian Studies Association.

Indra, Doreen. 1985. "Khmer, Lao, Vietnamese, and Vietnamese-Chinese in Alberta." In Howard Palmer and Tamara Palmer, eds., *Peoples of Alberta: Portraits of Cultural Diversity*, 437-63. Saskatoon, SK: Western Producer Prairie Books.

Kiljunen, Kimmo. 1984. *Kampuchea: Decade of Genocide*. London: Zed Books.

Muecke, Marjorie A. 1983. "In search of healers: Southeast Asian refugees in the American health care system." *Western Journal of Medicine* 139: 835-40.

Oberg, Charles N., and Amos Deinard. 1984. "Marasmus in a 17-month-old Laotian: Impact of folk beliefs on health." *Pediatrics* 73: 254-57.

Pickwell, Sheila M. 1983. "Nursing experiences with Indochinese refugee families." *Journal of School Health* 53: 86-91.

Royle, Peter. 1980. "Laos: The prince and the barb." In Elliot Tepper, ed., *Southeast Asian Exodus: From Tradition to Resettlement*. Ottawa, ON: Canadian Asian Studies Association.

San Duy Nguyen. 1984. "Mental health services for refugees and immigrants." *Psychiatric Journal of the University of Ottawa* 9: 85-91.

Tung, Tran Minh. 1980. *Indochinese Patients: Cultural Aspects of the Medical and Psychiatric Care of Indochinese Refugees*. Washington, DC: Action for Southeast Asians.

Contributors to the first edition

Chansokhy Anhaouy, Immigrant Services Society, Vancouver
Kate Frieson, Monash University, Melbourne, Australia
Soma Ganesan, Vancouver General Hospital
Nay Sim Ke, Vancouver
Heng Khauv, Vancouver
Madeline Lovell, University of British Columbia, Vancouver
Lily Tham Phranchanah, Vancouver
Banh T. Prom, Vancouver
Donna Shareski, Vancouver Health Department, Burrard Unit
T.K. Sihalathavong, Burnaby
Duang Thavonesouk, Langley
Khamvanh Xaygnachack, Langley

Contributors to the second edition

Somchay Khousakhoune, Mechanical Engineer, Calgary
Maureen Minden, Nurse-Midwife, Health Care and Epidemiology, University of British Columbia
Phangsy Nou, Cambodian Community Family Support Services, Vancouver
Savon Pen, Family Services of Greater Vancouver
Donna Shareski, Vancouver Health Department, Burrard Unit
Keo Simpraseuth, Ministry for Children and Family Development, Vancouver
Kham Simpraseuth, Dental Therapist, Saskatoon

4
People of Iranian Descent

Afsaneh Behjati-Sabet and Natalie A. Chambers

Iranian immigrants are a steadily growing ethnic group in Canada, living mainly in Toronto and Vancouver. The flow of people from Iran began in 1979, during and after the Islamic Revolution. By the 1990s about 5,000 immigrants from Iran were arriving in Canada annually. In addition, by 2000 about 1,500 Iranian refugees a year were also coming, making Iran the fourth- or fifth-largest source of refugees to Canada. Today most adult Iranians in Canada are first-generation immigrants who share many of the beliefs, values, and characteristics of their compatriots in Iran. Many now have Canadian-born children.

Unlike the small number of Iranians who willingly migrated to North America, particularly to the United States, before 1979, the majority of Iranians who have come to Canada since the revolution left against their will and under tremendous pressure. Especially early on, their flight was from unbearable living conditions and religious and political persecution. Under these conditions it seems natural for the process of adjustment and integration to be slow. On the other hand, the majority of Iranians residing in Canada came from large urban areas, belong to upper- and middle-class families, and are relatively familiar with Western education and values. Many of these migrants come seeking a better education for their children. Hence, the transition is probably smoother for this group of immigrants than for most. The Iranian immigrant and refugee population of Canada is probably in a relatively advantageous position when dealing with Canadian public services, particularly medical and health services.

Geography of Iran

Iran, formerly called Persia, is almost as large as the three westernmost provinces of Canada combined. It is mountainous in the north and west and low-lying in the centre and south. Bordering Iran to the north are Armenia,

Azerbaijan, the Caspian Sea, and Turkmenistan. To the west are Turkey and Iraq, and to the east, Afghanistan and Pakistan. The Persian Gulf and the Sea of Oman separate southern Iran from Kuwait, Saudi Arabia, the Arab Emirates, and the Arabian Sea.

Iran's overall climate, affected by two large deserts in the central and eastern regions, is dry with high summer and low winter temperatures. The northern region bordering the Caspian, however, has a mild and humid climate with long rainy seasons. The southern coast is also very humid, but with much higher temperatures, far less rain, and longer summers.

Tehran, the capital, is situated in a dry area at the southern foot of the Alborz Mountains and is known for its four distinct seasons. Many Iranian immigrants in Canada come from Tehran.

Iran has been classified as a developing country and is basically an agricultural society that produces rice, wheat, tea, cotton, citrus fruits, and dried fruits. It is one of the world's largest oil producers and a powerful member of OPEC.

The very rapid growth of the oil industry since the turn of the century and its nationalization in the 1950s dramatically increased per capita income in Iran and encouraged swift technological growth. Large urban areas developed, and migration to cities occurred on a considerable scale. This in turn deepened national class divisions.

In 2002 Iran had a population of approximately seventy-two million, mainly Indo-European. However, a large population of ethnic Turks, Kurds, and Arabs lives in the northern, western, and southern border areas. Also, many minority tribes are spread throughout Iran and support themselves by sheep- and cattle-raising. While these tribes retain most of their cultural heritage, some have become well educated and have travelled abroad for higher education. In addition, large numbers of Afghans flooded across Iran's border during the recent wars in Afghanistan, and some Iraqis, notably the "Marsh Arabs," escaped to Iran when persecuted by their government.

History of Iran

Persian culture goes back many thousands of years, and a written account of the history of Persia dates from 559 BC. During the course of its history, Iran (or Persia) has experienced several invasions and absorbed various cultures that have laid the basis of modern Iranian society.

Islam Established in Persia in the Seventh Century

The most important invasion was the Arab conquest in the seventh century, which put an end to the last of the pre-Islamic dynasties and extinguished the predominantly Zoroastrian society. The Islamization of Persia took place very rapidly, and Islam has since been the major religion of the country. Persia experienced several centuries of strict Islamic governance in which religious rules became the governing laws of Iran.

Constitutional Monarchy, Twentieth Century

Though a constitutional monarchy was established around the turn of the twentieth century, the constitutional system remained largely nominal, and Iran was governed by the undisputed power of the Shahs (kings). The last monarch was Muhammad Reza of the Pahlavi dynasty who reigned for thirty-seven years (1942-79). During these years some attempts at modernization were made. Universities were established and students were sent abroad by the government for higher education. The Unveiling Act of 1937 was the first step towards the emancipation of women, who were given voting rights in the 1960s. Western lifestyles and values became more common.

Islamic Revolution, 1979, and the Iran-Iraq War

In 1979 the last Shah was overthrown in the Islamic Revolution led by Ayatollah Khomeini, and the Islamic Republic of Iran was established with a strict fundamentalist regime in control. Since that time the government has attempted to entrench a much more traditional and religious lifestyle. This has made living conditions generally unbearable for a majority of the rapidly emerging educated and Westernized upper and middle classes, and for modern women in particular. Moreover, the lengthy and bloody war between Iran and its neighbour Iraq exacted unbelievable human casualties and economic destruction and evoked the constant fear of conscription in thousands of young boys and men. Added to this have been the persecution of various political, ideological, and religious groups and well-documented violations of human rights. All these factors constitute the most important reasons for Iranian migration to Western countries, especially to Canada and the United States, since 1979.

Towards the end of the twentieth century, many Iranians, especially women, have become more aware of their rights, and the *hijab* (or headscarf), formerly in black or dark blue, has become a "fashion statement" in bright colours. Women are now allowed to attend university, and even rural people want both boys and girls to get a good education. Some have noted that "even servants are willing to assert their rights." As more Iranians question the policies of the fundamentalist government and the absolute authority of the clerics, the government has become somewhat less harsh and the society more secular. However, the Republic of Iran today still prohibits freedom of speech, opposition parties, and all forms of entertainment considered to be un-Islamic.

Waves of Migration to Canada

Prior to 1979

Before 1979 small numbers of Iranians, mostly professionals and business people, migrated to Canada and the United States, and some who came for higher education remained in these countries.

The Islamic Revolution, 1979, and Onward

The major exodus from Iran took place after the Islamic fundamentalist government took over. Supporters of the Shah were persecuted, educated professional women were excluded from many jobs, including government and banks, and coeducation in universities was abolished. The latter policy excluded women from higher education since female-only universities were not immediately established. All women were required to wear the hijab, husbands were given the right to ban their wives from taking employment, and the age of marriage for women was reduced from eighteen years to thirteen. Many of these new policies threatened the livelihoods and lifestyles of middle- and upper-class urban Iranians and persuaded them to migrate to Canada and the United States. Those who had money to move and resettle arrived as independent and business-class immigrants, while others came seeking asylum.

After they became established in Canada some Iranian families sponsored relatives, mostly their parents, for admission to Canada. Even though the social situation in Iran has improved today, the economy has stagnated, making it more difficult to earn a living there; as a result some Iranians have begun to come to Canada largely in the hope of a better income. Finally, there was some shift away from the earlier pattern of middle- and upper-class migrants to more working-class Iranian immigrants, largely from urban areas.

Refugees, 1979 Onward

By 2000 about 1,500 Iranian refugees were arriving annually in Canada, many of them escaping religious persecution because they belong to the Baha'i faith. At the beginning of the Islamic Revolution, the Baha'i religion was banned and followers of the faith were executed. Under more moderate presidential rule today, executions have become rare, but there are still many restrictions. Baha'i cannot gather freely, cannot attend university or hold government jobs, and the religion's administrators are kept under surveillance. However, Baha'i are now quietly allowed to leave the country and even to return to visit if no mention is made of their religious membership.

In addition, some very devout Muslims, such as the Mujjahedin, have come to Canada. They were victims of the Shah's regime and were persecuted there. This group has some fundamental differences from the majority of Iranians in Canada, such as style of dress (particularly for women), strict adherence to Islamic religious practices, and political ideology. Overall, many of the refugees who have come to Canada are less educated and from the lower and middle classes.

In general, refugees from Iran prefer not to have their refugee status known among members of the Iranian community. Most Iranians in Canada are likely to assume that a refugee from Iran is a "political" refugee, and they usually want no association with Iranian politics because of the trouble it has caused in so many lives. For an Iranian in Canada, the question "Why did you come here?" is a very personal one, which should be avoided unless a great deal of trust has already been established.

Temporary Iranian Students in Canada

Some Iranians come to Canada solely for advanced education and intend to return to Iran upon completion of degrees. This group is rather small, and, after 1979, its members may have a stronger attachment to the more traditional lifestyle of their homeland. Females in this group generally wear the hijab and sometimes other body covering and adhere strictly to Islamic laws. Some of these women may insist on seeing a female physician.

Return to Iran from Canada

Like many other immigrants who have very high, sometimes unrealistic, expectations about how they will live in Canada, some Iranians are disappointed when they arrive. Many middle- and upper-class Iranians begin to see that they will not be able to obtain the same kind of employment or to earn as much as they did in Iran. As a result some return home permanently after a few months in Canada. A few return after several years.

The majority remain in Canada. Many older parents would like to return to Iran, especially since life now seems to be improving there in many ways, but they will not leave their children who have grown up in Canada. Some remain in Canada mainly out of a sense of pride. They long to return home to Iran but are ashamed to admit to themselves or to relatives that they have not "succeeded" abroad.

Language

Language in Iran

The spoken and written official language of Iran is Farsi, or Persian, a language that is over 1,000 years old. The Farsi script is Arabic. Since the Arab conquest and the Islamization of Persia in the seventh century, Farsi has been profoundly influenced by Arabic, although it has remained a distinctly different language. The Arab population on the Iran-Iraq border and near the Persian Gulf speaks Arabic, and the Turks along the border with Turkey speak a dialect of Turkish. Each tribal group speaks its own dialect. Because some people from Afghanistan also speak Farsi, Iranian health professionals in Canada sometimes provide health services to Afghanis.

Language in Canada

The extent to which Iranian immigrants know English upon arrival in Canada is associated with their level of education and social position in their home country. A few may be very fluent, some may have basic English, and some very little. In the latter case, school-going children may serve as interpreters for their parents. Children born or educated from an early age in Canada have little or no problem with English.

However, some Iranian health professionals in Canada have noted that large numbers of Iranian adults, especially non-working women but also many men, continue to have English-language problems years after their arrival. The large size and residential clustering of the Iranian immigrant populations, such as on Vancouver's North Shore, may contribute to this fact by making day-to-day English unnecessary for some people. Limited skills in English can be further compounded by very strong cultural values of appearance and pride that make it difficult for many Iranians to ask questions that suggest they do not understand the language. An English-speaking professional working with Iranians must use tact to discover whether a client has understood important information. Instead of asking "Do you understand me?" the professional can repeat the information using simpler vocabulary or say "I'm not sure I made that very clear" to permit questions with dignity.

Structure of Iranian Society in Canada

Iranians in Canada tend to confine their interaction to their own social class as defined by affluence and education, to their own religious group, and to persons of their own political persuasion. These social divisions are likely to be less noticeable in future generations. However, health professionals today will find it much easier and more effective to work with Iranian clients if they are sensitive to the existence of distinct subdivisions within the society.

Sensitivity to the subgroups of Iranian society may help avoid the kind of problem recounted by one health professional. She once tried to establish contact between two of her female Iranian patients in order to help one of them overcome severe isolation and loneliness. The patient immediately asked, "Which political group does this other woman belong to?" The answer was crucial to the patient, but the physician could not help. Similarly, a female Baha'i counsellor recalls trying to establish rapport with a depressed male Muslim client who had been referred to her by a Canadian professional solely on the basis of shared homeland and language. The client did not return after the first interview, and the counsellor's attempts to establish further contact failed completely.

Socioeconomic Status

The majority of Iranians residing in Canada belong to the more modern, educated, and affluent urban classes. A smaller group who arrived later, mainly in the 1990s, are from working-class, sometimes rural, backgrounds. Iranians are a very class-conscious people, for whom class is a central factor in Canada as well as in Iran. Accent, dialect, last name, and family history are markers of socioeconomic status. Families attempt to maintain social boundaries in Canada even though interaction of all classes occurs among children in the public schools. Individuals from wealthy classes in Iran who experience unemployment or underemployment in Canada continue to be respected for their previous status in Iran. However, working-class Iranians who acquire "new money" in Canada may be accepted by middle-class Iranians.

Today, free education at all levels has become accessible to larger numbers of Iranians of all social ranks. In 2000, 98 percent of children were enrolled in primary school. As a result, class mobility through education has become common.

Religious Subgroups

Approximately 98 percent of the population of Iran is Muslim, of whom 93 percent belong to the Shi'ite sect. It is Shi'ism that differentiates Iranians from most of the Muslim world, which is Sunni.

The 2 percent of the population of Iran that is not Muslim generally belongs to the more modern middle class. In this group are the Baha'i, the largest minority in Iran with about half a million members, but also Zoroastrians, Jews, and Christians, the latter comprising Armenians and Assyrians. Some intolerance exists towards all these groups, but the Baha'i have been severely persecuted.

The Baha'i faith is the only one among those mentioned above that is not officially recognized in Iran, and many members came, and continue to come, to Canada as refugees. Baha'u'llah founded the faith in Persia in 1882, and since that time the religion has spread around the world. Central to the faith is the idea that all of humanity has a single faith and that Baha'u'llah is the most recent in the line of messengers from God, superseding Buddha, Christ, and Mohammed. The Muslim clergy responded with hostility to this challenge to Islam, banished Baha'u'llah from Persia, and continues to ban the practice of Baha'i.

Generally, the Baha'i form a separate social group in Canadian Iranian society. They often adjust to Canada more easily than other Iranian immigrants in part because many were educated in Western institutions since they were and are excluded from universities in Iran. As well, from the time of the faith's founding, the Baha'i have been excluded from much of Iranian society and have relied on help from their own community. That support continues in Canada.

Political Subgroups

In Canada there are numerous subgroups based on political experiences in Iran. Supporters of the deposed Shah, of opposition political leaders (including those of the Islamic group the Mujjahedin, who led the Islamic Revolution), and of the more liberal movements in Iran are all represented. Some social interaction among the groups may occur, but members of each political persuasion strongly tend to associate with those of similar views.

Basic National and Cultural Characteristics

Regardless of the diversity of regional, ethnic, religious, and social class elements among Iranians, all have some cultural characteristics in common. These were perhaps developed to ensure Persian self-preservation in the face of political turmoil and instability over many centuries. Though Iranians have absorbed cultural traits from successive waves of invaders, they have managed to maintain their own sense of uniqueness and identity.

But these cultural characteristics may be modified over years, and generations, of residence in Canada, so professionals should still expect to find considerable diversity among Iranian clients.

Pride

A strong sense of Persian identity is a source of much pride, and Iranians are nostalgically tied to the past. For many Iranians, the loss of Persian identity is shameful. This strong sense of uniqueness and pride makes for a people who dislike admitting their smallest mistakes for fear of losing face. For example, it is very common for Iranians to deny material losses or financial needs. North Americans are often deceived by the well-groomed appearance of an Iranian and find it difficult to believe that this person may indeed be suffering financially. Yet, most Iranians, including those professionally trained, are actually working in low-income jobs in Canada.

Distrust outside the Family

Iranians have described themselves as suspicious, distrustful, and somewhat cynical in their dealings outside the circle of family and close friends. In the midst of the 1979 Islamic Revolution, Iranians were turned against one another and "ordered to spy on each other and report any misbehaviour." Cynicism and distrust also typify the Iranian's dealings with government authorities and the Western world, both of which are believed to have exploited the Persian nation. Underlying all this is a sense of insecurity associated with years of political unrest and upheaval.

Trust and submission are openly expressed and exercised only towards God and one's family and friends. Family members and close friends will literally sacrifice for one another. Family ties are strong, and it is one's duty to keep the good name of the family at all times.

Submission to God's Will

The deep-rooted cultural belief in fate or "taghdir" remains strong in all classes, though it is waning among the educated, who are more likely to assume individual responsibility for their own lives. Iranians traditionally expected to accept life's events and consequences with grace, based on the belief that "all is in the mighty hands of God." Because of pride and competitiveness, many Iranians residing in Canada suffer greatly from a sense of lost status and social rank. Canadians may notice that Iranian immigrants enjoy boasting enthusiastically about their glamorous past – which may sometimes be an attempt to be accepted and understood by the mainstream of society. Moreover, many Iranians in the West, in part to satisfy their pride, struggle to conceal losses, which they are expected to accept gracefully, and, as a result, develop various psychosomatic disorders.

Punctuality

The Western preoccupation with punctuality is not shared by Iranians, who almost always take their time to socialize and establish personal relationships before getting down to business. An Iranian patient may prefer to spend the first five or ten minutes of a medical appointment exchanging informal and personal information with the doctor. Iranians conduct their business affairs along similar lines, and many contracts are initiated and informally closed during social gatherings. This social ritual may sometimes annoy hurrying health and social service professionals. Keeping appointments is another potential area of conflict with Iranian patients.

Compromise

Many Iranians are reluctant to compromise or to recognize the validity of others' points of view and instead try hard to convert others to their opinion. It is often difficult for an Iranian, especially a man, to admit that he may be wrong.

Gestures

Touching, embracing, and kissing are very common among persons of the same sex, and conversational distance for Iranians is usually less than for North Americans. Eye contact may be less than is typical for North Americans, sometimes to show respect but also out of shyness.

Family Structure

The family is the most important element in Iranian culture, and life is usually dominated by family values and relationships. Family connections are still relied on in all classes for influence, employment, and security. Iranians in Canada who are unfamiliar with Western individualism find it difficult to adjust to the loss of their family connections.

The extended family has traditionally been the basic unit of society and has retained its social and psychological bonds despite the recent relative growth of nuclear families in urban areas in Iran. In fact, the word "family" in Persian refers to the extended family, and an Iranian is usually judged by the family name shared with grandparents, aunts, uncles, and cousins.

Iranian families can nevertheless be divided into two major groups, traditional and modern. In Iran, traditional family life is more commonly found in poorer and rural communities, and modern family life in urban and middle-class communities.

Traditional Family Structure in Iran and Canada

Among Iranians currently living in Canada, few belong to traditional families, except for the small number of fundamentalist Muslim families and, in some cases, the temporary postgraduate students. However, the traditional family structure provides a broader perspective on Iranian society and indicates the original lifestyle of the few traditional families that do exist in Canada. Most of the original practices and living arrangements disappear when these families move to the West, but many of the values persist.

The traditional Iranian family is a strong patriarchal unit whose head is the oldest male of the extended family, all of whose members live together in the same household. The family consists of husband and wife, unmarried children, married sons, and their wives and children. (While Islam allows a man to have four wives, very few Iranian men have more than one.) The father has authority over the entire family and is responsible for the discipline of all his children and grandchildren, although actual authority depends on the personalities of those involved. The wife's role is to submit to her husband. However, she is very close to her children and usually intervenes if conflicts arise between father and children.

Boys and girls are treated differently. It is assumed that girls do not need much education, since they are expected to become good mothers and homemakers and to learn by helping their mothers. Boys are not expected to help at home. As mentioned earlier, many of these traditional patterns are beginning to change.

By 2004 some immigrants of working-class or lower-class background have begun to arrive in Canada. These families, as some professionals have noted, encounter more individual freedom than they have been used to or expect. The new freedom leads to confusion and stress for all. In particular, men begin to experience a loss of power in the family when their wives begin to think about their rights and when children want more freedom.

Modern Family Structure in Iran and Canada

Modern families from middle- and upper-class urban Iran make up the largest proportion of the Iranian immigrant population of Canada. These immigrant families hold many Western values and follow some Western life patterns, notably in the weakening of parental authority, the greatly increased freedom of marital choice, and the development of the nuclear family. Single men continue to live with their parents, but married men are expected to live in separate households with their wives and children. Father continues to be the major breadwinner and head of the household, but has diminished power and authority.

In Iran, women's roles in the modern family have changed drastically since the 1960s. Many women then entered the workforce and more women sought higher education; these opportunities were greatly diminished after the Islamic Revolution. Yet they are improving again. More and more single women from modern families postpone marriage for better education. These women typically marry between the ages of twenty-two and twenty-five, whereas in traditional families most women marry between fifteen and eighteen.

The breakdown of the extended family, greater employment opportunities for women, increased marriage age, higher living standards, and the preoccupation with better education have all led to a decrease in the number of children in nuclear families to two or three. Women have become emancipated and educated and have acquired more decision-making power both inside and outside the home, but even the modern family remains a patriarchal unit in which sex roles are almost immune to change. Some women may expect their husbands to share household chores, and in some younger families in Canada this does occur, particularly in highly educated families. However, feminist ideology is uncommon and even unpopular among most women. This means that modern Iranian women are expected, and expect themselves, to take on most household responsibilities and as well as to maintain outside jobs.

In the family the mother is the centre of caring. While many Iranian women in Canada do stay home, those who are employed find themselves overburdened with responsibilities, including providing emotional support to others, overseeing family health care, and doing most household chores. Many women continue to cook homemade food for three meals each day to ensure that family members remain healthy and are not tempted by "fast food." Women may sacrifice their own health, especially their mental health, for their families.

Two major characteristics shared by families of all kinds are the respect and dutifulness shown the elderly and the value placed on the advice and support of members of the extended family for major problems, such as illness. For example, the health professional may be called by not just one but several of the patient's relatives to explain the results of a medical test. If an operation is recommended, the physician should expect to be consulted by several members of the patient's extended family before consent is given. The deep sense of duty towards the elderly includes responsibility for the care of old and dying family members.

Marriage

In Iran

In the traditional Iranian family, marriages are usually arranged. The couple's fathers negotiate the exchange of dowry, property, and jewellery, and the prospective couple has very little say in the matter. Chastity is highly revered, and unchaste single women are stigmatized. Girls are usually married between ages fifteen and eighteen. The daughter-in-law living in her husband's family must defer to his mother and to any older sisters.

In modern Iranian families, by contrast, marriage is generally the personal choice of the couple, and the bride is usually in her early twenties and educated.

In Canada

Dating is becoming more acceptable, but with limitations. Boys are usually given more freedom to date than girls, and dating generally begins at a later age than for Canadian youth. Iranians prefer their sons and daughters to date and mingle with those they know well and trust, preferably other Iranians from the same social class. Marriages are not arranged, but parental consent is essential to the decision. Family reputation, affluence, education, and physical appearance are the most important considerations in choosing marriage partners, and parents prefer their children to marry within their own social group. Iranian women are usually five to ten years younger than their husbands, although in Canada this gap is gradually closing.

Moreover, intermarriage with non-Iranians is becoming more common among all classes.

Domestic Violence

As in all cultures, domestic violence occurs in Iran, usually in the form of abuse of the wife by her husband, but it is hidden. A wife may go for help to her parents who will then organize brothers or other male family members to intervene to ensure that violence does not go too far. Some parents may advise their daughter to accept her situation since, according to Iranian law, her husband may take custody of the children.

The extra stresses of adapting to Canadian society often trigger family violence. For example, a husband may be unemployed or underemployed while his wife has been able to find a job. His loss of the traditional role of breadwinner and his dependence on his wife's income is an insult to his self-esteem. An Iranian man may feel helpless in this situation and may attempt to establish superiority by abusing his wife. This situation can be exacerbated when wives, discovering the greater independence of women in Canada, become aware that Canadian law protects them against spousal abuse.

An abused wife may decide to accept her situation. She may fear losing her children if the marriage breaks up. She may worry about being deported if she is dependent on her husband's sponsorship of their immigration status. Whether abused wives do seek help depends on their jobs or financial independence, their education, how long the abuse has gone on, their social and family network in Canada, and the ages of their children.

Women who disclose violence to someone outside the family are likely to talk to trusted women friends. Some reveal the problem to trusted Farsi-speaking family doctors. Many women wait a long time before they call the police, even when encouraged to do so by teenaged and adult children, who know the family situation and are often more conversant with Canadian law and sources of help. Some go to shelters for safety. Most prefer an Iranian domestic violence counsellor to whom they can talk easily and who will understand the Iranian family and social situation without needing further explanation.

As is true of many abused women in Canada, most Iranian women prefer to return to their husbands and children even after counselling and temporary separation. Counsellors who understand and support them in these decisions can be helpful by educating them about safety, perhaps encouraging them to know where their personal documents (passport, etc.) are and to have some money available if they must leave home. Those who do decide to leave the marriage may require help from a psychotherapist or psychiatrist to deal with loss and grief.

Separation and Divorce

In Iran

A bond of marriage is considered a strong unifying tie between two families and is never to be broken. Divorce is very rare and carries a great deal of stigma, but it does exist and the woman usually returns to her own family. According to Islam, men take custody of the children, who are then raised by the father's family.

In Canada

The stresses associated with migration, that is, lack of extended family support, change in family roles, and financial problems, along with a general increase in the women's awareness of their rights to independence, have led to a drastic and steady increase in the rate of separation and divorce in Iranian families in Canada. Divorce is somewhat easier in Canada than in Iran because extended families are generally absent and need not be consulted. However, especially for women in Canada, lack of financial independence and loss of face in the community make divorce much harder to accept. The tradition in Iran that women from broken marriages are supported by their original families is maintained in Canada, but few have families here. As a result most women who are divorced or separated live on their own after having achieved some financial security through employment, court rulings, or social assistance.

Children and Adolescents

Many Iranian parents came to Canada for the sake of their children's education and often they have made great sacrifices to do so. However, children generally have little part in major family decisions, and most children were not asked if they wanted to migrate to Canada. They often find it difficult to leave their own culture, extended family, and friends to start a new life, especially when they had no part in making the decision. As a result many children and adolescents experience depression following immigration.

However, once children are in school they may be the first in the family to learn English well and to understand aspects of their new culture. They may also begin to lose their mother tongue and start to grow apart from their families. Communication breakdown in the family, especially at adolescence, is common. The parents' tendency to shelter and protect children from Western influences and values is strong, so they expect their children to avoid integration into the larger society. At the same time, however, many parents expect that their children, both male and female, will achieve high marks in school. The conflicting standards sometimes result in family discord and adolescent rebellion. The longer the family resides in Canada, the more likely it is that parents will adapt and adjust to Canadian ways and allow their children more freedom. Discipline (for example, spanking) is usually administered by the father (and may be harsher than the Canadian norm) since the mother is considered to be the more loving, caring, and protective figure in the family. Verbal abuse of children may also be common.

Children may have some non-Iranian friends to play with, but many Iranian parents describe their children as forming meaningful and intimate friendships only with other Iranian children with whom they share language and cultural values. Young boys born in Iran may initially feel lonely and lost in Canada and may feel an acute need to connect with others. In Iran, boys are used to living close by one another, and they usually play in large groups. This social pattern is replicated in Canada when they live in a large Iranian community. In this case joining a large friendship group, especially for boys who feel excluded from the mainstream community, serves to strengthen a sense of belonging and identity. Adolescent "gangs" involved in illegal activities are not very common in the Iranian community, but media attention has sometimes served to exaggerate their presence.

In Iran, young adults do not leave home until marriage. However, in Canada, Iranian parents do not pressure their children to leave the nest; in fact, children are usually welcome for as long as they wish to stay. In Canada most adult children leave home in their early twenties, though the decision to attend university may involve leaving home earlier.

Work

The major problems faced by Iranians in Canada, particularly in their first years here, are unemployment, underemployment, loss of status, and financial loss – in short, downward socioeconomic mobility. Many families experience great disillusion following their initial excitement and discovery. The degree of disillusion depends in part on levels of education, language ability, and financial resources and seems to be more common among men over age thirty or so who were already well established in professions and business. Younger men not yet established in Iran seem to have an easier time adapting to Canada.

Many Iranian men hold university degrees, some at the doctoral level, and come from various professional backgrounds. Those with business backgrounds may not be as highly educated. Those who have come with investment capital have established small businesses, particularly in real estate and restaurants, and many Iranians in Canada have earned respect from their community for their success here. However other Iranian men and their families live and work in conditions poorer than they expected or were used to in Iran, and many are shocked that they cannot get the same work that they had at home but must accept a white-collar or even a manual labour job. Engineers work in gas stations, and persons with MA degrees are employed as security guards. Some professionals who cannot continue in their professions because their Iranian qualifications are not recognized in Canada may also be denied white-collar employment because they are overqualified. Many men do not earn enough money to care for their families' needs, so both parents must work.

Women, on the other hand, generally have a somewhat lower level of education, having usually finished high school or bachelor's degrees. The younger generation of Iranian women in Canada (aged late twenties to early forties) has usually obtained postsecondary degrees and been employed in Iran, mainly in the traditional areas of nursing, teaching, administration, and the arts. There are a number of female medical doctors residing in British Columbia, very few of whom practise medicine. Women tend to find employment more easily, in part because many are willing to accept positions that have less status than those they held in Iran. For example, a registered nurse from Iran may take a nurse's aide job in Canada, although she may not reveal this to her relatives and friends in Iran but instead say "I have a job in a hospital." This tends to perpetuate the unrealistic expectations of women in Iran for the continuation of their careers in Canada. Women who have never worked in Iran can fairly easily find a low-paid job.

For both men and women, obtaining a job commensurate with their Iranian experience and education is made more difficult if they cannot communicate easily in English with non-Iranians, as in employment interviews. Iranians may not have the native-English-speaker's understanding of the implicit connotations of spoken messages. Over the years in Canada some Iranian immigrants report experiencing a "glass ceiling," that is, they cannot move to the top positions in their place of employment and feel compelled to start over in another place, losing status and money in the process.

Iranians are very proud and attempt to keep face even in extreme financial difficulty. In particular, because parents often want the best education for their children when they come to Canada, they may select a location to live in that is more affluent than they can afford, simply so their children will reside in the catchment area of the "best" school. This creates great strain on family resources.

After 1984 most Iranians who arrived as refugees (government-sponsored or otherwise) have received social assistance. This can be very degrading for many proud Iranians and may partly account for the physical and emotional problems that health professionals frequently encounter.

Mrs. Farthi, from Iran

Mrs. Farthi, now fifty, came to North Vancouver from Iran seven years ago with her husband and young son, who was then twelve years old. She speaks English well and was able to describe her symptoms to their family physician. "For the past few months I've had trouble with my heart. My heart is very uncomfortable and it beats rapidly." Her doctor did a thorough physical examination, sent her for tests, and asked her to come back after the tests were completed.

When her physician told her that all the tests were normal, Mrs. Farthi insisted that her heart was still racing, "and I am afraid I am going to die." Her doctor leaned back in her chair and asked, "Are there things going on at home that are upsetting you?" At first she hesitated to say much, but then she admitted that since they arrived in Canada her husband had had difficulty finding work. He knew a little English and so had worked occasionally but had not found a steady job. They were fairly well-off when they came from Iran but had now used up most of their savings and depended on the income from her steady job as a clerk in a copy centre.

Neither her husband nor her son helps with the housework. Her son, now nineteen, lives at home and has not tried to find work. She said, "In the last couple of months my husband and I have quarrelled almost constantly. I think our son should find a job and contribute to our expenses; if he won't do that he should move out and live on his own. My husband just won't hear of that. There is a lot of friction at home."

Ways of Settling Conflict

In Iranian culture, problem-solving and conflict resolution usually occur in stages and according to a certain pattern. Every effort is made to keep a problem private. Should the parties involved (e.g., marriage partners, in-laws, business partners) fail to resolve the conflict, perhaps because of the extreme emotionalism of those involved, a third party is asked to intervene impartially. This person will be trusted and respected by both sides, usually an elderly man well known and respected in the community. If reconciliation happens, it is on the basis of "forgive and forget," and the problem is never mentioned again whether resolved or not. Professional help, be it from a counsellor, physician, lawyer, or the courts is only reluctantly sought as a last resort. This attitude may account for the delays, at times extreme, in the reporting of incidents of family violence, attempted suicide, or mental and emotional problems. However, if Iranians do seek professional help for serious conflicts, they generally prefer to be referred to non-Iranian professionals to preserve confidentiality and face.

Leisure

In Iran, community sports were not very common, and costly activities such as skiing, swimming, or tennis were available only to the elite. Iranian children in Canadian schools may be less active in sports and other extracurricular activities since the family usually emphasizes academic achievement. The school system will more easily involve Iranian parents in their children's academic work than in their extracurricular activities. The longer they reside in Canada, the more Iranian parents begin to value physical and social activities for their children. At the same time, the families themselves become more active physically and socially.

Leisure time, for the most part, is spent as family time. The commonest way of socializing is to visit relatives and friends, mostly Iranian, for many hours at a time and to eat extravagant Persian dishes, with children almost always present. Hosts are expected to have twice the amount of food necessary to feed the guests because it is considered extremely embarrassing if food runs out. Traditionally the food is made by the hostess, although this is changing as potluck dinners become more common. An Iranian party usually consists of three or four generations gathered together. Babysitters (and daycare, for that matter) are rarely used, and children are usually kept up until late at night.

Hospitality is one of the most important features of Persian culture and a source of much pride. Persian hospitality is characterized by extreme generosity in the sharing of food and tea, even for a casual visit. Guests are treated with great respect. The offering and receiving of food (or gifts) is done according to a certain ritual called *taarof*, which symbolizes courtesy and good manners. Once an Iranian is offered something, he or she is expected to reject it gracefully for a few times before finally accepting it from the other party, who is in turn expected to persist in making generous offers. Refusing food causes offence and may be perceived as rejection.

Reciprocity is very important. It is expected that all invitations will be returned. This can cause a strain on Iranians experiencing financial difficulties in Canada. Iranian women who feel unable to provide tea and food to guests may cease visiting others and consequently become very isolated.

Health professionals who are offered dinner invitations or gifts of specially prepared Persian dishes should regard them as tokens of appreciation and respect and, whenever possible, should accept them after some *taarof*. However, they should be aware that once they have gained the trust of their Iranian patients, they may be called upon for minor favours, as is done in Iran.

Relations with Mainstream Canadian Society

When Iranian families arrive in Canada, they may be fearful of Western influences, especially on their children. They do not approve of the permissiveness they see in mainstream Canadian society. Many are nostalgic about their past and their cultural identity; they fear change and distrust outsiders. Consequently, Iranian immigrants tend to isolate themselves from non-Iranians, especially at first, to protect themselves and their youngsters. Older Iranians tend to socialize mostly with Iranians; Canadian-born Iranians tend to mix cross-culturally. With a longer stay in Canada it is common for all Iranians to socialize with other Canadians, although some feel that "the door is closed to them" when they seek Canadian friends. Some religious subgroups, the Baha'i and Christians, for example, are known to be generally more open to socializing with others.

Some Iranians experience discrimination from the dominant society, especially with regard to being hired for certain jobs. The language barrier also tends to create misunderstandings and confusion and thus may increase the feeling of being discriminated against. Since September 11, 2001, some Iranians worry that anti-Muslim feelings in the West might affect them.

Early in their stay, many Iranians are not familiar with mainstream Canadian patterns of life and work, and sometimes they are unaware of their rights and the services available to them. For example, they may know nothing about rights of workers, such as the minimum wage, or that free legal aid services, unemployment insurance, and other social services may be available to them. However, Iranians trust and use most branches of the health services in Canada, with the exception of mental health services.

Health Beliefs and Practices

In the past forty or fifty years the Iranian people, particularly the urban populations, have rapidly become familiar with Western medicine and health care and have generally trusted and respected it. Nevertheless, some folk beliefs and traditions are retained and occasionally practised.

Iranian immigrants generally do not refute scientific theories about underlying causes of diseases. However, coming from a fatalistic society, they may place such theories side by side with their strong belief in the will of God, especially in the event of death. The belief that "all is in the mighty hands of God," though, does not prevent most Iranians from seeing a physician for help when needed.

Food and other natural substances are believed to play a role in health, and Iranians are known to seek constant guidance from physicians about their children's diets. To keep their children healthy and robust – for thin children are not considered healthy – Iranians tend to overfeed them, and they become overly concerned about poor appetites. The use of "hot" and "cold" foods to prevent or cure minor illnesses is also common. Consuming too much of one and too little of the other is believed to cause stomach upsets or other minor disorders. When minor ailments occur, such as low fever or cold symptoms, an effort is made to cure them at home with the help of food and herbs. Should the illness persist, the doctor is called. Delays in seeking medical help, with the exception of psychiatrists, are not a major problem among Iranians.

While traditional healing with food may not be as prevalent in Canada as in Iran, food remains a very important part of Iranian culture, and physicians have found that it is difficult to convince a patient to change eating habits in order to prevent further health problems. Iranian physicians have pointed out the importance of involving the woman who does the shopping and cooking in their consultations with other family members. Just recommending to a middle-aged man alone that he must change his diet to help prevent another heart attack is not enough; his wife must also be included since she is in charge of the family diet.

Pain is stigmatized in Iranian culture, and many people do not like others to know about the pain in their lives. They may only feel comfortable discussing pain with very close family members whom they completely trust, or with a trusted physician.

Health Services and Disease in Iran

In 2000 Iran had one physician for every thousand persons, and in contrast with pre-revolutionary times about 90 percent of the rural population had access to a Primary Health Centre. However, there is considerable discrepancy between rural and urban areas and between rich and poor, both in services and in health. About half of Iranians, mainly middle-class and urban people, pay privately for their health care, either out of pocket or through health insurance, and the rest are served by government agencies and private charities. Government health services sometimes lack quality, but working-class Iranians are reluctant to seek help from private physicians because of cost.

Those who can afford private services, the middle and upper classes, mostly urban residents, choose one general practitioner whom they and their relatives know and trust and with whom they establish close relations. Family doctors become the confidantes of their patients and have detailed knowledge of their patients' personal lives. In Iran, in contrast with Canada, patients do not need the family doctor's referral to make an appointment with a specialist. Appointments to see a physician are often made by the individual patient, or by the patient's mother in the case of young children. An elderly person is usually accompanied by his or her child.

Due to the expansion of free vaccination services, encouragement of breastfeeding, greater access to primary health services, and 95 percent access to safe water, the infant mortality rate in Iran has dropped from fifty-one deaths per thousand in 1984 to thirty-four in 2002, and by 2002 life expectancy was sixty-nine years. An aging population has been accompanied by a shift from deaths caused by infectious and parasitic diseases to deaths caused by coronary heart disease, trauma (vehicle accidents and suicide, for example), and cancer, most commonly for women, breast and vaginal cancer, and for men, skin, stomach, lymphatic, blood, and esophageal cancer.

Prevalence of Disease in Canada

Health consciousness is a rather important feature of the Iranian population in Canada. This may be accounted for by the fact that Iranians as a group do not present the health professionals with typical Western diseases. Physicians working with Iranian immigrants and students have recounted many cases of psychosomatic disorders and stress-related depressions, which are known to be more common among women and middle-aged men. Major reasons for the phenomenon seem to be loss of career, of status, or of extended family support. Because Iranians residing in Canada are often proud people and come from predominantly professional, educated, and affluent backgrounds, they find it difficult to cope with the losses they experience in Canada. These stresses lead to physical and mental symptoms.

Mental Illness

Iranians generally resist seeking help from psychiatrists and other professionals in mental health agencies, mainly because of the stigma associated with mental illness. Many are concerned that a psychiatric illness in the family will affect their children's chances of marriage. Thus, as a result of stigma, they often delay seeking help until the person is very sick indeed and the illness has become chronic, making treatment more difficult. Highly educated Iranians are likely to be much less resistant to timely treatment.

Especially in the educated middle and upper classes, mental illness is often attributed to heredity or physical dysfunction such as nervous system disease. It is important for health professionals to know that Iranians usually describe and experience mental illness somatically, often in the form of stomach problems, headaches, and backaches. Some may complain of "distress of the heart," the sensation that the heart is being squeezed, accompanied sometimes by fainting and palpitations. Professionals treating Iranians often associate many of their mental illnesses with the move from Iran to Canada. Grief for their lost home and stress over what they feel is an insoluble situation in Canada, exacerbated by lack of extended family support, may be associated with depression. The grieving process may last for many years.

The first reaction of many Iranians to a diagnosis requiring mental health treatment is denial. When faced with the necessity of treatment, they think in physical, not mental, terms and often are more comfortable with help from a neurologist than from a psychiatrist. For the same reason, they will more readily accept medication than "talk therapy." In general Iranian patients are extremely compliant in taking medication because they believe the medicine will cure, but some professionals have noted that they are very likely to stop taking medication at the first sign of side-effects. They may become frustrated if told that the mental illness can be controlled but not cured. Sometimes failure to cure the illness is attributed to a doctor's incompetence.

A small minority of Iranians with emotional problems may prefer counsellors and psychotherapists to medical doctors. But most are resistant to this form of treatment, which they see as unhelpful for dealing with "real" problems, and many are resistant to suggestions that they may need to change some of their behaviour.

Iranians in Canada may prefer to be treated by Iranian physicians because of difficulty in expressing themselves in English and because the physician and patient share cultural understandings. This is especially true if diagnosis and treatment involve discussion of the person's immigration experience and his or her reasons for leaving Iran. Mental health professionals note that Iranian patients are more likely to reveal political reasons

Mr. and Mrs. Momen, from Iran

Mr. Momen, his wife, and their two small children came to Canada in 1998 as convention refugees. Eight months ago Mr. Momen lost his job as a salesman in a carpet shop, so the family must live on Mrs. Momen's wages from work in an Iranian restaurant. Though they have great difficulty making ends meet, they are reluctant to ask for social assistance, and they don't want people in the Iranian community to know about their financial hardship. Both of their children are now in school, and Mr. and Mrs. Momen want the best for them, but they are worried. How can they save for university expenses? And how can they "keep up" with other parents who seem to spend a lot of money on their children?

Late one night his wife brought Mr. Momen into the emergency department because he was having very painful headaches. Neither Mr. Momen nor his wife speak much English, so the physician talked with them through an interpreter, an Iranian Canadian nurse who happened to be on duty.

Mr. Momen said he had not been able to sleep well for at least six months and almost every night had frightening nightmares. He also said, "People are telling me they are going to get me. I think it's the neighbours who live upstairs."

When the physician spoke further with Mrs. Momen, she said, "I took him to another emergency department about three months ago and the doctor there gave him pills but my husband stopped taking them because he said they were upsetting his stomach. As soon as he stopped using the pills, his headaches became much worse and tonight they were very bad. He started yelling about the voices and the neighbours and I got very scared. My children were very frightened and began to cry."

for coming to Canada if they converse with a professional in Farsi, and such information may be important in working through their mental health problems.

The Doctor-Patient Relationship

In general, Iranian patients seek a more personal or intimate relationship with their doctors than do mainstream Canadians, and some professionals feel that the lack of a close relationship may impair their patients' recovery. The patients may expect their physicians to listen to long stories about their health and personal problems, and they like to be given time to discuss their past accomplishments. They expect a great deal of understanding since they regard family doctors as confidantes.

The choice of a family doctor is usually made on the basis of personal recommendations from more experienced friends and relatives, and patients may be willing to travel a great distance to a doctor that they feel patients can trust.

A Canadian physician, in order to gain an Iranian patient's confidence and trust, must take the time to listen and respond sympathetically, undertake full and thorough examinations, and devote undivided attention to the patient during an appointment. Trust can be established during the first few visits, and once this is achieved, the patient becomes a "believer" in his or her doctor. This is a notion commonly held by Iranians, and once fulfilled, will very likely cause the patient to follow the physician's advice. Trusted and "believed in" doctors are regarded as definite authorities, or parental figures, and older male doctors are more readily trusted.

Iranians in Canada prefer to see health professionals who can speak Farsi. Shared language and culture seem to create a sense of understanding and trust. They may have difficulty communicating with professionals where each must speak English as a second language; these interactions seem to create frustration for both parties. Since Iran is a patriarchal society, male physicians are naturally trusted and esteemed more than their female counterparts. Moreover, the older the physician, the greater the trust and respect. But female doctors are trusted and even preferred in certain areas of medicine. Women obstetricians, pediatricians, and eye specialists are preferred, whereas female neurosurgeons, for example, tend not to be trusted. Iranian men prefer seeing a male physician rather than a female one. Of course these preferences tend to soften the longer Iranians live in Canada.

A trusted doctor may be offered gifts and invitations. If these are accepted, which is the polite thing to do in Iranian culture, the doctor may be called upon for minor favours, as is normal in Iran. For example, pediatricians in Canada sometimes find that parents ask for help and advice about their own minor health concerns or problems while the doctor is busy examining their child.

Trust and respect sometimes lead to further problems. Iranians may delay asking for a second opinion for fear of offending their family physician even though delay may cause anxiety for the patient. Those who have not followed the physician's advice, such as abstaining from certain foods, might at times try to conceal the truth to keep the respect of the doctor.

Iranians often are very frustrated and impatient with the Canadian medical appointment and referral system and feel they have little or no part in choosing the medical care they receive. They become impatient if they have to wait for appointments, and they often telephone immediately to obtain laboratory test results from physicians, expecting thorough explanations of results. In Iran no referral is needed for appointments with specialists. Thus, many Iranians worry not only about lack of choice in specialists but also about delayed diagnosis and treatment, with increased risk of complications, due to the waiting period for appointments.

Since preventive care is generally not practised in Iran, many patients complain that "the doctors didn't do anything" when medication is not prescribed. Pills and injections are most popular; injections are believed to render faster results. A physician residing in Canada who had practised for over thirty years in Iran recounts several incidents in which his Tehran patients refused to pay for the hour-long visits on the grounds that he had "only talked" and had not prescribed any kind of medicine. Expensive and rare drugs are preferred to ordinary pills, and doctors who prescribe the most expensive ones are regarded as the most skilled. Many young families in Canada, however, have changed their attitudes about medicine, and traditional views are weakening steadily.

Hospitalization

Iranians are very sociable, and hospital visits to friends or relatives are considered a moral duty. Visitors come in large numbers, bringing sweets, flowers, and gifts. It is a time to socialize and to keep the patient company, and most hospitalized Iranians enjoy having large numbers of noisy visitors. In Iranian culture it is considered shameful to leave a loved one alone in the hospital without visitors. For this reason, Iranians attempt to provide the patient with company at all times.

Iranians say they tend to disregard hospital visiting hours. Some like to stay with the patient overnight or bring forbidden food, remembering it is possible to do so in Iran if the family gives the staff money. Hospital staff may feel that close family members, a mother, say, or a spouse, are making extraordinary demands on hospital workers and interfering with their handling of the patient. An Iranian mother whose child is hospitalized might ask to stay with her child at all times, protest at the quality of food, and request and expect special treatment for her child. Or she may want to bathe the child and change its linen herself. These situations must be handled tactfully by staff, who should recognize that "people rely on their cultural styles of coping in such threatening situations as illness and hospitalization" (Lipson 1992, 20). If such problems arise, the most effective solution may be to ask the family doctor or a trusted specialist to intervene gently. Wherever possible, Iranian patients prefer to stay in private hospital rooms.

Iranians regard nurses highly, though they give them little respect in the presence of a physician. Messages that come from a doctor are much more readily obeyed. Iranian women may experience great discomfort in the presence of male nurses, so female nurses should be used with female patients whenever possible.

Iranians may be somewhat distrustful of social workers in hospitals and elsewhere. Social work is a new profession established only following the revolution in Iran.

Medication and Treatment

Iranian women consider that they practise preventive health care through their attention to the nutrition and diet of their families. Most Iranian women and children are used to daily exercise, especially in rural areas, and many women attempt to continue daily exercise in Canada by walking to and from the school or the grocery store. However, physicians find that asking an Iranian to exercise regularly or to cut down on certain foods may be a different matter. Patients often promise to follow their doctors' advice but seldom succeed in doing so. It may be very important to explain the advantages and disadvantages of following the recommended preventive methods. For example, Iranians with high blood pressure may be reluctant to cut down on salt and would prefer to rely on their medication to alleviate the symptoms. Because doctors in Iran offer little advice on prevention, professionals in Canada may need to help their Iranian patients build up an awareness of prevention.

In Iran most people use a variety of home treatments for minor illnesses and seek doctors' help only for serious illnesses, a practice that continues when they come to Canada.

Drugs are the preferred means of treatment among Iranians. Canadian physicians will have little difficulty in convincing their Iranian patients to take prescribed medications. In Iran expensive and rare drugs are preferred to ordinary pills. However, medication in Canada is much more expensive than in Iran, and some Iranians may not be able to afford even the least expensive generic brands. For this reason people sometimes offer unused medicines to other family members and friends who appear to have the same symptoms. Making the high cost of medicine in Canada even more frustrating is the fact that in Iran it is possible to return unused medicine to the pharmacy in exchange for another kind.

Iranians in Canada are generally very well groomed, so it is not obvious who may be suffering financially. For this reason physicians should attempt to discuss the cost of medications before they are prescribed and to involve the patient in the decision making. A shorter course of medications may be prescribed if finances are a problem, allowing the patient a choice about whether more is needed. Building up trust with the patient in these ways will increase compliance when a long course is required, since Iranians may otherwise be in the habit of discontinuing medication as soon as they feel better, sometimes creating complications and recurrence.

Family Planning

Families in rural Iran are much larger (up to twelve children) than those in urban areas. In fact, the average number of children in modern middle-class families in Iran had shrunk to two by 2002, by which time 73 percent of couples in Iran were using some form of modern birth control.

In Canada, most young Iranian families do not have more than two or three children. Couples may be financially pressed and concerned about their children's education. Birth control, although forbidden by Islam, is practised by almost all Iranian families in Canada. The favourite methods of contraception, generally chosen by women, are birth control pills and the IUD.

Couples generally plan to have their first child within the first three years of marriage. Since children are regarded as blessings, and procreation is considered the major reason for marriage, family pressures on couples increase when the first pregnancy is delayed. The second child usually follows within two to three years, but it is not uncommon for couples to wait for many years before having a third child. Male children are generally preferred.

In Iran, abortions are illegal except for medical reasons in an attempt to save the life of the mother. Before the revolution, many abortions, legal, illegal, professional, and non-professional, took place in hospitals, clinics, and homes. The frequency of abortions among Iranian women in Canada may not be as high as that among other Canadian women, but Iranian women from all religions and social backgrounds seek help to terminate unwanted pregnancies.

Since premarital sex is considered taboo, a pregnant single woman may be harshly ostracized, particularly in rural Iran. Educated middle-class families often seek abortions in complete secrecy. Illegitimate infants are usually put up for adoption or placed in an orphanage. Pregnancies out of wedlock cause intense crisis and turmoil in Iranian families, regardless of class.

Pregnancy and Prenatal Care

Pregnancy is considered a blessing, and expectant Iranian women become the focus of much attention and care. The traditional belief among all classes of Iranians is that pregnant women must abstain from heavy physical work, rest frequently, and eat rich and healthy foods. Extensive weight gain often becomes a problem. Exposure to Western medicine has changed this trend to a certain degree. Nevertheless, health professionals in Canada may encounter difficulty in convincing pregnant Iranian women to exercise regularly.

In Canada, the majority of pregnant Iranian women and their husbands attend prenatal classes. However, men are typically very uncomfortable in this situation. Language problems are also a barrier to attendance.

Because of the relatively high level of education among younger Iranian women in Canada, they generally recognize first signs of pregnancy and therefore go to the doctor at an early stage. The husband and mother of the pregnant woman are the first family members to be informed. Advice about managing the pregnancy is passed on from mother to daughter or daughter-in-law, usually immediately after the onset of pregnancy.

Childbirth and Postpartum Period

Childbirth in Iran takes place in hospitals, private clinics, and homes, and delivery is attended by physicians and certified midwives. Close female relatives keep mothers company at childbirth. In Canada, more and more Iranian fathers are now present in delivery rooms.

Iranian women express their pain and anguish in labour more freely and loudly than Canadian women. Screaming and sobbing are considered normal when giving birth. In fact, women are encouraged to scream loudly and freely. Some Iranian women may find the pain unbearable, and it is common for them to ask for an anesthetic.

In Iran infants are brought to their mothers only to be breastfed, since new mothers are believed to need rest and quiet. Extended family members are always available to help in the early weeks after birth, and the new mother is either taken to her parents' home or joined by her mother. Certain foods, such as barley and water drained from boiling rice, are considered good for increasing the milk flow, and mothers are fed these and other rich foods. In Canada, breastfeeding usually lasts for nine months to a year. The length of this period, however, may change according to the mother's work and health. Iranian mothers have no difficulty in using substitute formulas.

Visiting the new mother and her baby is common practice among Iranians. The mother and infant are not secluded and usually begin socializing outside the home within two or three weeks of childbirth. Regular visits by public health nurses in Canada are highly valued by Iranian women, who, although unfamiliar with the idea, fully appreciate the information and support they receive. Most new mothers need and use this education about childcare in Canada and the resources available to them.

Sexuality

In both Iran and Canada, discussion of sex in the family is definitely taboo. Premarital sexual activities, although not uncommon, are considered sinful in modern families, whose attitude towards chastity is only slightly more open than that of traditional families. Sex before marriage is more acceptable for men and much less common among young women. By 2004, the tolerance of premarital sex seems to have increased slightly among Iranians residing in Canada. Young Canadian Iranians may engage in premarital relations, but it remains a very personal issue, not to be freely discussed even among friends.

The official prevalence of HIV in Iran among young people aged fifteen to twenty-four is very low, about 0.05 percent for men and much lower for women.

Drug and Alcohol Use

In Iran, opium is used casually, rather like marijuana in the West, though it is prohibited by law. It is used across all social classes, usually by men, and it may be offered to guests along with other refreshments as a sign of hospitality. Young people may use opium to deal with the frustration of cultural restrictions on personal freedom. Although it is widely used as a recreational drug by many young adults, it has the same long-term effect as heroin. Addiction occurs quickly and will be concealed from family members. Addicted Iranians may be especially liable to isolate themselves from loved ones to prevent the family from discovering their problem.

Some Iranians may use drugs in Canada as a relief from the disillusionments of immigration. They have come with high expectations, anticipating the best of everything, and they can become frustrated, angry, and resentful when faced with downward mobility in Canada.

Cultural barriers often prevent Iranian drug addicts from seeking help in Canada. Men are raised to believe that they should solve their problems within themselves and should not show vulnerability by crying or discussing pain. Many addicted Iranians do not attend mainstream services because of the language barrier, but they may attend groups run by other Iranians.

Alcohol is prohibited in Iran. But many people, mostly men, drink homemade alcohol or buy it on the black market. Some educated Iranians in Canada drink alcohol, especially young people, and older people might drink as well, though not in front of the young. In Canada alcohol abuse does exist, but the incidence is not very high. Again, Iranians needing treatment often avoid Alcoholics Anonymous because of language problems.

Nutrition and Food

Iranians eat well and plentifully because food is the major medium for socializing. Family members eat together, and mealtimes are for enjoying one another's company. In Iran, lunch used to be the most elaborate meal of the day, usually followed by a siesta. Since living conditions in Canada do not allow for elaborate lunches, dinner has replaced lunch as the main meal. Iranians sit at the table and use cutlery.

A staple in Iran is rice, and Iranians boast about their many rich and lovely rice dishes and spend much time preparing them. Meat is an essential part of most Persian dishes; lamb, veal, beef, and chicken are the most popular. Fish is eaten in moderation, but other seafood such as crab, lobster, and oysters is not commonly eaten. The consumption of pork is forbidden by Islam, and Iranians have generally not developed a taste for it. Oily food is preferred, and animal fat remains popular. The use of herbs is common, but spices are employed in moderation, with the exception of saffron. Persian food is not hot or spicy.

Iranians follow customary practices regarding the balance of foods served at a meal. "Hot" foods must be accompanied by "cold" foods. The actual temperature or spiciness of the food is unrelated to its classification as hot or cold. For example, honey and walnuts are hot, and cucumbers and yoghurt are cold. Iranians in Canada have maintained their traditional diet and continue to enjoy their homemade dishes. Fresh food is preferred, and the majority tend to "avoid canned, frozen or otherwise processed foods" (Lipson 1992, 18). The consumption of junk food among children, however, has increased. Sugar consumption, especially in tea, which is often drunk throughout the day, is rather high, possibly accounting for early tooth decay in children.

Dental Care

In the past, dental care was a secondary concern for Iranians and was largely neglected. More recently, many Iranians have become aware of its importance. For financial reasons, many persons may be hesitant to visit a dentist in Canada, but when they choose to do so they are very selective. Some Iranians "shop around" for the best price for a specific service, and they may bargain for a discount. In Iran, bargaining displays intelligence and is an acceptable and expected part of the culture. Some Iranians have commented, "They expect the best treatment at the lowest cost." There are many Iranian dentists practising in Canada.

Many Iranians want to take an active role in deciding their own treatment, and they may expect detailed explanations about decisions made by the dentist. Some Iranian newcomers are unfamiliar with flossing, but they may insist that they have done so to avoid offending the dentist.

Rehabilitation

Like mental illness, mental and physical handicaps are stigmatized in Iran. Most kinds of prenatal and perinatal disabilities are viewed as hereditary and hence are concealed from the eyes of the public. Although this trend is changing among the educated middle classes, all Iranians become uncomfortable in the presence of persons who are physically or mentally disabled. Many fear that the disability may run in the family and pity the victim and the family. This attitude, combined with the shame and pity felt by the victim's own family, almost always results in depression in the victim, isolation, and sometimes suicide.

In Iran, the deaf and blind are the least stigmatized and the developmentally delayed the most. Persons disabled later in life suffer less stigma but probably just as much pity. There may be more acceptance of disability as a result of the war with Iraq, which left many people disabled. After that war some programs to involve disabled persons in sports were developed.

Because of Iranian attitudes to disability, and the scarcity of rehabilitation and self-care services in Iran (with the exception of those for the blind), mentally and physically disabled persons lack the motivation to adapt. In Canada, rehabilitation professionals may find it extremely difficult to work with Iranian clients and their families, though the greater public awareness of disability and the extensive services available in Canada may help some Iranians become more accepting.

Care of the Elderly

Most Iranian families residing in Canada are nuclear families. Nevertheless, when grandparents do join their children in Canada they usually live with them, at least initially, for reasons of financial and emotional support. This is especially true for very old persons. However, many families live in very small suites, so well-off seniors may eventually wish to live apart, although perhaps still in close proximity. Some professionals have noted that sponsorship arrangements may make elderly parents vulnerable to enduring abuse or neglect since they fear being deported if they complain or if their child withdraws support.

Many Iranian seniors become very depressed in Canada. They feel useless and disrespected and are often confused and challenged as they observe their children and grandchildren adapting to new ways. Many seniors do not have and do not learn usable English or French, so they find it difficult to visit others and make friends.

The deep sense of duty towards the elderly in Iran includes responsibility for the care of old and dying family members. There are very few nursing homes in Iran and it is considered disrespectful and cruel to send elderly people to them. If families do place their elderly in Canadian nursing homes, they often want to be closely involved in the senior's care and thus tend to interfere with the nursing home's management of the old person.

Death and Dying

"God gives life and God takes life." This belief is commonly held by almost all Iranians, even those who do not practise religion. For this reason, members of a dying person's family do not plan for death, nor do they ever give up hope, not even after doctors have pronounced that the patient is dying. Grief is not permitted in the presence of the dying patient for fear of weakening the person's will to live. Death, as near as it may be, is never openly discussed.

Iranians prefer a diagnosis of a terminal illness to be initially withheld from the patient. Canadian physicians may find it most acceptable if they call in one family member, preferably a male, to reveal the diagnosis to him tactfully and gradually. That person can then consult the rest of the family on how to proceed. The family usually prefers to inform the patient gradually about the illness, always emphasizing the possible positive outcomes and the possibilities for treatment. Iranian families feel that much harm can come from bluntly confronting the patient with a poor prognosis; they complain that doctors in the West are insensitive to this issue and condemn a physician's directness in presenting the bad news. Physicians should be aware that the death of the father of a family will be felt by the whole family as the loss of its very centre. Breaking the news to young children and to close family members not present at the time of death is done gradually and tactfully, often in stages.

Plans for the funeral and mourning are made only after death has occurred. It is believed to be best to die at home in the presence of the whole family and that dying in loneliness and solitude is disgraceful.

Muslims in Iran do not use coffins to bury their dead. Because of this, some Muslim Iranians have difficulty with burial practices in Canada. Most Iranian religious sects prescribe certain bathing rituals for the dead, and most Iranians in Canada ask to bathe their dead accordingly. Funerals may be held on the same day as the death or several days after. It is often preferred that the body be kept in the hospital before burial. Cremation is most uncommon among all Iranian subgroups, who bury their dead according to their own religious ceremonies.

Once death occurs, mourning is typically loud. In fact, men and especially women are expected to sob loudly. Visits of condolence are a moral obligation for all relatives, friends, and even acquaintances. Memorial services are held at the time of the funeral as well as several days later; for example, Muslims hold memorial services on the fortieth day after death. Annual anniversary services are also very common. Grieving and mourning are expected to be lengthy, often lasting several months after the death, but the dead person is usually not openly discussed for fear of upsetting close family members. Women wear black – often for months after the death – and men generally wear black ties at the funeral and memorial services. Prayers and religious chants for the deceased's soul are common practice.

Working with Iranians

Some issues are considered by many Iranians to be very personal, and questions about them should not be asked unless the information is medically necessary. In particular, Iranians will be very reluctant to discuss their reasons for leaving Iran, the conditions of entry to Canada (whether as an independent immigrant or as a refugee), and their political and religious allegiances.

Many Iranian professionals in Canada have noted that Iranians often have language problems. Though many speak and read some English upon arrival in Canada, many others do not perfect the language over time and seem to reach a plateau; this is especially true of women who do not work and older people, but also some working men. Professionals should be aware that even middle-class Iranians may not fully understand medical instructions or may be reluctant to ask questions in English lest they reveal their ignorance. As with other non-native speakers of English, it is important for professionals to speak simply and clearly and to check indirectly whether the person has understood. Some doctors routinely write the important information such as diagnosis, recommended treatment, side-effects, and so on, to hand to the patient to take home. Having this concrete information reassures the patient and may increase compliance.

No one knows all there is to know about persons from Iran. The contents of this chapter should be used as background information to be verified and elaborated upon by personal interaction with each Iranian patient and his or her family. The Iranian community is extremely diverse: people have different points of view, different experiences, varied social class memberships, educational levels, and religions, and have come to Canada under a variety of circumstances. Professionals must find ways of learning about each client in order to understand how best to help that person and avoid the hazards of generalizing and stereotyping.

Further Reading

Aghajanian, Akbar. 1995. "Husband-wife conflict among two-worker families in Shiraz, Iran." In M. Singh Das and V.K. Gupta, eds., *Gender Roles and Family Analysis,* 203-8. New Delhi: M.D. Publications Pvt.

Aghajanian, Akbar, and Ali A. Moghadas. 1998. "Correlates and consequences of divorce in an Iranian city." *Journal of Divorce and Remarriage* 28: 53-71.

Arasteh, A.R. 1964. *Man and Society in Iran.* Leiden, The Netherlands: Brill.

Bonine, M.E., and K. Keddie. 1981. *Continuity and Change in Modern Iran.* Albany, NY: State University of New York Press.

Fathi, Asghar. 1991a. "The 1979 Revolution and its aftermath." In Asghar Fathi, ed., *Iranian Refugees and Exiles since Khomeini,* 4-7. Costa Mesa, CA: Mazda Publishers.

Fathi, Asghar. 1991b. "Theories of involuntary migration and the Iranian experience." In Asghar Fathi, ed., *Iranian Refugees and Exiles since Khomeini,* 8-20. Costa Mesa, CA: Mazda Publishers.

Graham, R. 1978. *Iran: The Illusion of Power.* London: Croom Helm.

Hanassab, Shideh, and Romeria Tidwell. 1996. "Sex roles and sexual attitudes of young Iranian women: Implications for cross-cultural counselling." *Social Behavior and Personality* 24: 185-94.

Jalali, B. 1982. "Iranian families." In M. McGoldrick, J.K. Pearce, and J. Giordano, eds., *Ethnicity and Family Therapy.* New York, NY: Guilford Press.

Korshidi, Mehrangiz. 2001. *Seniors Working to Prevent Abuse of Seniors in the Iranian Community.* Vancouver, BC: BC Coalition to Eliminate Abuse of Seniors.

Lipson, J.G. 1992. "The health and adjustments of Iranian immigrants." *Western Journal of Nursing Research* 14: 10-29.

Lipson, J.G., and A.I. Meleis. 1983. "Issues in health care of Middle Eastern patients in cross-cultural medicine." *Journal of Western Medicine* 139: 854-61.

Mackay, Sandra, and W. Scott Harrop. 1996. *The Iranians: Persia, Islam and the Soul of a Nation.* New York, NY: Dutton Books, Penguin Group.

Malek, Mohammed H. 1991. *Iran after Khomeini: Perpetual Crisis or Opportunity?* London, UK: Research Institute for the Study of Conflict and Terrorism.

Mesdaghinia, A., O. Ameli, Sh. Khatibzadeh, and F. Hajebi. 2003. "Health and welfare systems in the Islamic Republic of Iran." In *Country Studies in Health and Welfare Systems: Experiences in Indonesia, Islamic Republic of Iran and Sri Lanka,* 3-47. Kobe, Japan: WHO Kobe Centre.

Moallen, Minoo. 1991. "Ethnic entrepreneurship and gender relations among Iranians in Montreal, Quebec, Canada." In Asghar Fathi, ed., *Iranian Refugees and Exiles since Khomeini,* 180-204. Costa Mesa, CA: Mazda Publishers.

Moghissi, Haideh. 1999. "Away from home: Iranian women, displacement, cultural resistance and change." *Journal of Comparative Family Studies* 30: 207-17.

Momen, Moojan. 1991. "The Baha'i community of Iran: Patterns of exile and problems of communication." In Asghar Fathi, ed., *Iranian Refugees and Exiles since Khomeini,* 21-36. Costa Mesa, CA: Mazda Publishers.

Nyrop, R.F. 1978. *Iran: A Country Study.* Washington, DC: American University Press.

Omid, Homa. 1994. *Islam and the Post-Revolutionary State in Iran.* New York, NY: St. Martin's Press.

Shafii, Rouhi. 1997. *Scent of Saffron: Three Generations of an Iranian Family.* London, UK: Scarlet Press.

World Book Encyclopedia. 2000. "Iran." In *The World Book Encyclopedia,* 10. Chicago, IL: World Book.

Zonis, M. 1976. *The Political Elite of Iran.* Princeton, NJ: Princeton University Press.

Contributors to the first edition

P. Boustani, Physician, Vancouver
Tali Conine, School of Nursing, University of British Columbia
Carol Herbert, Physician, University of British Columbia
F. Mirhady, Physician, Vancouver
K. Mirhady, Physician, Vancouver
G. Partovi, Vancouver
P. Partovi, Vancouver
A. Raseky, Physician, Vancouver

Contributors to the second edition

Mr. Bagheri, Drug abuse support worker, Vancouver
Mishi Campbell, Domestic violence counsellor, Vancouver
Tali Conine, School of Nursing, Emerita, University of British Columbia
Roshi Gomshi, Family counsellor, North Vancouver
Sedi Hendizadeh, Settlement worker, Vancouver
Maheen Khodanbandeh, Translator, North Vancouver
Mehrangiz Khorshidi, Psychiatrist, North Vancouver
Amir Mirfakharaie, University of British Columbia
Jamaluddin Mirmiran, Psychiatrist, University of British Columbia
Homa Mogiry, Psychiatrist and holistic nutritionist, North Vancouver
Senira Sadedhi, Dentist, Vancouver

5
People of Japanese Descent

Karen Kobayashi, with Teruko Okabe, Kazuko Takahashi, and Elizabeth Richardson

Japanese Canadians differ from a number of immigrant groups described in this book because two-thirds were born in Canada (in 2001, 65 percent). In contrast, three-quarters of Chinese Canadians resident in Canada in 2001 were foreign-born. The majority of Japanese Canadians are the descendants of immigrants who began arriving in Canada as early as 1877. Immigration from Japan has dwindled since 1960, and by 2000 about 1,000 persons were immigrating from Japan each year.

In the 2001 census about 85,000 persons in Canada identified themselves as having Japanese ethnic background. A large majority of them lived in either British Columbia (44 percent, mainly in Vancouver) or Ontario (34 percent, mainly in Toronto), with the remainder in Alberta, Manitoba, and Quebec. Their places of residence result largely from the government-imposed dispersal of Japanese east of the Rockies following their internment in the BC interior during the Second World War. Those who went to Ontario to do farming or forestry eventually moved to Toronto to improve employment and education opportunities for their Canadian-born children. A second group who went to the Prairies to farm returned to Vancouver after the settlement ban was lifted in 1949 to work in fishing or logging.

Because of the large proportion of Japanese Canadians who are Canadian-born, it is not surprising that 60 percent of them use English as their first language. Very few of the *issei* (first generation) learned English, because they suffered profound social and political discrimination from the time they arrived in Canada, but by now most of this generation has passed away. Those who speak Japanese at home are most likely to be *shin-ijyusha* (postwar immigrants) and temporary residents such as businessmen and students. The largest group using Japanese as its first language lives in British Columbia.

Karen Kobayashi wrote this chapter. Teruko Okabe, Kazuko Takahashi, and Elizabeth Richardson wrote the chapter for the first edition; some of the earlier information is included in this revision.

Focus on Most Recent Immigrants and Temporary Residents

This chapter is focused primarily on new immigrants and temporary residents because, as relative newcomers, they may experience the most difficulty with the Canadian health care system. Problems can arise because of differences in cultural belief systems, unfamiliarity with Western practices, and lack of fluency in English. These difficulties can also occur to a lesser degree for some of the older *nisei* (second generation) and *kika nisei* (Canadian-born but educated in Japan).

Third- and fourth-generation Japanese Canadians, referred to as *sansei* and *yonsei* respectively, are unlikely to differ from other Canadians. They usually have few ties to a local Japanese community beyond their own families, and most of what is presented here does not apply to them.

And yet traditional beliefs and cultural practices are often adhered to by Japanese Canadians whose families have been resident in Canada for several generations. For example, a Japanese Canadian woman may be English-speaking and married to a Caucasian but still avoid bathing when she has a cold or flu without being aware that this practice is related to traditional Shinto beliefs. Even among the *sansei* (third generation), who are highly acculturated, there is a great deal of cultural diversity. Thus it is important not to make assumptions based on generalizations but to assess each person individually.

Waves of Migration to Canada

Early Immigration, 1877-1920

The first immigrants from Japan in 1887 (pointedly referred to as "sojourners") were farmers and fishermen, often second sons, who left overcrowded Japan for economic opportunities in Canada. Some stayed a few years and then returned home or moved on to the United States. As was true with South Asians and Chinese, the Japanese were victims of the extreme discrimination that eventually erupted in anti-Asian riots in Vancouver in 1907. After that, immigration was limited by government, but wives, including "picture wives" chosen at long distance, and children were allowed to join men already in Canada. The community began to grow slowly until immigration came to a standstill in the 1920s with changes in the immigration laws. The Japanese who arrived in this wave are called the *issei*. Their children, born mainly from 1920 to 1940, are the second-generation *nisei*. The *kika nisei*, a subgroup of this second generation, were born in Canada, educated in Japan, and then returned to Canada.

The Second World War had a profound effect on the Japanese Canadian community. After the Japanese bombing of Pearl Harbor in December 1941, all persons of Japanese ancestry, the majority of whom were Canadian citizens, were forcibly removed from the coastal areas of British Columbia. All men between the ages of eighteen and forty-five were immediately separated from their families and sent to road camps along the Hope-Princeton, North Thompson, and BC-Jasper highways. Older men and all women and children were sent to a temporary centre at Hastings Park in Vancouver and eventually to internment camps in the BC interior. The disruption of the traditionally strong family unit, where the father and older sons had dominant positions, caused great anguish. To add insult to injury, all property and possessions (homes, fishing boats, farms, and so on) were confiscated by the government and sold with minimal compensation. At the end of the war, after almost three years in the camps, the internees received an ultimatum from the government: either resettle east of the Rockies or be sent back to Japan. Once resettled, the vast majority of families had to begin the long and arduous task of rebuilding their lives from the ground up as many had lost everything. Not until 1949, four years after the war had ended, were Japanese Canadians allowed to return to the west coast.

Postwar Immigration, 1960-2004

Most postwar immigrants, referred to as the *shin-ijyusha*, have come to Canada to find freedom, both social and economic. Some, mainly professionals, have come to break away from the lifetime employment with the same company that until recently was typical of Japan, as well as to improve their quality of life. Some are retired couples who may divide their time between Canada and Japan. A significant number are temporary residents, mainly employees of Japanese companies or university researchers, in Canada with their families for a few years. In this group as well are the working-holiday and English-language students, mainly young women, who arrive annually for work-study for six months to two years. Finally, a number of young Japanese women have come as wives of Canadian men who may or may not be of Japanese background; some of these women have little or no family support of their own in Canada.

Work and Economic Status

The *nisei* (second generation) are today mostly in their sixties and seventies. They were educated in Canada, usually (but not always) have fluent English, and generally attained a higher level of education than their parents. For the most part they are a middle-class generation. In early adulthood many *nisei* men struggled to further their education and find a job and eventually worked in large businesses, took up fishing or farming, or owned a small business. *Nisei* women often juggled the demands of marriage, family, and secondary employment and thus moved in and out of paid jobs. Many have now retired.

Their children, the *sansei* (third generation), having benefited from educational and job opportunities not accorded their parents' generation, are an upwardly mobile group now in their thirties and forties. Many have postsecondary education and successful careers in areas such as business, health care services, and education.

The postwar Japanese immigrants and temporary residents are usually from middle-class backgrounds with some postsecondary education. They tend to be relatively young, independent, and confident at the time of their immigration. Eventually, many become involved in small business ventures like restaurants, trade in textiles/food products, or language and cultural translation services. Although English is part of the high school curriculum in Japan, the majority find that they are unable to communicate effectively when they arrive.

Many postwar immigrant women stay home until their children are older and then find work; those with no young children at home find paid employment. The type of work they obtain is often dependent on their fluency in English. Typical occupations include hostesses or servers in Japanese restaurants, travel agents or tour guides, clerical staff in Japanese companies, factory workers, and employees in small businesses.

Religion

The principal religions in Japan today are Shintoism, Buddhism, and Christianity. Most people in Japan are tolerant of religious beliefs and do not regard simultaneous involvement in several religions as being incongruous. For the most part, birth and marriage rites follow Shinto traditions, while end-of-life beliefs and funerals are Buddhist. This is also true among Japanese immigrant populations in North America.

As in the general Canadian population, only a small percentage of Japanese Canadians today actively practise any religion. The majority of Japanese Canadians however, report Buddhist or Shinto religious affiliations, while an increasing number, particularly among the *sansei* and their children, the *yonsei* (fourth generation), are Christians. A small number of prewar immigrants are Catholic, in part the result of the strong missionary presence in the Greenwood camp during the Japanese Canadian internment. In addition, there are three "new religious movements" from Japan with churches and fellowship centres in Canada. These are *Seicho-no-Ie* (House of Growth), *Konkokyo* (The Teaching of the Glory of the Unifying God), and *Tenrikyo* (Religion of Divine Wisdom). *Konkokyo* and *Tenrikyo* are two of the thirteen modern sects of Shintoism brought to North America by Japanese missionaries in the early twentieth century.

Shintoism

The indigenous religion of Japan has ancient origins. It is polytheistic in that spirit gods, *kami,* are worshipped at shrines. The word "Shinto" is written as two Chinese characters: *shin* is the character for *kami,* meaning divinity or god; *to* is the character for *michi,* meaning way or path. Thus, Shinto literally means the "the way of the gods." All natural objects and phenomena are considered to have *kami,* so that the gods of Shinto are innumerable.

Shintoism is largely concerned with obtaining the blessing of the gods for future events. Ceremonies are held to bless babies, children, weddings, and the start of new enterprises. Talismans (*omamori*), which can be purchased at Shinto shrines in Japan, serve a variety of health-related functions, such as the delivery of a healthy baby, speedy recovery from illness, or successful surgery. In Shintoism, the emphasis is on purity and cleanliness. Terminal illness, dying, and death are considered "impure" and akin to "contamination" of the body. This belief can initially hinder open and frank discussions with recent immigrants and temporary residents about informed consent procedures, treatment options, and advanced care directives.

Various types of Shintoism exist. They range from the belief that the Japanese emperors are direct descendants of the Sun God, *Amaterasu,* to the state Shinto that was once forced upon all Japanese, to the domestic Shinto that many practise in their own homes, to the numerous Shinto sects that emerged in the nineteenth century during a period of increased religious freedom. Although there are no Shinto shrines in Canada, the two sectarian Shinto organizations, *Konkokyo* and *Tenrikyo,* both have pre-war and post-war immigrant congregations in Toronto and Vancouver. The larger of the two organizations, *Tenrikyo,* offers organized Japanese language programs in these cities as a way of introducing the religion to Canadians.

Buddhism

Buddhism reached Japan in the sixth century via China and Korea. It holds that the ultimate state is one of self-enlightenment, attained by waking to the truth. There is no god in Buddhism; the emphasis is on ridding oneself of hate and jealousy through infinite love. Fanaticism is rejected and tolerance is desired.

Buddhism is a major presence in the contemporary life of people in Japan. Even if they are non-believers, they go to temples, are buried according to Buddhist rites, and after death are given posthumous Buddhist names. Memorial services are held on the first, seventh, and forty-ninth days after death, corresponding to the believed dates of departure from the body of the three souls – vegetative, animal, and spiritual. After that, services for the extended family and friends are held at specific intervals through the fiftieth year. During the annual *O-bon* season (July or August), it is believed that the souls of the deceased return to visit. In Japan, this event is marked by the return of family members to their ancestral homes.

Traditionally, an altar (*butsudan*) with pictures or artefacts of deceased family members is maintained in a household's place of honour, and every morning and evening family members greet their ancestors with prayer. This ritual ensures that individuals who pass away in their later years remain a significant part of the daily lives of their families for many generations.

Among Japanese Canadians, Buddhism is the religious affiliation with the largest following. There are Buddhist churches in every major urban centre in Canada, including two in the Greater Vancouver area. In addition, Buddhist churches exist in smaller rural communities in Southern Alberta (Picture Butte, Taber, and Coaldale), places where pre-war Japanese Canadian families have settled and remained.

The Buddhist ministry to Japanese Canadians began at the request of the *issei* living in Vancouver in the early 1900s. The first Buddhist temple was established in the Powell Street area of Vancouver known as Japantown in 1905. In the early days of settlement, services were social occasions as well as religious events, and provided respite from hard labour and loneliness for the predominantly male Japanese community. Buddhist temples, or churches as they later came to be called, formed an important part of the social network of the local Japanese community, much as in a Christian parish. Today, congregations in most cities are made up of the descendants of the early *issei* pioneer members, a testament to the perseverance, diligence, and devotion of the large community of Japanese Canadian followers of Buddhism.

In Japanese immigrant populations, as in Japan itself, Buddhism has exerted a tremendous influence on every aspect of culture, from art, literature, and architecture to morals and modes of thought. With regard to contemporary health beliefs and practices, Buddhism teaches that all illness and disease have spiritual, mental, and emotional components. This belief contradicts conventional Western medicine, which refers to illness or disease originating in the mind as "psychosomatic" and which has traditionally focused on the physical origins of illness. Given this emphasis, psychosomatic illness is often regarded in a very negative light. Many alternative healing practices, however, utilize a Buddhist system of health care beliefs by treating the mind, body, and emotions as one.

Language

Canadian-born Japanese have fluent English, except for small numbers of elderly *nisei* (second generation) who use Japanese as their first language at home and are unable to communicate easily in English. In contrast, new immigrants and temporary residents often have language difficulties in their early years in Canada, though all have studied English in high school in Japan. Many do not understand or speak English well. Many take ESL courses, try to learn English in their jobs, listen to English radio and TV, and socialize with English-speaking Canadians. They usually find it easier to read English than to speak it, and some physicians working with them have found it useful to write down important information, such as complicated drug regimes, to reinforce understanding.

Family Structure

Living Arrangements

A key influence on the Japanese family and its way of life has been Confucianism, a code of ethics with origins in China. For many generations this code has dictated that the Japanese live together in extended families, though in recent decades in Japan this practice has been declining rapidly. Urban apartments are common in Japan today, and they are not large enough for multigenerational households. Accompanying this downsizing of space has been a decreased desire among adult children to have parents and parents-in-law live with them. In Japan this is often seen as indicating a weakening of *oya koh koh* (filial obligation), a cornerstone value of Confucianism. In Canada most households are two-generation nuclear families.

Family Values

The first generation, *issei,* maintained traditional Meiji-era Japanese values: strong ties to the family unit, respect for and obligation to elders, a dominant position for the father and an inferior position for women and children, and emphasis on thrift and hard work. Given the economic hardships endured by the Japanese during this early period of immigration, it was economically necessary for most women to work outside the home. Nowadays many of the remaining *issei* and older *kika nisei,* those born in Canada but educated in Japan, have retained basic customs such as Japanese food consumption and the practice of traditional medicine. These customs are often much more "traditional" than those followed in contemporary Japan.

Many feel that the traditional values of family loyalty, honour, and obligation have been lost in the younger generations.

Despite their elders' belief that the *sansei* (third generation) and *yonsei* (fourth generation) have very little understanding of or adherence to the traditional *issei* value system and the fact that they do not usually identify strongly with their Japanese origins, these younger people do feel a strong obligation to the family, particularly to parents and grandparents.

Family Roles in Health Decisions

In *nisei*- and *sansei*-headed families, that is, families born in Canada, health decisions are based on the urgency of the medical situation. These decisions are not the special prerogative of the elders or family head.

But the families of postwar immigrants and temporary residents are more traditional. The husband's role in these families is to work diligently at his job and provide for the family. In return, the wife is to respect, honour, and care for him. Her primary responsibility is to manage the household and raise the children, including their education and discipline. In some cases other family members are consulted before a decision is made. In making a health-related decision, such as whether to take a child to a physician's office, weight is often given to an older family member's opinion, and the final decision is the husband's.

Child-Rearing Responsibilities

Japanese Canadian parents are devoted to meeting the physical and emotional needs of children, and children are expected to respect, honour, and obey their parents. While women have prime responsibility for raising children, in more traditional and recent immigrant families a woman's mother-in-law may assume responsibility for ensuring that her daughter-in-law performs all her household and child-rearing duties properly. This is unusual in Canada, however, because in-laws usually live far away.

Postwar immigrants and temporary residents believe that it is their duty and obligation to take an active part in finding suitable marriage partners for their children and to teach children proper conduct. Among the *nisei*, these issues are not solely decided by parents but instead are negotiated between generations.

Role of Women in Health Care

Japanese Canadian women, particularly the more traditional women among the older *nisei* and among recent immigrants, play key roles in the care of ill family members. A traditional wife will see it as her responsibility to attend to the health care needs not only of her children but also of her husband, her parents, and sometimes her in-laws. Her role in health care is not limited to times of illness but is also preventive. These women assume primary responsibility for the maintenance of their family's health through diet and close attention to body states and functions, not unlike Canadian-born Japanese women. Although they nurture their husbands and children through illness, when they themselves become more than mildly sick they typically must depend on their own parents and siblings for assistance because their husbands are traditionally not socialized to care for their wives. In Canada, severe illness may therefore cause additional stress for recent immigrant women who do not have at hand the support of their mothers or an extended family network.

Lifestyles of Postwar Immigrant Women

These women have been brought up to marry and have children, so they tend to consider employment temporary and accept relatively low-status work with low pay. And yet, unlike earlier immigrant women who had limited elementary school education, the majority of postwar immigrants have completed junior college before marrying or joining the workforce. Whereas pre-war immigrant women married in their late teens or early twenties, in modern Japan women tend not to marry until their late twenties or early thirties. With a later age of marriage, these postwar immigrants are in their fifties before their children are no longer a responsibility or have left home. At this point, they may take up hobbies or attend classes in the community to fill the gap created by their children's absence. Some women find it a difficult period of adjustment because they have devoted so much of their lives to raising their children.

Family Problems

Common to all Japanese Canadian immigrant families is the expectation that family members stand together when dealing with outsiders. Within the family, the moods and feelings of others are highly respected, and much interaction is indirect and non-verbal. The well-being of the collective unit takes precedence over individual desires, and marital or familial problems are usually worked out among family members without any outside assistance.

Conformity to rules of conduct and etiquette is an important aspect of Japanese Canadian culture, regardless of immigrant status, and family problems tend to be hidden from outsiders as shameful (*haji*) for the whole family. Examples of such problems include chronic unemployment, mental illness, pregnancy out of wedlock, breaking the law, and dropping out of school. Financial problems and alcohol abuse may lead a man to aggression and to beating his wife or children. But it is important to the family that outsiders remain unaware of and uninvolved in these difficulties. Family issues are dealt with first within the family. If this is unsuccessful, the family may seek an arbitrator, someone discreet whom the family respects, to assist without causing the family loss of face. It is very unlikely that the person chosen for this role will be a professional or stranger.

Respect for Elders

In more traditional pre-war and new immigrant families, respect is automatically given to the primary wage-earner, to men, and to older adults. Within the family hierarchy, the father has the most authority, followed by the grandfather, the eldest son, the mother, and finally the daughter. In general, however, older adults are revered and respected, and the eldest son is typically responsible for his aging parents. In Canada, however, the firstborn, regardless of gender, generally takes the initiative, or an unmarried daughter may assume responsibility for the care of parents in later life.

Stress in New Immigrant Families

Among recent immigrants, family members often suffer stress and depression due to language and cultural differences. Conflicts can occur, for example, when women attempt to maintain the traditional roles of wife and mother while holding down full-time work outside the home. Women who are not employed after immigration may feel a loss in status because the housewife's role in Canada does not enjoy the high esteem that it does in Japan. Contacts with non-Japanese women outside of the home and at work lead her to become more independent. If a man comes to Canada with fluent English or acquires it quickly, he is able to retain his role of authority within the family. However, if he depends on his children to translate, his position will be weakened. His authority may also be undermined if his wife becomes more independent, particularly if she takes on full-time employment.

Marriage, Intermarriage, and Domestic Abuse

Intermarriage with non-Japanese Canadians was almost non-existent for the *issei* and was extremely rare for the *nisei*. It has become normal, however, for the third generation, the *sansei,* who for the most part have had very limited contact with other Japanese while growing up. In fact, the intermarriage rate for *sansei,* over 90 percent, is the highest of any ethnic minority group in Canada, an indicator of their nearly complete acculturation.

Among postwar immigrants, men tend to seek out wives in Japan where they look for more culturally and linguistically compatible partners, whereas young, recent immigrant women and working-holiday women often find marriage partners in Canada. These women look widely for prospective partners, who may be non-Japanese Canadians, *sansei,* or postwar Japanese immigrants.

A few young Japanese women have in the postwar years been brought to Canada from Japan as wives either for Japanese Canadians or for non-Japanese Canadian men, some of whom have worked in Japan as English teachers. Some of these men may believe that Japanese women are more obedient and caring for men, though recent social changes in Japan have enabled women to become more independent. Some of these women arrive with little or no usable English, few skills, and no relatives in Canada. They can be very vulnerable, as when an abusive husband threatens withdrawal of support during the immigration process. Domestic abuse sometimes occurs, and women without family support and with few linkages to the Japanese Canadian community are more likely to appear in social agencies and clinics than are abused women in other Japanese Canadian families.

Child-Rearing

In Japan, the mother, sometimes with the assistance of one or both grandmothers, assumes primary responsibility for raising the children, a highly valued occupation in contemporary Japanese society. Once in Canada, new immigrant and temporary resident mothers continue in this role, preparing for their children's education, arranging tutoring, attending parent-teacher conferences, and so on. For the most part, new immigrant fathers have more time to spend with their children in Canada because working hours tend to be shorter than in Japan and after-hours socializing is not as prevalent. Despite an increased presence in their children's lives, however, they may still be reluctant to become involved in school-related activities, which they regard as part of the mother's domain.

In new immigrant and temporary resident families, infants are encouraged to be passive, and crying is discouraged out of deference to neighbours. This belief is carried over from Japan, where the vast majority of the population live in small dwellings closely crowded together. Some may believe

Yoko Okamoto, from Japan

Jim was a twenty-eight-year-old Canadian teaching English in Yokohama for two years when he met his wife, Yoko, an eighteen-year-old student in his class. He was attracted to her because she seemed so caring and accommodating, and she was excited and flattered that he wanted her to marry and return to Canada with him. She was pregnant when they arrived in Toronto.

Almost immediately Yoko realized that even though she had studied English in Japan she could not understand clerks in stores or even her doctor. She was totally dependent upon Jim not only for money but also for accompanying her to shop or take the bus to the Buddhist church. She had no friends or family members in Canada who could help her out. She was sad when she realized that life in Canada was not what she had envisioned.

Their daughter was born not long after they settled in Toronto, and for some time Yoko's life was centred on caring for her. Eventually Yoko asked Jim if she could take ESL classes to improve her English so that she could shop on her own and perhaps find a part-time job to help with the family's finances and earn a bit of money for herself. Jim absolutely refused, fearing her attempt to be independent. He thought she might meet other men or even leave him. Their arguments sometimes escalated into physical violence, especially if he had been drinking.

Then one day, as Yoko was pushing her child in a stroller near their home, a car ran up over the curb and hit them. They were not badly injured, but the ambulance took both of them to the hospital. The doctor saw a large bruise on Yoko's face and several on her arms which were obviously not the result of the accident and tried to inquire about them, but Yoko did not understand the questions, and there was no one available to interpret. When Jim finally arrived two hours later, another physician asked him about his wife's bruises and accepted his explanation that Yoko had fallen on an icy sidewalk. Jim then helped Yoko, carrying the baby, into a taxi, and they went home.

that keeping quiet is also better for the child's health. Children are breastfed for the first year. Toilet-training begins at seven to ten months by placing the child over the toilet, but there is no pressure for the child to succeed immediately.

Generally, new immigrant parents are very permissive, making very few demands of young children up to the age of about six or seven. Once they start school, however, discipline is increased. This involves the mother demanding consistency and teaching consideration for others. Instruction tends to be by example rather than verbal, in the belief that children learn best by imitation. Light spanking is not uncommon, and punishment is exercised by threatening the child with abandonment or exclusion from the family, or by means of embarrassment or shame.

Children in new immigrant families are taught early on to respect elders and those in authority, to distinguish between relatives or close friends (insiders) and others (outsiders), to develop *giri,* or a sense of obligation to others (parents, family, community), and to be modest and considerate. Children also learn that it is appropriate and acceptable to depend on others and to ask for favours (*amaeru*). Initially this dependence is on the mother and later is transferred to the group. This fostering of dependence is in stark contrast to the North American style of child-rearing, which promotes independence in the early stages of development. Another important notion taught to Japanese children is that of *gaman,* the need to be stoical and endure adversity patiently without complaint.

Children of postwar immigrant parents often attend Japanese school after English school hours or on weekends because there is a strong desire for the Japanese language to be preserved across generations. In the case of temporary resident families, school-age children are expected to attend intensive Japanese classes on Saturdays to ensure they are able to re-enter school upon their return to Japan. There is also pressure from these parents for children to go to tutorial classes to advance their math skills while in Canada.

In adolescence, new immigrant children are expected to be diligent in their school work and generally are not given many responsibilities. In many families, there continues to be a strong emphasis on scholastic achievement, and studies take priority over friends. Part-time jobs are allowed if academic achievement is not compromised. Compared to their North American–raised counterparts, teenagers in new immigrant or temporary resident families may appear immature and sheltered, as independence from parents has not been emphasized to this stage.

Names

Customarily, the family name comes first and the given name second. Adults generally call each other by their family or surname and add the suffix -san, meaning "Mr." or "Mrs." or "Miss." An example is Tanaka-san. Adults call children by their first names, adding -kun for boys and -chan mainly for girls. Examples are Takeshi-kun or Midori-chan. Children do not call older siblings by their first names but instead use special terms meaning older brother (*oniisan*) and older sister (*onehsan*).

Women typically change their surnames when they marry. Recently in Japan some have chosen to keep their own names, but this is considered very modern and unconventional. Another more contemporary phenomenon is the dropping of the "ko" ending from women's names, such as in Teruko or Akiko.

Gestures and Body Language

In both pre-war and postwar immigrant communities, bowing indicates respect and is used for greeting or taking leave of others. The depth of the bow is generally a measure of the rank or status of the recipient. Handshakes are not common between newer immigrants but are acceptable with Westerners. The physical expression of affection is open towards children but between spouses occurs only discreetly or in private.

Avoidance of eye contact traditionally denotes respect among new immigrants and temporary residents. However, most recognize and accept that eye contact is a feature of Western communication. In conversation, head nodding indicates attentiveness and understanding but not necessarily agreement. Similarly the statement "I understand" means "I understand what you are saying" but does not always imply agreement or compliance. Smiles may reflect a variety of emotions from joy to confusion, embarrassment, or politeness. Women especially are acutely aware of and sensitive to nonverbal reactions, such as facial expressions indicating hesitancy. They are quick to adjust and restore the comfort of the other person.

Conflict and Communication

From childhood, the expression of strong emotions, especially anger, is discouraged in Japanese Canadian families. Interpersonal harmony and cooperation are valued highly. Indirectness is used when revealing moods and feelings, and conflict and confrontation are avoided. Thus, agreement may be outwardly simulated in an attempt to maintain harmony. In such instances, a person may express disagreement indirectly by looking doubtful or remaining silent. This behaviour is typical of older *nisei* and new immigrants, but less evident in the *sansei*. Outside the family, conflict resolution and negotiation is occasionally accomplished by using a mediator (perhaps a minister or respected friend) to assist in the process. When this is not achieved, indirect modes of aggression may occur, such as gossip or avoidance.

Sleeping Practices

In the past, the preference in Japan was for more crowded and intimate sleeping arrangements rather than isolation in separate rooms; sleeping alone was considered pitiful and lonely. Moreover, separate bedrooms were often not possible due to the small size of Japanese homes. In fact, new immigrant children up to the age of five may still share a bed mat (*futon*) with a parent, and even the sharing of a room by preteenage siblings of both sexes is not uncommon. For the most part, however, new immigrant and temporary resident families adopt Western-style beds and, if adequate space is available, separate rooms for children.

Clothing

In Japan, people wear Western clothing in their everyday life, but traditional clothing is still popular as formal attire for events such as weddings. This is less the case in Canada, where new immigrants have fully adopted Western-style attire for all occasions. Shoes should be removed when entering a home, and slippers are worn indoors. In Canada, both pre-war and postwar immigrants continue this custom.

Unlucky Numbers and Ages

At birth, an individual is already considered to be one year old. Moreover, New Year's Day, or January 1st of the calendar year, marks the transition to the next chronological age (*kazoedoshi*), not the individual's actual date of birth. For example, a child born on December 30th becomes two years old on New Year's Day, though only two days old by Canadian reckoning.

The numbers four, nine, and thirteen are considered unlucky. The word "four" in Japanese is *shi,* which also means "death"; the character for "nine" is associated with a word meaning "suffering." Certain ages are believed to be potentially dangerous; for women these are nineteen, thirty-three, and thirty-seven and for men twenty-five, forty-two, and sixty-one.

Recreation and Leisure

Traditional sports (judo, karate, aikido) as well as modern ones (baseball, tennis, golf, curling) are enjoyed by both pre-war and postwar immigrants. Since the pre-war period, sports clubs and leagues have been organized and established in Japanese Canadian communities across the country. Calligraphy, flower arranging, bonsai, tea ceremony, cooking, karaoke, folk dancing, and sewing continue to be common leisure activities for older *nisei* and new immigrant women. Sightseeing tours and visits to hot springs, locally and abroad, are popular among older adult immigrant populations.

To drop in unannounced is generally considered rude, and a home visit should be accompanied by a gift for the hostess. Guests are welcomed into homes and offices, and typically tea is served with fruit and sweets. This custom is practised by both older *nisei* and new immigrants.

The *issei,* or first generation, seldom mixed socially with non-Japanese. However, the *nisei,* or second generation, being able to speak English, have integrated well in sports and social activities with mainstream society. In middle and later life they have taken the initiative by organizing social-gathering clubs in many of the larger Japanese Canadian communities. The *sansei* and their *yonsei* children have little sense of being different from other Canadians and therefore fully participate in recreation and leisure activities offered to all Canadians.

Festivals and Holidays

Many festivals are celebrated in Japan. The New Year is the main holiday season, and many people return to their family homes at this time for a three-day celebration from 31 December to 2 January. People also return home during the summer holiday season of *O-bon* in order to visit the graves of their ancestors. There are also special holidays throughout the calendar year to celebrate children, the transition to adulthood, and respect for the aged. Japanese Canadians continue to celebrate New Year's Day, but other holidays are rarely celebrated, because Japanese traditions are integrated with Canadian culture, whose holidays such as Easter and Christmas have become the focus of celebration.

However, in many of the larger Japanese communities across Canada, particularly Vancouver and Toronto, local Buddhist church organizations hold *O-bon* festivals in August. Besides being times of remembrance for deceased family members, these events serve as social gatherings with food and folk dancing (*odori*).

Health Care Beliefs and Practices

The health care beliefs and practices of contemporary Japan derive from three main sources: the indigenous Shinto belief system; *kanpo,* the medical tradition brought to Japan from China in the sixth century; and Western medicine.

Shinto Health Care Traditions

Early beliefs in Japan were that illness was caused by evil spirits or by exposure to polluting sources, such as blood, sick people, and dead bodies. Treatment involved purification rituals like hot spring baths and herbal infusions. Very few Japanese Canadians continue to practise these treatments exclusively, preferring instead to combine these traditions with Western medical therapy.

Kanpo: Traditional Japanese Medicine of Chinese Origin

The *kanpo* system is based on a belief that illness results from an imbalance in certain areas to which a person must therefore give careful attention: diet, sleep, exercise, and interpersonal relationships. There is also a belief that the universe, both physical and social, exists in a dynamic state of balance between two polar forces: yin and yang. Yin represents what is female, negative, dark, cold, and empty, while yang contains what is male, positive, light, warm, and full. Yin and yang qualities are ascribed to everything, including parts of the body, symptoms, and diseases. Body organs are believed to have specific connections with one another; for example, if the lungs are weak, the kidneys will show a weakness also.

The abdomen (*hara*), referring to stomach and intestines, is important in the traditional view of health and illness. There tends to be a greater fear about diseases of the stomach than about other illnesses, as problems with the stomach are thought to affect the balance of the whole bodily system. Traditionally, a cloth was wrapped around the abdomen for protection from cold (*haramaki*), and this practice continues today in Japan, especially with children and the aged.

Also stemming from the classical Chinese medical tradition is the belief that human beings are affected by the natural environment, so attention should be paid to the effect of climatic changes on the body. Neither the parts of the body, nor the whole person, function in isolation. Rather, they are parts of a dynamic interdependent system.

A further belief is in the existence of a series of pressure points on the surface of the body. The stimulation of one point exerts an effect on another part of the body. Pathways called Meridians connect these points and allow for the transmission of energy.

Treatment in traditional medicine is aimed at restoring bodily balance and harmony. The primary methods are herbal medicine, acupuncture, and moxibustion (the burning of small balls of moxa, or dried mugwort, on appropriate pressure points). Therapeutic massage techniques (*shiatsu*) are also used for muscle or joint problems as well as for general body weakness and fatigue. Traditionally, the pressure point system was used in shiatsu, but there are now different schools with centres in North America, some of which have incorporated chiropractic techniques.

Diet is an important aspect of treatment, and corrective diets may be based on the classical concept of yin and yang foods. No synthetic drugs are used, and surgery is not a part of this medical tradition, because it is believed to upset the bodily imbalance further. Treatment should be mild and is simply intended to boost the innate potential of the body to heal itself, a process that is slow and gradual. Attention is paid to mild symptoms because it is believed that ignoring them will lead to a worsening of the condition, which will then require lengthier treatment.

In Japan, medicines are made from dried herbs, most of which are imported from China and are therefore expensive. The herbs are boiled and strained to make a bitter-tasting liquid. Herbal medicines are believed to work gradually over a period of time, and small, mild, and frequent doses are believed to be more beneficial than larger and stronger doses that are taken less often. Herbal medications are either prescribed and sold by Japanese doctors practising traditional medicine or purchased prepackaged at pharmacies. Their use has become more common in recent years in Japan with increasing concern about the side-effects of synthetic drugs.

Both acupuncture and moxibustion use the Meridian and pressure point systems. In the case of acupuncture, needles are inserted into the body at appropriate points. With moxibustion, heat is the source of stimulation, and the small balls of ignited moxa, or mugwort, are left on the skin until it becomes hot. In some methods, another substance, such as ginger, is placed between the moxa and the skin for protection. In others, the moxa is placed directly on the skin, causing blisters and scarring. Acupuncture and moxibustion are used most often to treat musculo-skeletal problems. In Japan, both are practised by licensed practitioners, although moxibustion is also commonly used by people themselves at home to treat minor symptoms.

The involvement and cooperation of patient and family in the treatment process is considered an important part of therapy, and traditional practitioners spend time developing trust and rapport with patients.

There are several Japanese immigrant practitioners with offices in Vancouver and Toronto who offer moxibustion and acupuncture. Recent immigrants and temporary residents in Canada may turn to traditional medicine for chronic and degenerative illnesses but use Western medicine for acute episodes or may combine both types. Women tend to be more familiar and comfortable with the practice of traditional medicine than are men.

Western Health Care in Japan

Western medical facilities in Japan are excellent. There are large public hospitals as well as many small private hospitals and clinics that are owned and operated by doctors. Medical facilities are accessible to local communities, even in rural areas.

Almost all Japanese are covered by health insurance, either through the national government program or through their employers. The coverage is extensive and includes dental care, pre-, peri-, and postnatal care, as well as drugs, which are dispensed by physicians themselves. Large hospitals have on-site pharmacies where patients can get prescriptions filled immediately following examination and diagnosis.

Although Western medicine is by far the dominant system in contemporary Japan, the influence of traditional medicine may still be seen in its practice. Patients are encouraged to consult physicians for mild symptoms and conditions, such as coughs, colds, or general feelings of fatigue. People are very sensitive to the possible side-effects of drugs, which tend to be less potent than those prescribed in North America but are taken more frequently. After consulting a doctor about a complaint, a patient is asked to return for frequent check-ups, sometimes daily, when medication may be reviewed and reissued. In general, patients expect to receive some medication or treatment when they visit a doctor. Sometimes a family member will remain with a patient during an examination, and occasionally, if a patient is unable to keep an appointment, a relative or close friend will attend in order to report on the patient's progress or receive medication or test results.

Disease Prevalence and Life Expectancy in Japan

General health standards in Japan are very high. In 2002, infant mortality was among the lowest in the world at 3.8 per 1,000 live births (5.0 in Canada), and the life expectancy for Japanese men was seventy-eight years (seventy-six in Canada) and for females eighty-five years (eighty-three in Canada). In the 1990s, life expectancy for men and women increased by one and three years respectively.

The major causes of death in Japan are cardiac disease, stroke, and cancer, the most common among the latter being stomach cancer. The high incidence of stomach cancer is believed to be related to the consumption of a diet high in nitrites and sodium (e.g., cured meats and fish). Beginning in the 1990s, HIV and AIDS have become major public health issues in Japan.

According to longitudinal health studies conducted in the United States, Japanese Americans are at a lower risk of heart and cardiovascular disease than their Caucasian counterparts, but at a higher risk of stroke, stomach cancer, Type II diabetes, and vascular dementia. Although similar studies have not been carried out in Canada, research into the "healthy immigrant effect" indicates that with increasing adaptation to a Western diet and changing health practices over time, Asian immigrants are more likely to develop disease profiles similar to those of their North American–born counterparts.

Relationship between Physician and Patient

Physicians enjoy very high status in Japanese society. Patients defer to them and will comply readily with medical directives. At a medical consultation, a patient expects to have a thorough examination, to be asked about subtle body changes, and at the conclusion to receive medication and an explanation of the condition or illness.

Doctors in Japan are generally hesitant to inform patients of a diagnosis of cancer, except in cases where there is a high probability of successful treatment. As cancer is popularly believed to lead to inevitable death, informing the patient is thought to be too depressing and anxiety-inducing, and thus to lead to a worsening of the patient's condition. As a rule, the family is informed initially and decides whether or not to tell the patient. Many patients eventually infer the diagnosis by themselves.

In Canada, finding a Japanese-speaking physician is a high priority for postwar immigrants and temporary residents, who tend to be reluctant to discuss health, family, or social problems with non-Japanese physicians, feeling that they will not understand the cultural context. However, in Canada there are not many Japanese-speaking family physicians and very few Japanese-speaking specialists. Anyone can make an appointment to see a specialist in Japan, and many find the Canadian system of referral by physician inconvenient and a waste of time. As in other Asian cultures, women tend to prefer female obstetricians and gynecologists. In general, new immigrants find the Canadian patient-physician relationship more friendly and familiar than in Japan, where it tends to be distant and formal. Canadian physicians for their part find that these new immigrants tend to be stoical.

In Japan, health care professionals who are not physicians have lower status. Nurses, for instance, function more like receptionists or secretaries

Mrs. Nishimura, from Japan

Mrs. Nishimura came to Canada from Japan after her husband died. She hesitated to leave her friends and home in a small coastal town, but her daughter and son-in-law in Victoria convinced her that she would be happy living with them, and they could help her as she grew older. When she first arrived, at age seventy-six, she did much of the cooking and worked in the small garden, a useful contribution because her daughter and son-in-law both spent very long hours in their corner store. She sometimes visited her son, who lived in Vancouver. Once a week when the family went to the Buddhist church, she was able to chat with other older women, some of whom lived nearby and came to see her. One friend convinced her to go to English classes at the church, where she learned enough to carry on a very basic conversation.

Then, four years after she arrived in Canada, she became ill with cancer and required nursing care that her daughter could not provide unless she stopped working, something the family could not afford. When Mrs. Nishimura moved to a palliative care home, she quickly gave up hope. There were no familiar Japanese foods, no daily hot baths, no Japanese-speaking staff. Her daughter came every day after work, but those visits, and the food that she brought, were not enough to relieve Mrs. Nishimura's sadness.

As Mrs. Nishimura's health declined, her non-Japanese physician asked the family to come to the care home. After reviewing her illness, he told Mrs. Nishimura directly that they could continue to make her comfortable but that she should prepare for her death. Later, her daughter and son and her daughter's husband agreed that a Japanese doctor speaking in Japanese would not have said it that way. The Canadian doctor seemed cold and not very considerate. They wondered if they had made a mistake in convincing Mrs. Nishimura to come to Canada, and for a while they even thought of going back to Japan when their own time came to die.

With permission of Yuko Shibata

than qualified health care practitioners. In Canada, new immigrants and temporary residents sometimes have to learn to accept care from a nurse whom the physician has authorized.

Medication and Treatment

Japanese immigrants are sometimes concerned that Western drugs are too strong and cause side-effects. However, compliance is usually good if regard for the physician is high, that is, if the patient perceives the physician as competent and appropriately formal in his conduct. Family members can also influence compliance. For example, if an older parent has a negative reaction to a prescribed medication, a son or daughter may discourage continued use by saying, "That medicine is too strong for you."

Some older *nisei* (second generation) as well as postwar immigrants use traditional medicines for both chronic and acute conditions. Herbal medicines may be purchased in the Chinatown areas of major urban centres and are considerably cheaper than in Japan. They are taken for allergies and stomach and bowel problems, as well as for general health maintenance. A small number of these immigrants also use moxibustion as a home remedy for a variety of problems including back pain, shoulder stiffness, and general tension. In addition, practitioners of acupuncture and shiatsu may be consulted, although in Canada these specialists are not as common and may often be regarded as underqualified.

Hospitalization

The average length of stay in Japanese hospitals is longer than in Canada. This is due at least in part to a belief that during illness and recuperation, people should receive extra care and attention as well as bed rest. Family members play an active role in providing care during hospitalization, washing clothes, bringing meals, and staying with the patient for long periods of time.

In Japan, there is an expectation that friends and co-workers will also visit a hospitalized patient. Not visiting is likely to be interpreted as an expression of negative feelings. Visitors are expected to bring gifts, preferably of a perishable nature such as fruit or cut flowers, which symbolize the temporary nature of the illness and betoken a speedy recovery. Potted flowers, for example, would inappropriately suggest a lengthy or permanent illness. Postwar immigrants in Canada continue this custom of hospital visiting, while pre-war Japanese Canadians are more likely to base their decision to visit on the closeness of the relationship with the patient.

Generally, new immigrants prefer to use their own nightwear because hospital gowns are considered to be impersonal and wearing one's own clothes is thought to strengthen an individual's sense of control. They may also dislike wearing clothes that other patients have previously worn. Gowns with ties at the back compromise feelings of privacy, and many Japanese Canadians feel uncomfortable during stays in Canadian hospitals where the use of such gowns is mandatory.

In Canada, older *nisei*, postwar immigrants, and temporary residents are generally considered by health professionals to be "ideal" patients: stoical, cooperative, grateful, uncomplaining, and unquestioning. However, there may also be a communication problem. Patients who have difficulty with English may be afraid of not understanding hospital staff, and recent immigrants may be unfamiliar with hospital routines or expectations, and both may be too embarrassed to ask for clarification and so agree to everything.

Hospital bathing routines can present a problem for older Japanese because many prefer a bath to a shower and almost all prefer the water to be much hotter than is normally used in Canada.

Mental Health

In Japan, traditionally, there is a general stigma associated with mental illness. A child of marriageable age, for example, may be discouraged from choosing a partner with a personal or family history of psychiatric treatment. Families may hide members experiencing mental health problems and be ashamed to seek professional help. Thus treatment, especially institutionalization, is likely to be delayed until the family can no longer deal privately with the problem. These attitudes are slowly starting to change as mental health assistance and resources become available in communities across Japan.

As in other Asian cultures, mental illness among Japanese immigrants in Canada tends to be expressed through somatization rather than by psychological complaints. Excessive sensitivity to the social and physical environment (*shinkeishitsu*) is a common culture-bound neurosis related to the inability to satisfy dependency needs (*amaeru*). Individuals suffering from this syndrome tend to be perfectionist and highly self-conscious; they are also believed to be intelligent and creative. Physical symptoms include fatigue, sleeplessness, stomach aches, and headaches. This condition is believed to stem from a childhood syndrome and is characterized by frequent crying, irritability, and temper tantrums. It is held to derive from overindulgent and overprotective mothering, and to occur more commonly in boys than girls. For such conditions families often seek traditional treatment, acupuncture, and moxibustion.

Among Japanese new immigrants or temporary residents, young men and women may resort to suicide when the pressure to succeed in academic endeavours is so great that failure represents a loss of face for the family. In elderly adults, suicide attempts may occur when role changes (e.g., wife to widow) lead to feelings of unworthiness and alienation.

In Canada, depression is a common mental health problem among middle-aged housewives in the postwar immigrant community. They lack the cultural support for the traditional roles of wife and mother, particularly after their child-rearing years are over. If they have been influenced by the more liberated values of Canadian women, but are still part of a traditional, male-dominated marriage, they may experience conflict and depression. Husbands and children generally adapt more quickly than wives to Canadian society as a result of exposure at work and school. Housewives, by contrast, can be left behind in linguistic and cultural isolation. These women rarely seek professional help of their own accord and endure with what support can be provided by friends or extended family members.

The forced internment and property loss of Japanese Canadians during the Second World War continues to be a potential source of mental health problems among the pre-war immigrant community. With suppressed anger, problems of identity, and depression, many of these older Japanese Canadians have been unable to obtain appropriate mental health treatment because of language (*issei*) or cultural barriers (*nisei*). Despite their rapid acculturation after the postwar dispersal, many *nisei* still feel embarrassed or ashamed to discuss such problems outside the family.

For many postwar immigrants and temporary residents, talk therapy is not considered appropriate treatment for mental health problems. It is regarded simply as a means to elicit information about "real" physical symptoms, whose treatment and elimination will prevent the later development of mental symptoms. The cultural values of interpersonal harmony and fulfilment of social roles, including service to the family, may provide the best therapeutic goals for mental health problems. In general, it may be more effective to help the individual accept the illness and adapt to it within the social environment rather than try to cure it.

In Canada today there are very few Japanese-speaking mental health professionals. Most of the small number of Japanese-speaking psychiatrists have trained, or are being trained, in Japan or abroad and have little knowledge or experience of mental health services in Canada. Many of these professionals do not see patients on a regular basis in medical offices but rather consult with individuals in outpatient clinics or at community centres. Due to the stigma attached to mental health problems among Japanese Canadians, the public nature of consultation venues is often the biggest deterrent to seeking help. In the end, many new immigrants and temporary residents with minimal fluency in English are referred to English-speaking psychiatrists. For patients who have difficulty expressing themselves in English and who feel that the professional does not understand the cultural implications of their problem, this can be very frustrating. With their lack of experience and trust in Canadian mental health services, many new immigrants from Japan avoid seeking help until the problem becomes debilitating.

Family Planning

Most new immigrant couples try to start their families within the first two years of marriage, and the preference is for two children. Although traditionally boys were favoured as first-born, many couples now have no special preference for the sex of offspring. Generally, the husband uses a condom, because oral contraceptives are not widely prescribed for women in Japan.

In Japan, although abortion is not sanctioned – traditional Buddhist beliefs hold that all life is sacred – it is in fact quite common and accepted. The procedure is generally performed in a gynecologist's office. Premarital sex is not condoned for women but is acceptable for men. If an unmarried woman becomes pregnant, she brings shame to the whole family. Commonly her family hides the problem by sending her to stay with relatives until she has had an abortion. A birth out of wedlock is strongly disapproved of; the status of the child is low and the family loses face. An illegitimate child in Japan is usually kept and raised by the mother's family, but in Canada until recently it has usually been given up for adoption, especially if it is of mixed race.

Pregnancy and Prenatal Care

Customarily, a woman tells her husband and family as soon as she knows that she is pregnant. Pregnancy and birth are viewed as joyous events for women, who are pampered and well taken care of during this period. Some new immigrant and temporary resident women may even return to their hometowns in Japan during the second or third trimester to give birth. By doing so, parents guarantee Japanese citizenship for their child.

Japanese women are expected to eat well-balanced meals during pregnancy. After the fifth month, salty and spicy foods are restricted, while milk, seaweed, and soy products are stressed. Fruit and vegetables are recommended to avoid constipation. In Canada, more emphasis is placed on vitamins, dental care, regular medical visits, and prenatal classes.

In Japan, visits during pregnancy may be made to a Shinto shrine to pray for a healthy baby. In the past, during the fifth month of pregnancy, on a day considered auspicious for easy delivery, a long white cotton sash was often purchased at a temple or shrine. This was worn wrapped around the abdomen under the outer clothing for the remainder of the pregnancy and usually for about one month after delivery. It was believed to ward off illness by keeping the abdomen warm and to prevent the fetus from moving around too much and becoming too large, which would result in difficult delivery. Today, this custom is rarely practised, and pregnant women are not overly concerned about the size of the fetus.

Childbirth

It is traditionally a mother's role to care for her daughter at the time of childbirth, and in Japan it is not uncommon for a woman to return to her family home for the birth of the first child. For this reason, the doctor who sees a woman during her pregnancy is often not the one who delivers the baby. For subsequent births the wife's mother usually comes to her daughter's own home to help her. For new immigrant and temporary resident women who choose to deliver in Canada, the arrival of the wife's mother is usually timed for the period right after birth when she can assist her daughter during the initial period of adjustment to parenthood.

In Japan, childbirth is usually at a neighbourhood hospital with a doctor and midwife attending. Generally the husband is not present at the birth. Gowns are not supplied by the hospital, and women wear their own clothing in labour. The preferred position for childbirth is in bed with the head raised. Anesthetics are available but decorum during painful bouts is considered important, so women are stoical. Infants are taken to the nursery immediately after birth and given glucose water. Circumcision is not performed.

In Japan, pregnancy and childbirth belong exclusively to the realm of women. However, in the case of new immigrants to Canada, husbands, although perhaps embarrassed and uncomfortable, are usually interested in attending prenatal classes and in being present at the birth, if only to interpret for their wives. Often the wife's mother (or the husband's mother) does not arrive to provide the customary care and support until after the birth.

Postpartum Period

In Japan, it is traditional to present the infant's umbilical cord (*heso-no-o*) to the mother when she is discharged from hospital. Preservative is sprinkled on the cord, and it is enclosed in a wooden box tied with a ribbon. This custom continues in some, but not all, hospitals in Japan but is not practised in Canada.

In Canada, the postpartum period may be difficult for new immigrant or temporary resident women, particularly if their mothers or mothers-in-law are unable to come to assist with caregiving. For the first month, a new mother is not expected to go out or do anything except breastfeed the baby. During this period, the family receives visitors, unless the baby is premature or abnormal, in which case people may be too embarrassed to visit.

In Japan, a newborn baby, especially a first-born, is taken by parents and grandparents to a Shinto shrine for blessings and prayers for a long life. When a baby is born to Japanese immigrants in Canada, family members in Japan may visit a local shrine and send talismans commemorating the visit.

Weaning takes place later in Japan than in Canada, and breastfeeding for a full year is not uncommon, especially as most women are not employed outside the home. In Canada, where many new immigrant women have to return to work after a period of maternity leave, infants are weaned earlier, although generally breastfeeding is preferred to bottle-feeding.

Women do not discuss postpartum depression openly with physicians or specialists, because mental health problems tend to be hidden or ignored in Japanese Canadian families.

Childhood Health and Illness

In Japan, the common childhood diseases are colds, influenza, chest conditions, ear infections, and stomach aches. There is a traditional belief that leaving a crying child unattended is unhealthy and may result in hernia or a protruding navel from overexertion. During mild illnesses, feeding, bathing, and massaging by the mother reinforce the family bonds and are considered important in preventing more serious health conditions. Home treatments, most often prepared and administered by the mother, include herbal remedies for colds and general malaise. Families accept vaccinations since prevention of disease is welcomed. An ill child arouses great concern because the child must be given extra care and because its condition may reflect negatively on the family. Consequently, children are often kept home from daycare or school until they feel better. These practices continue when immigrants come to Canada.

Disability and Chronic Disease

Although Japanese Canadian families are concerned for physically and mentally disabled members, they may also feel shame and embarrassment about these conditions. As a result, they may be reluctant to discuss problems or seek support and may tend to avoid or conceal treatment or institutionalization.

Children under the age of fifteen who have chronic diseases, such as asthma, eczema, or nephrosis, are primarily under the care of the mother. In general, a family's compliance with physician-directed treatment depends on the degree of satisfaction with the physician. Lack of compliance may be due to poor explanation by the physician, lack of understanding by the family, incorrect diagnosis, overprescription of medication, or apparent lack of concern by either the physician or family. When and if problems do arise, postwar immigrant patients, not wanting to challenge the physician's authority, may be reticent to inform the doctor about difficulties with treatment regimens, such as side-effects.

Hygiene and Bathing

Traditional Shinto notions of impurity and pollution classify aspects of the world as either clean, pure, and safe or dirty, polluted, and dangerous. The "outside" is associated with impurity, and so the Japanese remove their shoes and wash their hands upon returning home. Within the home, the toilet is considered the least clean area, and in Japan it is always separated from the bathing area. The lower body, from the waist down, is believed to be less clean than the upper half. This division is reflected, for example, in the separate laundering of clothes worn on the upper body from those worn on the lower half of the body. Because of a traditional belief in the contaminating qualities of blood, menstruating women may consider themselves unclean.

The Shinto belief system stresses the importance of expelling poisons from the body, so that enemas, frequent bathing, hand washing, and gargling are considered basic to good health. In Japan, people do not use baths simply to wash themselves; in fact, the actual washing and rinsing are done outside the tub. The bath itself is a long, leisurely soak in a deep tub full of very hot water. Family members use the same bath water in turn, and the tub is emptied after the last person has finished. Customarily, bathing is done at night. For both older *nisei* (second generation) men and postwar immigrants, a deep bath is preferred to a shower because the purpose is not only cleanliness but also relaxation. Bathing is associated with good health and is usually avoided during periods of illness, especially fevers or upper respiratory infections. Thus a resumption of bathing signals recovery. Women often avoid hot baths while menstruating and prefer instead to take showers. When in hospital or nursing homes, older Japanese Canadians and new immigrants often complain that the bath water is not hot enough.

Dental Health

Until the 1950s, before dental insurance was generally available in Japan, people usually went to a dentist only when they had a toothache. Now that dental care is provided through a national health insurance system, fillings tend to be favoured because dentures and orthodontics are not covered under the national plan. Since insurance coverage does not include preventive dental care, such as cleaning or polishing at regular intervals, people tend to develop dental caries early in childhood. As a result, many Japanese dental offices operate on an emergency basis, treating dental problems after they occur. It is not surprising, then, that new immigrants and temporary residents tend to view dental work more as a cure and than as prevention.

Similarly, the *issei* and older *nisei* generally regard preventive dental care as unimportant. Where they lived dental care was relatively inaccessible, and most of them could not afford it. Later generations, the younger *nisei* and the *sansei,* have increased access to dental insurance plans through their employers, recognize the importance of good oral hygiene, and generally have check-ups on a regular basis.

Recent immigrants and temporary residents, two groups usually lacking comprehensive dental coverage, may continue to avoid dental visits because of the high cost and because they are not used to preventive strategies. Some may assume that a dentist who encourages regular check-ups is desperate for business, not attempting to prevent further dental problems.

Food and Nutrition

The traditional diet in Japan consists of white and brown rice, soybeans, fish, salted pickles, fermented soybean paste (*miso*), noodles, soybean curds (*tofu*), green onions, spinach, yam, Japanese radish, eggs, seaweed, bamboo, mushrooms, greens, grapes, oranges, and other fruits. This diet is low in fats but high in salt. A traditional breakfast is rice, fish, pickles, and soup, although it is more common now to have toast and coffee. Typically, lunch and dinner include rice, fish, vegetables, and clear soup. Between meals, the Japanese may have some kind of sweet. Women are responsible for the majority of shopping and food preparation. Japanese Canadians may use chopsticks (*hashi*), forks, and spoons. To slurp while eating noodles in soup is acceptable and indicates appreciation.

Egg in *sake* (Japanese wine) is consumed for head colds, and some people eat hot noodle soup to induce sweating in cases of mild fever. Hot, soup-like steamed rice (*okayu*) is eaten for diarrhea or when recovering from surgery or serious illness. Ginseng tea, garlic, garlic wine, green onion, mushrooms, and salted plums are taken to maintain good health and prevent illness. These food rituals are generally followed by both the *nisei* and new immigrants.

It is extremely difficult for people to give up soy sauce and salted pickles, two mainstays of the Japanese diet, when a low salt diet is prescribed. Older adult immigrants, in particular, may complain that there is nothing left for them to eat, although low-sodium soy sauce and other sauces are now available on the market.

With the increasing Westernization of the Japanese diet and the infiltration of American-based food outlets into Japan, however, it is now common for young people to eat fast food lunches and dinners (McDonald's, Kentucky Fried Chicken, Mister Donut, Starbucks Coffee) rather than traditional-style meals. After moving to Canada, new immigrants tend to eat more foods that are high in sugar, fat, and animal protein, and low in nutritional value. As a result, the health status profiles of longer-term immigrants (those who have been in Canada ten years or more) begin to resemble those of their Canadian counterparts as their diets become more Westernized. For example, older people commonly have oatmeal and toast for breakfast.

Use of Alcohol and Tobacco

Drinking alcohol on a regular basis is more acceptable for men in Japan than it is in Canada; in fact, drinking is very much a part of the business culture in contemporary Japan. Wives and others tolerate moderate overindulgence because they believe it relieves work-related stress. While occasional drunkenness is not uncommon, chronic alcoholism is rare. Men usually drink after work in bars or at home. Although Japanese women traditionally drank very little, this is less true of young women, especially in Canada.

Traditionally, smoking was a man's domain. Among the younger generations in Japan however, women are now more likely to take up smoking. This habit tends to be curbed somewhat among working-holiday or student-visa students who find the cost of tobacco products in Canada to be double that in Japan.

Care of Older Adults

Given the immigration trends from Japan since the 1970s, there are relatively few older postwar immigrants compared to *nisei*. The small numbers of older immigrants who have arrived in the recent past have generally come to join families already settled here. Occasionally, families are unable to adjust to this situation, or the aged parent becomes a burden and has to be placed in a mainstream care facility. In such cases, the older parent may experience extreme culture shock and social isolation, being unable to communicate well in English, unfamiliar with the culture, and unused to Western food. Bathing regimes, in particular, are unacceptable because bath water is much cooler than they are used to.

Despite having a number of chronic health conditions, many older *nisei* continue to live independently in self-contained apartments; an increasing number of older, widowed women in particular live in low-income housing in large urban centres. Most have families, but prefer living independently to being a "burden" on their adult children. Many live near other older *nisei* who form their social network. Consequently, they are less isolated and lonely than if they were scattered in the suburban homes of their families.

Because of the history of social and governmental discrimination in Canada, some older pre-war Japanese Canadians carry with them a fear and distrust of any type of formal authority. This attitude creates problems in care facilities and hospitals and often results in a high degree of stress and anxiety for older *nisei*. Differences in food and lack of fluency in English (for the *kika nisei*, born in Canada but educated in Japan) are also significant problems for those living in residential care settings. Moreover, prior to the 1990s when there were few alternatives for ethnospecific care, older Japanese Canadians were placed in many different mainstream care facilities throughout large cities, further contributing to their loneliness and alienation.

Generally, both pre-war and postwar immigrant families feel some guilt and shame about placing aged parents in institutions, and some may wish to keep the fact hidden from friends and anyone outside family members. At the same time, adult children and their spouses are often employed full-time outside the home and therefore unable to provide the necessary care for a frail or disabled parent.

Until the early 1990s, there were very few seniors' housing developments or long-term care facilities designed to accommodate Japanese Canadians as they aged. In 1992, the Momiji Seniors Centre, an assisted-living residential complex for elderly Japanese Canadians, opened its doors in Toronto. The Momiji Health Care Society, in addition to running the centre, also operates a forty-bed unit exclusively for Japanese Canadian seniors in a municipally run extended care facility in downtown Toronto. A more recent development, the Nikkei Seniors Home Project in Burnaby, offers both independent and assisted-living accommodations for Japanese Canadian seniors in the Lower Mainland of British Columbia. Both developments offer pre-war and postwar immigrant seniors a continuum of care, including support services and activity programs, in a culturally and linguistically sensitive environment. Funding for these projects has come from all three levels of government and from an enormous amount of community fundraising support nationwide. In 2003, there were waiting lists for both complexes.

Death and Dying

The Buddhist belief in reincarnation and the established commemorative rituals for the deceased provide comfort and reconciliation. After death, a Buddhist is given a name (*ho-myo*) by a priest, in a ritual attended by the family. A wake is held on the evening before the funeral, which is by cremation. Additional services are held on the seventh and forty-ninth days, and services for the happiness of the dead are held on the first, second, sixth, and twelfth anniversaries. According to Shinto beliefs, the recently deceased are contaminating, so funerals, memorial services, and associated rituals serve to counteract the essential pollution associated with death. For example, salt is sprinkled over those returning home from a funeral as an act of purification. In the Buddhist tradition, many families maintain an altar in their homes where offerings to deceased members are made at special celebrations.

It is considered better to die at home than in hospital, and in cases of terminal illness in Japan, physicians may advise willing families to take the patient home. However, this is the ideal, and many families feel unable to cope with a dying patient at home. When someone is dying, the family is responsible for contacting relatives and friends, who are expected to pay their last respects. Family members decide on the treatment of the body after death. This holds true for both pre-war and postwar immigrant families. Because of the stigma associated with cancer and dementia, more recent immigrant families are oftentimes reluctant to acknowledge these as causes of death.

Use of Health and Social Services

Strongly affected by their experiences during the Second World War, older *nisei,* like their *issei* parents, tend to be more conservative in attitude and lifestyle than younger generations of pre-war or postwar immigrants. In general, they have a difficult time fully trusting non-Japanese Canadian professionals and so may not welcome outsiders' involvement in personal health or family issues. Instead, this group prefers to rely on family and community support networks to manage and resolve health-related problems. Postwar immigrants for the most part are receptive to professional input and support in health care, but they prefer Japanese-speaking practitioners. The tendency for new immigrants to seek outside help is largely due to their having little if any family support or close social networks in Canada.

Delivering Culturally Relevant Health Care

Postwar immigrants and temporary residents often do not have a high enough level of English comprehension to fully understand health care information related to diagnosis and treatment even if they seem able to converse in the language. Some physicians have found that writing down instructions in note form is a good way to confirm information relayed verbally because there is a strong likelihood that the patient will have it checked by family members or friends.

In many cases, *kika nisei* (born in Canada but educated in Japan), new immigrants, and temporary residents rely on family members or friends to translate for them during medical or social service appointments. This raises several important issues. First, family members or close friends may screen information, feeling that it is in the "best interest" of the patient; for example, they may not give "bad news" to a patient (as with cancer diagnosis). Second, though family members or friends have an increased sensitivity to cultural issues and a personal history with the patient, the ability to translate health information accurately varies greatly among individuals. In some cases, preteen children may be called upon to translate for immigrant parents concerning a diagnosis of serious illness or spousal abuse, and such serious family issues can leave children emotionally traumatized. For these reasons, it is important to ensure that fully trained interpreters who are neutral parties are available whenever possible when the information being given is of a highly sensitive nature.

For all health care practitioners dealing with older or new immigrant Japanese Canadian patients, it is best to avoid direct confrontation regarding health issues because it may cause embarrassment and fear of losing face. Furthermore, it is important to be aware that sexual matters, mental illness including dementia, and family issues are difficult areas for open discussion because they are considered extremely private. Given this, the family's preferred solution may be to call in a respected friend or relative, not a professional.

Further Reading

Kobayashi, K.M. 1999. "Bunka no tanjyou (emergent culture): Continuity and change in older nisei (second generation) parent-adult sansei (third generation) child relationships in Japanese Canadian families." PhD diss., Department of Sociology, Simon Fraser University, Burnaby, BC.

Kobayashi, K.M. 2000. "The nature of support from adult children to older parents in Japanese Canadian families." *Journal of Cross-Cultural Gerontology* 15: 185-205.
Lebra, T.S. 1979. *Japanese Patterns of Behavior.* Honolulu: University of Hawai'i Press.
Lock, M. 1983. "Japanese responses to social change: Making the strange familiar." *Western Journal of Medicine* 239: 25-30.
Nakane, C. 1970. *Japanese Society.* Berkeley, CA: University of California Press.
Shibata, Yuko. 2003. "Overlapping lives: cultural sharing among five groups of Japanese Canadian (nikkei) women." PhD diss., Department of Anthropology and Sociology, University of British Columbia, Vancouver, BC.
Smith, A., and K.M. Kobayashi. 2002. "Making sense of Alzheimer's disease in an intergenerational context: The case of a Japanese Canadian nisei-headed family." *Dementia: The International Journal of Social Research and Practice* 1: 213-25.
Tempo, P.M., and A. Saito. 1996. "Techniques of working with Japanese American families." In G. Yeo and D. Gallagher-Thompson, eds., *Ethnicity and the Dementias,* 109-22. Washington, DC: Taylor and Francis.

Contributors to the first edition
Kouichi Asano, Physician, Vancouver
Ruth Coles, Mount St. Joseph Hospital, Vancouver
Diane Kage, AMSSA, Vancouver
Tatsuo Kage, Tonari Gumi, Vancouver
Rose Murakami, Health Sciences Hospital, University of British Columbia
Reverend Gordon Nakayama, Vancouver
Diane Nishi, Vancouver
Sakuya Nishimura, Burnaby
Fumitaka and Masako Noda, Physicians, Vancouver
Ken Shikaze, Tonari Gumi, Vancouver

Contributors to the second edition
Ruth Coles, Nikkei National Heritage Centre, Burnaby
Roderick Hashimoto, Konko Church, Vancouver
Setsuko Hirose, MOSAIC, Vancouver
Cathy Mikihara, Nikkei National Heritage Centre, Burnaby
Kenji Shimizu, Dentist, Burnaby
Takeo Yamashiro, Tonari Gumi, Vancouver

6

People of South Asian Descent

Shashi Assanand, Maud Dias, Elizabeth Richardson, Natalie A. Chambers, and Nancy Waxler-Morrison

South Asians are people with cultural origins in the Indian subcontinent, which includes Pakistan, India, Sri Lanka, Bangladesh, and Nepal. Although most South Asians in Canada have come from these countries, people of South Asian cultural heritage have also immigrated to Canada from other parts of the world, notably the South Pacific (Fiji) and East Africa.

South Asians in Canada, though sharing a British colonial heritage, represent great social and cultural diversity. Differences are introduced by variations in urban and rural background, in levels of education, and especially in the length of time they or their families have lived in Canada. Immigrants from an educated, urban background arrive with prior knowledge of the English language and of many aspects of Western culture, whereas those from rural areas often find the cultural gap very wide.

The general cultural and social diversity among South Asians is mirrored by the great variety in health beliefs, practices, and experiences, both at home and in Canada. It is impossible to document the range of detail, such as differences in childbirth customs between Fijian and Ugandan Asians or the differing health care expectations between a well-educated computer scientist from Bangalore and a farmer from India's Punjab. Instead, we present general patterns of practice and belief, indicating where possible how these may vary. We want to make practitioners aware of both the patterns and the great differences among South Asians, depending on country of origin, religion, class, degree of urbanization, and length of time in Canada. It is therefore important to investigate each individual's situation.

Main Emphasis on India and Pakistan

Most of our examples are from India, and the main focus is on new immigrants and people from less developed, often rural, communities, because they are the ones who have the most difficulty with the Canadian health system.

Immigrants from Sri Lanka have cultural backgrounds and beliefs similar to many other South Asians, but they are not discussed here. Most Sri Lankan immigrants to Canada came in the 1990s as civil war refugees, and unlike other South Asians they came from a country that has long had a comprehensive and free Western-style medical system.

Waves of Migration to Canada

1900-60, Sikhs from Rural India

The first South Asian immigrants to Canada arrived in British Columbia around 1900. Predominantly Sikh men from the northwest state of Punjab, they came here to earn money. Most found work in the forest industry, particularly in the sawmills of Victoria, Vancouver, and New Westminster. In 1909, South Asian immigration was banned, though the ban was modified in 1919 to allow wives and children to join husbands and fathers. Because of restrictions on immigration, there were only about 6,000 South Asians in Canada by 1942. The ban was lifted in 1947, and immigration then increased, mainly of Sikhs from rural areas in northern India who found employment as unskilled workers.

1960-90, South Asians from Many Countries

Changes in immigration regulations in the 1960s drew people from all parts of India and Pakistan, mostly highly educated technicians and professionals. In the 1970s there was significant migration of professionals and business people from East Africa, particularly Uganda, Kenya, and Tanzania, when political changes threatened residents of South Asian background. In 1987 and after, large numbers of South Asians from Fiji migrated to Canada to escape ethnic conflict and political tension. Throughout this period many South Asian families already established in Canada sponsored other relatives to join them.

1990-2004, Family Sponsorship and New Immigrants

During the 1990s India provided more immigrants to Canada than any other country except China. Pakistan was third, with 15,000 immigrants in 2001. In 2001 about 28,000 persons arrived from India, half of whom were immediate family members joining relatives already here. Many sponsored family members were from the Punjab, mainly from rural farm families. Some were young brides coming to join husbands of Indian background resident in Canada; young men and their families sometimes arrange marriages to girls from India and Pakistan in the belief that they are less "modern" and can more easily accept life in an extended family than can those who have grown up in Canada. Immigrants in the independent category were highly educated professionals seeking further specialist training, more lucrative work, and better education for their children. Included in this category were wealthy persons, some of whom retained their properties at home but preferred life in Canada.

South Asians in Canada Today

In 2001 about 504,000 persons living in Canada were born in South Asia. In addition to these first-generation immigrants are many more South Asians whose families have lived in Canada for two or more generations. Many live in urban centres. While they work in a very wide range of occupations, ranging from members of Parliament and medical specialists to unskilled labourers, the majority have white-collar and skilled blue-collar jobs.

Home Countries and Reasons for Migration

Most immigrants with South Asian cultural backgrounds have come from India, Sri Lanka, Pakistan, East Africa, and Fiji. While they have many basic beliefs and practices in common, other characteristics and experiences are peculiar to each country. For that reason, it is important to know something about each country, especially the quality of life there and the conditions under which South Asians left home and moved to Canada.

India

After gaining independence from Great Britain in 1947, and following the prompt separation from Pakistan, India's democratic government took on the enormous challenge of social and economic development in a country of great diversity. The presence of jungles, a desert, plains, tropical lowlands, and high mountains suggests the variety of ways in which people in India live and work.

Cultural diversity mirrors geographic diversity. There are eighteen recognized languages and several hundred dialects in India. In addition to speaking their own local language, some persons speak Hindi, the official language, and relatively small numbers of more educated people speak English. About 83 percent of the population in 2000 practised the Hindu religion, and 11 percent were Muslims. The remaining 6 percent were Christians, Sikhs, Buddhists, and Jains.

Until recently India experienced relatively slow economic progress, held back by a rapidly growing population that needed food, clothing, shelter, and education. Since the early 1900s the Indian population has grown by several million a year and in 2002 had reached one billion, the second largest in the world. India is about one-third the geographic size of Canada but has thirty-three times as many people, giving it one hundred times the population density. Three-quarters of the population live in rural areas, but pressure on agricultural land has forced many rural villagers to crowd into the cities looking for work. Economic development since independence has placed India among the industrial nations in the world. By the end of the millennium India had become known around the world for its high-tech computer centre in Bangalore. However, the benefits of rapid economic development have been unevenly distributed, so that a small urban elite enjoys a high standard of living while very large numbers of Indians live at or below subsistence level.

However, in general, the quality of life in India has improved in recent years. Life expectancy has risen from about thirty-two years in 1950 to sixty-five in 2002. But health still remains a significant problem. The infant mortality rate, sixty-five deaths per thousand live births, contrasts with Sri Lanka's twenty. Even in 2002 fewer than half of births, 42 percent, were attended by skilled midwives or doctors. However, 88 percent of households had safe water supplies, mostly from private or communal wells.

As a result of expanded education programs, in 2002, 41 percent of women and 68 percent of men were literate. Education is legally required for all between the ages of six and fourteen, but many villages have no schools or teachers. Moreover, even where they can attend, children of poor families often leave school to work to supplement the family income.

Conflict between Hindus and Muslims occurred when India and Pakistan separated in 1947 and has flared up between Sikhs and the central government since 1982 and more especially since 1984 when the government launched a military attack on the Sikh Golden Temple. Hindu-Muslim conflict in 2002 reflected ongoing religious tensions. Control of Kashmir has long been contested between Pakistan and India and continues in 2003. All these conflicts, and others, have fuelled immigration to Canada.

By 2000 the Sikhs from northern India, particularly the Punjab, represented the largest group of migrants from India. Most have come to Canada through sponsorship by relatives already settled in the country. Many were farmers or landowners with relatively little formal education or English, although by the standards of India's villages they were relatively well-off. Most speak Punjabi. While the Sikh population in India is tiny compared to the majority Hindus, Sikhs form the majority Indian group in Canada. The largest Sikh population is in British Columbia's Lower Mainland and in Victoria, Duncan, and Nanaimo; many also live in the interior of British Columbia. There are also sizable Sikh communities in Edmonton, Calgary, Winnipeg, and Toronto.

The next largest group of South Asian immigrants in Canada is also from northern India and mainly Hindu. The majority of these immigrants were part of a large wave of South Asian professionals who came to Canada in the mid-1960s. In general, this group was highly educated, from the middle or upper class, and English-speaking. Many came to Canada from the United States, where they had been attending university, and most were independent immigrants who did not have relatives to sponsor them. Educated professionals and business people from northern India continue to migrate to Canada.

Immigrants from southern India form a smaller group, but one that is growing with the increased migration of computer specialists. Most are from urban areas, are either Hindu or Christian, well educated, and English-speaking. Some are trained teachers, health professionals, accountants, engineers, and the like. They are independent immigrants in search of economic advancement and better opportunities for their children.

Pakistan

Pakistan is about the geographic size of British Columbia and in 2002 had 149 million people of whom about 97 percent were Sunni Muslims. The country originated when the British withdrew from India in 1947. Muslims feared political and social domination by the majority Hindus and created Pakistan out of separated areas in the northwest and northeast of India. The two parts, called West and East Pakistan, had little in common except the Muslim religion, and the tensions erupted in civil war in 1971 when East Pakistan declared itself the independent state of Bangladesh.

Most of Pakistan (formerly West Pakistan) has a dry climate with hot summers and cool winters. The economy is based largely on agriculture and herding, and about two-thirds of the population lives in rural villages. Most city people are factory workers or shopkeepers, although the urban population also includes educated middle- and upper-class people who have adopted many Western styles and ideas. While the official language is Urdu, the majority speak various dialects of Punjabi as a first language. Urban professionals speak English as well.

Health and health services in Pakistan are considerably poorer than in neighbouring India. In 2002 the infant mortality rate was eighty-seven per thousand live births compared to India's sixty-five, and only about 20 percent of births were attended by trained attendants. There is an educational gender gap, with 59 percent of men able to read and write but only 30 percent of women.

In the late 1960s many Pakistanis came to Canada as independent immigrants, escaping the uncertainty and religious and political conflict that eventually culminated in the civil war. Most were urban, highly educated, of upper- or middle-class background, and proficient in English. These migrants are now middle-aged and have been joined by other family members. Since the early 1990s immigration from Pakistan has steadily risen, from 2,000 per year in 1990 up to 15,000 in 2001. Some of these are sponsored family members, but the majority are independent immigrants, many of whom have chosen to settle in Toronto. As well, Pakistan is a major source of refugees; more than 2,000 refugees arrived in 2001, making Pakistan the third-largest source of refugees to Canada that year. Some refugees are Christians who claim they have been subject to religious persecution in Pakistan.

East Africa

People of South Asian culture have come to Canada from three East African countries – Uganda, Kenya, and Tanzania. All three were British colonies until after the Second World War, and all have predominantly rural populations performing agricultural work. Black Africans compose the majority of the population in each country. While Swahili and other local languages were and are used in rural areas, English is commonly used in urban areas among middle-class people. Since they gained independence from British rule (Uganda 1962, Kenya 1963, Tanzania 1964), their economic and social policies have changed, and unrest and conflict have been common. These changes have caused many people of South Asian origin to leave.

From the late nineteenth century, many Indians had immigrated to the British colonies in East Africa in search of better economic opportunities. Most were traders and entrepreneurs, and they came to play a dominant role as middlemen in the colonial economies of Uganda, Kenya, and Tanzania and elsewhere. Most lived in urban areas and small towns.

Over the years the South Asians' economic success and prominence came to be resented by the indigenous African majority. Thus, as the East African countries became independent in the early 1960s, the social position of South Asians deteriorated. In 1972 the Ugandan dictator Idi Amin ordered the expulsion of all South Asians from the country, whereupon 6,000 of them migrated to Canada as political refugees. About 30 percent were professionals, and about 50 percent had been in business. Most of the rest were skilled workers. South Asians left Kenya after independence when the government took over many farms and businesses owned by non-Africans. At the same time, South Asians in Tanzania felt threatened and departed. Many immigrated to Canada, some directly, others via Britain. By the 1990s the annual migration to Canada from these three African countries had diminished to a few hundred, or at most a thousand.

The majority of South Asian immigrants from East Africa were Ismailis, a branch of the Shia sect of Islam, although some were Sikhs, Hindus, and Sunni Muslims. Their knowledge of English and education made settlement in Canada somewhat easier than for many South Asians. Many South Asians from East Africa are now involved in business enterprises, while others are professionals in the medical, legal, and commercial fields. In western Canada, the largest population is in the Greater Vancouver area, but many also live in Edmonton and Calgary.

Fiji

Fiji is a tropical South Pacific country made up of more than three hundred scattered islands. The economy is based on crops such as sugar cane and coconuts as well as on tourism. Fiji was a British colony until 1970 and continues to use English as its official language, while Fijian and Fiji-Hindi are the other main languages. In 2000 nearly half the population (49 percent) were native Fijians, of Melanesian and Polynesian descent, while nearly as many were of Indian descent (46 percent). There were also smaller groups of Chinese, Europeans, and others.

South Asian Fijians are for the most part descendants of indentured labourers who arrived from India before 1920 to work on the sugar plantations. Over the years they achieved prominence in retail trade and transportation and came to control much of Fiji's business and industry.

In the 1960s, a small number of South Asian Fijians entered Canada, and immigration increased significantly after Fiji became independent in 1970, with growing racial conflict and political and economic tension. However, political conflict between the South Asians, then in the majority, and the minority Fijians erupted in 1987, which accelerated the migration of South Asians from Fiji to Canada. In the 1990s about one thousand South Asian Fijians migrated each year.

Most people from Fiji are proficient in English, which is the language of instruction in the British-style education system. Quality of life in Fiji is generally excellent, and people are used to Western-style health services. In 2002 the infant mortality rate in Fiji was seventeen per thousand live births, and life expectancy much higher than in the other South Asian source countries, at sixty-eight years for men and seventy-one for women. The main waves of immigrants were largely skilled and semi-skilled workers, and most, unable to find comparable employment here, had to accept whatever jobs they could find, typically in small manufacturing plants and in the service industry. The majority of South Asians from Fiji are Hindu, and about 15 percent are Muslim. By 2002 there were about 14,000 South Asian Fijians in Canada. Roughly three-quarters lived in Vancouver and the remainder in Alberta.

Language

The languages most commonly spoken by South Asians in Canada are English, Punjabi, Fiji-Hindi, Gujarati, Urdu, and Fijian. Most South Asians in

Canada come from former British colonies where English is taught and used by some or all of the population. Thus, those immigrants with higher education are already proficient in English when they arrive, while immigrants from rural areas without much formal education may have little literacy in their first language and no knowledge of English.

Because the South Asian communities in Canada tend to be large and geographically clustered, daily life is often conducted in the home language. However, when they first arrive in Canada, South Asian men tend to acquire English more quickly than do women because of the men's daily exposure to it in the workplace and because English is necessary for job advancement. Some immigrant women are reluctant to learn English and tend to avoid formal language training unless it is required for employment or citizenship. They may also have difficulty integrating language classes with full-time jobs or home responsibilities. Many women cope by relying on their husbands or children to translate when necessary. Many elderly South Asians, especially those who have migrated to Canada at an older age, never learn English.

Contacts with Family at Home and around the World

Most South Asians in Canada belong to networks of relatives and friends that circle the world. For many of them, these global networks are just as important and contribute just as much to their identities as do their local networks in Canada. Ties to their home countries are particularly strong. When they can afford time away from work and the expense of travel and gifts, many persons originally from India, for example, travel home to visit relatives. Often South Asian families send home for special medicines, and a person in Canada thought to need special Ayurvedic treatment or certain protective ceremonies may return to his or her home country to get them.

Marriage arrangements are commonly made between South Asian families in Canada and families in their home countries. These arrangements often involve trips by the prospective husband to meet the woman and her family. In some cases immigrant families may send an adolescent or a young adult child, especially a daughter, to relatives in their home country in the hope of meeting a suitable marriage partner. These marriages further strengthen linkages between Canadian South Asians and their home communities.

South Asians are very likely to have relatives in the United States, Great Britain, Australia, and elsewhere around the world with whom they keep close touch, by letter and telephone and now by e-mail. Home videos also serve to keep a scattered family together. For example, when an elderly Indian patriarch died in Canada, a video of the cremation ceremonies was sent to his son in India, his daughter in Europe, and grandchildren in

Australia. Family members around the world often provide practical help as well: a Canadian South Asian family may provide a home for a nephew from India who is attending a Canadian university, or South Asians in Australia may help a brother from Canada find a job to advance his career in Australia.

Visits back and forth often mean that families in India, for example, learn about the West from the glimpse of Canadian culture brought by their visiting relatives. And South Asians resident in Canada may discover on their visits that many things have changed at home, even that some "traditions" kept by South Asians in Canada are no longer practised. Many South Asians become very skilled at shifting their identities when they move from one culture to another.

Religion

The most common religious groups in the South Asian communities in Canada are the Hindus, Muslims, and Sikhs although there are also some Jains, Christians, and Buddhists.

Hinduism

Hinduism has no single founder but rather denotes a broad range of cultural patterns that include religious rituals, family and social relationships, and general attitudes towards life. These patterns are sanctioned by reference to sacred scriptures and a variety of deities.

A feature of Hinduism is its tolerance of diversity. An ancient religion, it constantly absorbed and reinterpreted the beliefs and practices of the peoples with whom it came into contact. There is thus widespread variation among Hindus in, for example, food habits, styles of dress, and forms of worship.

There are, however, some fundamental notions common across Hindu culture. One is the concept of the unity of life, that all life is interdependent, both human and animal. Life is a continuous circle without beginning or end, so that death and birth are merely transformations of form. After death, the soul is reborn in another life form.

Two other aspects of Hindu culture are karma and caste. The law of karma states that the present is affected by past action, and the future by present action. All actions have consequences that must return to the actor. The fortunes of the soul in each rebirth are determined by behaviour in former lives. Also part of Hindu culture is the idea that society is organized into a hierarchy of social classes called castes, into one of which each individual is born. Each caste has its own rules about social contacts with members of other castes. For example, inter-caste marriage should not occur. Each caste also has rules about who may cook the food its members eat. Most Hindus will eat food prepared by members of their own or a higher caste; thus people of the highest caste may eat food prepared by fellow members only. While education and modern industrial life have weakened some caste barriers, the prohibition on inter-caste marriage is still strong.

Most Hindu religious activity centres on the home, and may involve the family, an individual, or perhaps a few friends. Most homes have a small altar, with a statue of a god and candles or lights, where family members may worship and make offerings. Many Canadian cities have Hindu temples as well. Rites mark important life-cycle transitions. For example, the birth ceremony traditionally takes place before the umbilical cord is cut, and about ten days later there is a naming ceremony. Among high-caste Brahmins, a rite is performed when a boy reaches puberty. At that time he is given a sacred thread which is tied across one shoulder and around his waist and is worn under his clothing for the rest of his life.

Sikhism

A relatively new religion, Sikhism was founded in northern India at the end of the fifteenth century by Guru Nanak, who sought to combine Hindu and Muslim elements in a single religious creed. His teachings embodied belief in a single God and the equality of all people, and he rejected the caste system. Sikhism includes Hindu concepts of reincarnation as well as karma. Unlike in Hinduism, the representation of God in pictures and the worship of idols are forbidden. Worship within the Sikh brotherhood, or community, is important. Guru Nanak was followed by nine gurus, or masters, the last of whom was Guru Gobind Singh. The writings of the early gurus were compiled in the Sri Guru Granth Sahib, the Sikh sacred book.

No specific birth rites are prescribed, although a newborn baby is taken to the temple to be named. The most important ceremony for a Sikh is that of baptism. Although there is no set age for this, it is believed that a person should be capable of assuming responsibility for his or her decisions before being baptized. Not all Sikhs, however, decide to be baptized.

Baptized Sikh men are enjoined to wear turbans and do not cut their hair or beards. They wear a comb, white undershorts (symbolic of chastity), and a small symbolic sword. In addition, baptized men and women should abstain from smoking or drinking alcohol. Most men and women, whether baptized or not, wear a steel bracelet on the right wrist. Some Sikhs are vegetarian, but this is a matter of personal choice.

The Sikh temple is a meeting place where both religious and social activities are held. There is no "Sabbath day" for the Sikhs, and prayer ceremonies are held every day. However, to conform to Canadian work schedules, a weekly religious service is held from Friday morning through Sunday afternoon. During this time, male and female members participate in the reading of the Granth Sahib, taking turns to read for two hours at a time until the entire scripture has been completed. People may attend the service at any time during the weekend, and at its conclusion a vegetarian lunch, prepared by members of the temple, is served. Many Sikh temples also provide a variety of social services to their community. There are Sikh temples in many cities in Canada as well as in small towns with substantial Sikh populations.

Islam

The word "Islam" literally means "submission," and a Muslim is one who submits to the will of God, rejects all other gods, and follows the teachings of the Quran, or Koran, the holy book which records the will of God as revealed to the prophet Mohammed (AD 570-632). The central belief of Islam is expressed in the phrase: "There is no god but Allah ["God" in Arabic] and Mohammed is his Prophet." This statement of faith is repeated on many ritual occasions.

Islam imposes a code of ethical conduct encouraging generosity, fairness, honesty, and respect. Muslims are required to pray five times daily, facing the direction of Mecca, after a ritual washing, and they should additionally attend a mosque to pray together on Friday. They are to abstain from food, drink, and sexual activity from dawn to dusk during the month of Ramadan, the ninth month of the lunar Muslim calendar. Since the months of the lunar calendar derive from the solar year, Ramadan falls at a somewhat different time each year. Adultery and gambling are forbidden, as are the consumption of pork and alcohol. Other meat and chicken must be killed in a prescribed manner.

Shortly after the death of Mohammed, Muslims divided into two major sects over the issue of who should succeed the prophet as religious leader. These sects are known as Sunni and Shia; Sunnis are by far the largest Muslim sect; Muslims from Pakistan and India are most likely to be Sunni. Many Ismailis, members of a Shia sub-sect, left the Indian state of Gujarat for East Africa after the late nineteenth century. In 2003 the Ismailis were led by the Agha Khan IV. Each Muslim sect forms a separate community with its own religious practices and mosque.

Festivals and Religious Holidays

Diwali, or the Hindu "Festival of Lights," is celebrated in October or November to give thanks for prosperity. Holi, a Hindu spring festival from northern India, is celebrated in February or March to mark the end of the cold weather. It is a day of fun when sweets and gifts are exchanged.

Baisakhi, the major Sikh festival, is celebrated by worship and dance each year on 14 April. These celebrations in Vancouver and Surrey are usually attended by tens of thousands of people who watch parades of floats from different temples and marvel at traditional sword fighting and enjoy free food.

Ramadan is sacred for Muslims as the month in which Mohammed received the first of his revelations from God and is observed by month-long fasting during daylight hours. Some Muslims are exempt from fasting, such as pregnant women or people travelling. The date of Ramadan varies from year to year. The end of Ramadan is celebrated with a festival that includes a feast, new clothing, and gifts. Eid-ul-Adha is an end-of-year celebration which traditionally involves the sacrifice of a sheep or goat; the meat is then shared with family, neighbours, and the poor.

Family Structure

Families in South Asia

In South Asian culture, the family is the most important social unit. It extends beyond the nuclear grouping of parents and children to include grandparents, brothers, sisters, and their families. Traditionally, the extended family lives together in one household, so that in the grandfather's household, his unmarried daughters, all his sons, and their wives and children live together. Traditionally, parents do not live with their married daughter. Often there are other relatives as well, perhaps a distant cousin who is attending a nearby college or an elderly aunt whose children have migrated abroad.

The extended family provides an identity for the individual as well as economic and emotional security. Interdependence is valued highly, and the lifestyle is collective rather than individualistic. Possessions are shared, and there are few secrets within the household. Ideally, earnings are shared, and the whole family prospers together.

Traditionally, South Asian culture is largely male-dominated, and gender roles are well defined. The man is leader as head of the family, provider, and major decision maker. His wife is in charge of nurturing and performing or organizing household duties. Her most important responsibility is to look after her family, and her training is totally geared towards her role in the home. An older woman has considerable authority in the management of day-to-day household affairs, and women's work in the home is accorded great respect. With the exception of poorer women in rural areas, most women traditionally did not work outside the home and were therefore financially dependent upon their husbands' families.

In traditional culture, a woman is seen as her husband's possession, and she is taught to be submissive and to obey him. In spite of this asymmetry, women and girls nevertheless have a high social and religious status. They are considered to bear the honour of the family, and traditional society is

Mrs. Gill, from India

Mrs. Gill, seventy-three, from India, was admitted to a nursing home directly from an Abbotsford hospital where she had been treated for a stroke that paralyzed her right side. She had no English, so staff could not talk with her directly. But they were intrigued and concerned because every day she propelled her wheelchair with one hand up and down the long corridors as far as she could go, seldom stopping and not talking with anyone. No one understood why, and some began to speculate that her mind had been affected by the stroke. Finally the staff decided to seek a Punjabi-speaking social worker to interview Mrs. Gill and then discuss her situation at a case conference.

At the staff conference the social worker reported that Mrs. Gill had been the household head in her son's home, making all the household decisions and organizing the work of others including her daughter-in-law. She had been very active. Suddenly, she could do nothing and was sent to a new place where she had no responsibilities and could not even speak with anyone. She believed that if she exercised vigorously by propelling her wheelchair, the paralysis would disappear and she would be able to go home to her proper position. When the social worker probed about depression and suicidal thoughts, Mrs. Gill said, "If I could die today, I would be happy."

very protective of them. The honour of the family depends largely on the purity of the daughter before marriage.

Within South Asian culture the elderly have authority and respect. They have an important role within the extended family, counselling the young, mediating family disagreements, arranging marriages, and helping to raise grandchildren. Institutional care and pension systems are essentially non-existent in the home countries, and the eldest sons become the guardians of aging parents.

South Asian countries, particularly India, have recently experienced rapid social and economic change. An expanding educated middle class has meant that many young people must move far away from their families to take promising jobs. They establish nuclear families in which husband and wife tend to take much more flexible roles than they would if living with an extended family, though they retain many of the earlier values such as respect for elders. These changes are common in urban areas but have yet to be felt in rural areas where the traditional family system remains.

South Asian Families in Canada

In Canada, the South Asian extended family is common, with brothers and their families living together with their parents. This family is a close-knit, interdependent unit. While married daughters do not generally live with their parents in India, this occurs in Canada when a daughter has sponsored her parents' immigration. Today many South Asians in Canada live as nuclear units although often near other relatives. Nevertheless, their sentiments and often their behaviour continue to be those of the extended family.

In the extended family, earnings are often pooled. In some families, income is given to the grandmother who is then responsible for the household finances and allocates money to her daughter-in-law to run the household. In other cases, the eldest son may manage the family's finances. Most decisions are made by the head of the household, who is usually the most established, financially secure male. On all important matters, close relatives are consulted and their opinions given considerable weight. Health care decisions, such as when to consult a doctor about an ill child, are made by the senior members of the family. Care for ill family members is the responsibility of the wife or mother. In Canada, just as in her home country, she is likely to be assisted by grandparents or other relatives.

With so many persons living in an extended family household, there is bound to be family conflict. Open expression of disagreement is not the norm; instead, discord may be signalled by withdrawal. In these cases an elder may try to mediate differences in an effort to get family members to adjust to, not change, the situation.

If the extended family unit is working together well, it is a highly supportive system. It is not necessary to find babysitters with grandparents or other relatives available to help. If a woman is sick, she is able to take a day off while someone else takes over the cooking, cleaning, and child care. However, if the family is dysfunctional, a daughter-in-law, for example, may find difficulty in taking time off from household duties because of family censure.

Some traditional gender relationships are changing in Canada just as in India, particularly in middle-class nuclear families. More mutual decision making between husband and wife may occur, and women often become more involved in family financial matters such as banking. Many parents give children more say about their futures, including marriage. However, other values, such as those involving religion or sexuality, are more resistant to change.

Marriage

Marriage in South Asia

A marriage is traditionally arranged by the bride's and groom's families and considered to be a union between families, not individuals. These arrangements are something like business contracts: the young woman is given to the groom's family, who receive her labour and potential for producing children in exchange for agreeing to care for her for the rest of her life. Marriages almost always bring together people of the same religion, caste, and economic position. Each family puts a great deal of effort into investigating the background and status – and with Hindus the horoscopes – of the prospective spouse and family. Parents are especially concerned that their children find a compatible spouse because marriage breakdown creates problems for the community as well as for the young couple. A girl is taught from the start that she is a temporary member of her own family, waiting to be given as a gift to a husband and become a member of his family. She is taught that once given in marriage she may never leave her husband's home, although many young wives do return to their parents' homes for extended periods for the birth of their children. There is a great deal of support from the families and the community to make a marriage work.

The dowry system, the giving of gifts by the bride's family to the bridegroom, is practised in South Asian culture. Because the man is the earner and will have to support his wife for the rest of her life, the dowry represents her contribution to the marriage and is considered to be her share of the inheritance from her parents. Depending upon the family's situation, the dowry can be anything from small household items and clothing to appliances, a car, an apartment, land, or gold jewellery. In some cases, the dowry system is abused and in-laws' demands are unreasonable, causing a major crisis for the bride and her family. In extreme cases this has led to "bride-burning," in which the groom's family threatens and then kills the bride.

South Asian men expect to marry a girl who is a virgin and who has not been out with other men. With the exception of very cosmopolitan urban families, girls are consequently well protected and not allowed to date; a girl who has dated is considered loose and not a suitable marriage partner. Traditionally, bride and groom did not see each other until their wedding day. However, nowadays many Indian families arrange meetings between prospective couples, usually in the company of other family members, where they may see and talk to each other. If one of the young persons objects to the marriage, the family will usually look for someone else.

Girls are married young in India, at an average age of twenty, while grooms are usually at least four years older. The belief is that the bride's adaptation to her husband's family's home will be easier if she has not developed her personality to the fullest extent. If she is young she will be more flexible and adaptable. Similarly, if she has not dated other men she will be more likely to accept the husband her parents have chosen for her. In general, a South Asian man does not expect to make any changes or adjustments when he marries, because it is his family and his life that his wife is entering.

As society has changed in South Asia, so have marriage patterns. In more educated and middle-class families it has become more common for young people to find their own spouses, perhaps at university or at work. These "love marriages" often reflect traditional patterns in that the couple is from the same religion, caste, and class. Eventually most parents, though not all, will find such a match acceptable.

Marriage in Canada

Marriage patterns of South Asians in Canada today vary according to the degree of acculturation of the families, their length of time in Canada, their religion, and the particular situation of the couple.

Some observers estimate that about one-half of South Asian marriages in Canada are arranged by parents. Arranged marriages typically occur among new immigrants and first-generation residents, but also sometimes in other families. Just as in South Asia, parents consider the social and economic position of the prospective spouse's family, the personal strengths and prospects of the groom, the reputation of the bride, and so on, and among Hindu families they may examine the couple's horoscopes. The young woman's family is likely to offer a dowry to the groom's family. In Canada most young people are given the opportunity to meet and get to know their marriage partners, and they may exercise their right to make the ultimate decision, although this depends on such things as the education and employment of parents and their children. Sometimes there are conflicts if parents believe they have chosen the best possible match. An arranged marriage usually implies that the new bride will join her husband's extended family.

Many families look for marriage partners, especially brides for their sons, in home countries rather than in Canada. It is felt that young women who have grown up here have had too much freedom to accept an arranged marriage and entry into a new extended family. There is also a belief that, because divorces are common in Canada, a marriage has a better chance of survival and stability if the bride has a more traditional background. Many young women who are recruited as brides in their home countries and come to join their husbands' extended families suffer from the lack of nearby support from their own families who remain in the home country. They miss the family support during the period of adjustment to their in-laws' homes and in the event of marital problems. Often these women are afraid of gossip and thus do not confide in anyone.

It is estimated that about half of South Asian marriages in Canada are "love marriages." Individual choice of spouse is more likely to occur in families with longer residence, more education, a better economic situation, and a greater level of acculturation.

Some South Asian families see dating as unacceptable. However, young people born in Canada may date in secret and seek their parents' consent only when they believe they have found a suitable marriage partner. Many parents have adapted in varying degrees to their Canadian-born children's expectations. Some middle-class young people are now using the Internet to search for marriage partners.

Although caste is generally said to be unimportant for Hindu South Asians in Canada, inter-caste marriages are still unusual. This can create family conflicts with young adults who have grown up here and do not respect the caste system. There is pressure from family and community to marry within one's own religious group as well. Parents fear the loss of their culture, and some may disown children who intermarry. However, marriages between Sikhs and Muslims are occurring, and marriages between Sikhs and Westerners are becoming more acceptable. In the latter case, couples may have two marriage ceremonies, one for each cultural tradition.

Dowries are often given in arranged marriages and may represent the bride's inheritance. However, many of the more acculturated South Asian families in Canada divide inheritances equally between all children regardless of gender, even when the daughters have already been given dowries.

Remarriage for widows and female divorcees is uncommon, although parents of a young widow under thirty may be able to arrange a marriage for her. There are few opportunities for these women to meet a suitable partner even if they wish to remarry. Widows with young children who return to South Asia in search of a partner are very likely to be taken advantage of by men looking for a way to emigrate. Widowers, however, may remarry by sponsoring a young wife from the home country.

The process of migration and adjustment to a new culture can impose stresses on marriages, particularly early in the couple's stay in Canada. Though the man is traditionally the breadwinner while his wife stays at home, economic necessity compels many South Asian women in Canada to find employment. This change can be threatening to a traditional husband and his family if they feel that his wife is becoming too Westernized and perhaps having too much contact with other men. The husband may react by attempting to increase his control over her, and she may respond by resisting. The experience of employment for women often makes them more independent and assertive, which husbands may find threatens their traditional dominance. A working wife's increased sense of independence may in turn reduce her patience with traditional marital and extended family conduct. Moreover, external employment places an additional strain on women who often must continue to shoulder the sole responsibility for the care of home and family.

Separation and Divorce

Separation and divorce are rare in traditional South Asian society. There is a strong cultural pressure on the couple, especially the wife, to stay together. A woman is brought up to believe that she should never leave her husband's home, and most of the responsibility of making or breaking a home is placed on her. The families of both husband and wife will become deeply involved if there are marital problems, because separation and divorce stigmatize both families. In traditional society, for example, the unmarried brothers and sisters of a woman who had left her husband and returned to her parents would find it difficult to arrange marriages with suitable families. Parents of the couple and sometimes a respected religious leader will try to resolve problems and decide who is at fault, and every attempt is made to reconcile the couple.

Separation and divorce among South Asians in Canada continue to be rare, though increasing. However, even for Westernized South Asians "falling out of love" is not an acceptable reason to dissolve a marriage. The dowry can sometimes cause the break-up of a marriage if the husband and his family feel cheated. For example, a woman who sponsors her husband's immigration to Canada may feel that no further dowry is necessary. However, his parents, when they immigrate to join them later, may begin to resent her family for not giving a bigger dowry. Or, a girl who comes from India to marry a man here may not bring household goods with her as she has to travel so far, and this may be held against her by her husband's family.

A South Asian woman who has separated from her husband is unlikely to initiate divorce proceedings, because she is singled out as the one who left the home or the relationship. It is more acceptable for a man to leave his wife and children and initiate a divorce. A woman who leaves her children with her husband is considered a bad mother, except among Muslims, where custody of the children is more likely to be given to the husband's family.

Domestic Abuse

In Canada the cultural constraints on a South Asian couple to stay together at all costs, combined with the stresses of living in an unfamiliar society, financial difficulties, and other family tensions, may lead to marital discord and sometimes abuse. Sikh women are more likely to come to the attention of professionals in this regard, perhaps because of their relative equality and freedom in the family, and the fact that Sikhs form the majority of South Asians in Canada. However, such marital discord is known to occur also in Hindu, Muslim, and other South Asian groups.

Abuse in marriage can take many forms. Husbands may confiscate their wives' pay-cheques or prevent them from attending English classes in order to maintain their isolation from Western society, and so on. Physical violence of all kinds may also occur and is often associated with men's use of alcohol.

If a wife is abused by her husband in her home country, her family may step in to protect and support her. If she leaves her husband, her parents might guarantee her safety and take responsibility for his conduct after her return to him. However, in Canada many women lack the protection of family nearby, and some have no family at all in Canada. This is especially true of young brides brought in from the home country. Some of these women may expect a social worker or counsellor to ensure their safety in the home. Sometimes in Canada friends from the same town or village in South Asia mediate for a woman in the absence of her parents and relatives, taking responsibility for her and deciding what is in her best interests. However, in this situation the woman becomes indebted to them and is often obliged to follow their advice.

An abused wife may nonetheless be encouraged by her own family to protect the family name by ignoring the abuse and submitting to her husband or to the will of the extended family. Families may sometimes continue to send their daughters back to abusive husbands until the abuse becomes life-threatening. Within the extended family the elders may encourage the abusive husband, rather than rein him in, leaving his wife with no protection.

Wives who do leave violent husbands, like many Western women in the same situation, usually return to the marriage to try again, especially the first time. Intense pressure from their husbands' families occurs. Some women are unaware of their rights in Canada; some are isolated from mainstream services because they lack English; many are afraid of reporting spousal abuse to their physicians, who may also be members of the South Asian community and, it is feared, may not respect confidentiality. Many women worry that they will lose their children, and almost all fear the poverty that will follow separation.

Immigration policies themselves serve to deter abused women from leaving their spouses. Until 2002, South Asian men who sponsored wives from the home country were financially responsible for them for ten years, so an abused wife feared deportation if she left the marriage during that time. Wives who hope to sponsor their own parents later are reluctant to leave their marriage because they are dependent upon their husband's income to qualify as sponsors. In 2002 the period of dependence on a financial sponsor was reduced from ten years to three years.

There is strong social pressure to keep matters of spousal abuse within the family and within the South Asian community. An in-law may accompany an abused wife to the doctor, supposedly as a chaperone or translator but really to ensure she will not reveal abuse. A physician who suspects abuse must therefore arrange to speak with the patient alone, using a third-party interpreter if necessary. Then the physician needs to build up a relationship of trust with the woman. South Asian professionals who attempt to educate families about women's rights to personal safety may be ostracized by the community for encouraging family break-up. Some South Asian women are more comfortable disclosing abuse to other women like themselves, a fact that underlines the importance of programs run by women. Moreover, many abusive husbands refuse to participate in counselling unless forced to do so by a probation officer.

Among more acculturated South Asians in Canada, it is becoming more acceptable for a woman to leave her husband if he is unfaithful or abusive. In general, however, most South Asian women do not want to break up their family even if they are experiencing abuse. Their security and identity are based in South Asian culture, and they do not want to adopt the Western cultural solution of separation and divorce.

Child-Rearing

There is a preference in South Asian culture for male children, who, unlike female children, will have important ritual functions, will raise the status of the family in the community, will enlarge the family through marriage, and will care for the parents in their old age. Boys are favoured and receive more attention than girls, with the eldest male being the most privileged. The eldest female sibling is given a great deal of household responsibility, which can be very demanding. Though girls are loved, they are more likely than boys to be disciplined and loaded with household chores.

Independence in young children is not encouraged, especially in girls, and young children may have little or no experience of being away from parents or relatives. When they live in a large extended family, young children are indulged by grandparents, uncles, and aunts and are held, comforted, and rarely punished. In South Asia, and commonly in Canada, there are no fixed schedules for young children; a child eats when hungry and goes to bed when tired. As boys and girls grow older, they are discouraged from playing together because of fear of sexual experimentation.

Children are generally taught by example rather than by instruction. Spanking is not uncommon, and parents may use threats of physical punishment to control behaviour. Children may be given treats to avoid tension and behaviour problems; a child may be given candy to avert a temper tantrum. As growing children learn about Canada, they have been known to deter parental punishment by threatening to call social workers or "help lines" to lay complaints of physical abuse. This behaviour frightens parents, both as a threat and as a demonstration of their loss of control over their offspring.

By the time they are of school age, children are expected to have some self-discipline and to respect the authority of parents and teachers. A child's obedience to elders may be taken as a measure of love of family, while disobedience brings shame and hurt.

South Asian parents, particularly those with few resources or no relatives here, must often work long hours and may thus "under-parent" their children, leaving older children in charge of younger ones. Other parents may neglect their children by focusing on economic advancement; they can give money but not time. Some children therefore become "latch-key kids" who are increasingly isolated from their parents and their cultural community.

Adolescence

A South Asian adolescent's experience depends a great deal on how long the family has resided in Canada. New immigrant parents coming to join relatives may expect their adolescent children to behave just as they would in India. Adolescents born in Canada of immigrant parents are more likely to experience an "acculturation gap" with their parents; the young people take on mainstream values and behaviours while their parents try to maintain the cultural practices they knew at home.

In many South Asian homes, teenage boys are given more freedom than girls on the ground that as future earners they must learn to deal with the outside world. Many boys may be expected to take part-time jobs after school to contribute to the family income. On the other hand, girls may be very protected and not allowed to date on the ground that they must be "pure" at marriage. In some families, a girl may be expected to come straight home from school and not have the freedom to go shopping with friends, use the local library, or participate in after-school activities. Girls may not be allowed to participate in school athletics, especially if travel with a team is part of the program. Some are expected to return home to care for younger siblings. South Asian teenage girls deprived of the freedoms enjoyed by their mainstream friends are torn between peer pressure at school and traditional parental expectations, creating conflicts that can lead to rebellion and depression.

In second-generation or more acculturated South Asian families, parents may allow their children much more independence. These parents may have second thoughts if they see their children are losing ethnic identity and might even marry outside the community. Such children may be encouraged to begin attending religious and cultural functions, and girls are sometimes pressured to return to the home country in the hope that a spouse will be found there (Prathikanti 1997, 90).

Traditionally, parent-child conflicts are resolved within the family or community and outsiders are not involved. Where a teenager is misbehaving and the immediate family feels helpless, another relative may be called in to help. However, in Canada, children may question the authority of family members who are not part of the nuclear unit: "What has my uncle to do with my business?"

Communication gaps between adolescents and parents may occur when children have been raised speaking English as a first language at school while parents continue to use their own language at home. In rare cases when the children cannot fluently speak the native language, they may have very limited communication with parents and elders.

Children and adolescents are sometimes used as interpreters by parents who are not fluent in English. This role can be demanding and stressful for an adolescent who, for example, accompanies his father to the bank to arrange a mortgage. Where he is unable to interpret through lack of understanding, he is likely to feel inadequate and depressed. A pattern of reliance on children for interpretation or for other tasks (such as filling out income tax forms) can lead to role reversal, where children lose respect for parents while parents lose authority and control.

As with any other cultural group, a very small minority of South Asian adolescents, caught between traditional cultural values and those of Canadian society, may become involved in illegal activities. Some may see quick but illegal money-making schemes as a way to confirm their own worth and identity in the new culture or as a means to rebel against the traditional cultural values of their parents. Young men who have become addicted to drugs and alcohol are vulnerable to manipulation and may find a sense of belonging and identity in gang membership. Adolescent boys who have low academic success may drift away from school when they realize that they can make money illegally without the trouble of pursuing a high school education. Young girls may be vulnerable to recruitment for the same reasons. In these cases parents preoccupied with providing for their families and establishing themselves in Canada may first learn about their child's behaviour from a school counsellor. Most parents are shocked to discover that their children are involved in such activities. In spite of the small number of South Asian youth who are involved in illegal pursuits, media exaggeration sometimes serves to stereotype the whole community.

Children's Experiences in Canadian Schools

Many South Asian parents want their children to be well educated and place a high priority on schooling. However, in home countries, schooling is done by the teacher with little or no parental involvement. South Asian parents new to Canada are not used to participating in school activities or consulting with teachers. Few may get involved in their children's homework. Some parents may consider extracurricular activities and social development unimportant and a waste of their children's time and expect teachers to take responsibility for disciplining children, as in the home countries.

New immigrants, both students and parents, are likely to find the Canadian school system very different from their experience at home. Here the atmosphere is generally much more lax and liberal. The fact that children receive sex education in Canadian schools may upset some parents, who believe that sexual matters should not be discussed in front of children or adolescents, especially girls. Whereas in South Asian culture children are taught that it is rude and disrespectful to argue with parents or teachers, in Canadian schools children are more ready to voice their opinions and in fact are encouraged to do so. As a result, South Asian school-aged children face a conflict between the values of Canadian society and those of their parents. Parents for their part may feel that their own values are being judged and found wanting by their adolescent children, as well as by the mainstream community.

Work

New South Asian immigrants often come to Canada to pursue economic and educational opportunities and have very high expectations and idealistic images of Canada. Migrants from rural villages who come to join relatives also may have inflated expectations because they have been led to believe that all Canadians are very prosperous.

However, most South Asians from rural backgrounds must begin work in relatively unskilled jobs because they lack English and the requisite training. Men may work in lumber mills, in construction, or as janitors. Women, whose income is required for basic family needs, take jobs as factory workers or on farms, in restaurants and canneries, and as cleaners.

Independent South Asian immigrants, such as teachers, college professors, physicians, nurses, and computer programmers, have obtained admission to Canada on the basis of their professional training but then find that the accreditation process can be lengthy and sometimes insurmountable. Many of the men must start with jobs far below their level of education, in construction or as taxi drivers, parking lot attendants, or janitors. Educated women may find a job more easily than their spouses. Perhaps being more flexible and willing to accept a drop in status, they may start work in nursing homes or as store clerks. At least at the beginning, fluency in English is more important than level of education in getting a job. Educated immigrants can be very distressed to discover that it could take ten years to return to the standard of living they had in South Asia.

Cultural Values and Behaviour

Names

South Asian names vary with religion and region. Women take their husband's surname at the time of marriage. Hindus may have three names: a personal name, a complementary name, and then a family name. Two names are more common, and in any case many women drop their middle name after coming to Canada. Sikhs typically have three names: a personal name, then a title (Singh for men, Kaur for women), followed by the family name. Examples are, Mohinder Singh Sandhu or Raminder Kaur Gill.

Clothing

Traditional clothing for women varies from one region to another. Many South Asian women wear a sari, a straight piece of cloth draped around the body like a long dress. Sikh and Muslim women from northern India and Pakistan typically wear a *salwar kameez,* which consists of gathered trousers beneath a long tunic, sometimes with a long scarf over the shoulders. Widows usually wear plain white clothing. In Canada, some women continue to dress traditionally, while others adopt Western clothing, especially in the workplace. Many women, particularly the elderly, prefer slacks to skirts or dresses, to ensure that their legs are covered. Originally, South Asian clothing indicated the wearer's regional background, but today the style is usually dictated by current fashion. The kind of clothing a South Asian person wears may not necessarily be a clue to the person's level of acculturation since adoption of Western dress may coexist with traditional values and behaviours.

Traditionally, South Asian women do not cut their hair; Sikh women especially do not cut it for religious reasons. Women who are of the second or third generation in Canada are more likely to cut their hair and wear Western-style clothing, particularly if they are educated and work in offices or in a profession. Many Sikh men wear turbans and are likely to have beards.

Courtesy

The traditional form of greeting for Hindus is with the palms of the hands pressed together in front of the chest. Muslims are more likely just to say "Salam" in greeting. Shaking hands is not common, particularly for women. Customarily, eye contact is considered rude and disrespectful, especially with elders.

Affection

Physical expressions of affection such as hugging and kissing are rare in public, even among family members and close friends. Indeed, displays of affection are considered extremely inappropriate between members of the opposite sex, even husband and wife. On the other hand, in India public hand-holding by men is common and is a sign of friendship, not homosexuality. The opinions of relatives and other members of the community are held in high regard, and gossip can be used to exert social control over these behaviours.

Recreation

Recreation tends to be centred in the family and community, especially for people who have come from rural areas. Men go out to meet friends, but very few women from rural backgrounds go out alone to socialize, except to meet other women at their homes or to visit the temple to prepare for weddings or other community celebrations. Gatherings in the home tend to be segregated by sex, with women in one room and men in another. Some wives may insist that their husbands consume alcohol only at social activities away from the home.

Sleeping

It is not uncommon for children in extended families up to the age of twelve to share a bedroom with their parents or with siblings of the opposite sex.

Traditional Beliefs about Illness

All over South Asia people view illness in quite similar ways derived from Ayurvedic medicine, the ancient Indian medical system. An illness is regarded as the result of an imbalance in the body humours, bile, wind, and phlegm, and the purpose of treatment is to re-establish the balance. An imbalance in humours can result from various sources, usually dietary. For example, a headache may result from eating too many eggs, which are believed to be "heating" foods. Other sources of imbalance include working in the hot sun, immorality, and excesses of alcohol, sex, or even study. Possession by a demon or the "evil eye" of a jealous neighbour may account for still other diseases, particularly mental illnesses.

A variety of traditional treatments exist to rebalance the humours. Most commonly, these are homemade herbal decoctions such as teas made by grinding herbs or spices and boiling them down in liquids. Specific foods may be used to re-establish bodily balance. Foods in South Asia are classified as "hot," "cold," or "neutral," not in terms of temperature or spiciness but on other grounds. (There is no universally agreed-upon classification; what constitutes cold food varies from one community to another.) Bathing (or its avoidance), massage, and rubbing oil on the body are other ways to rebalance and thus to cure.

Forms of traditional treatment may also be directed towards the supernatural causes of illness. In South Asian villages people in stressful circumstances may explain their troubles supernaturally. For example, a newly married girl, having left her own village to live with her husband and his parents, may fall ill with the stress of overwork and an unsympathetic mother-in-law. For such an illness, an exorcist or priest may be called in to perform a ritual chant. The ceremony may end with a symbolic action: the tying of a protective thread around the patient's wrist, the writing of a protective verse to be worn in a metal cylinder on a chain around the neck, or the inscribing of religious verses on the patient's hands. A sick person may also make promises of gifts to a temple god upon recovery. South Asians believe many avenues are available to treat illness. Traditional medicines, vows, rituals, and Western medicine may all work, and all may be used for the same illness.

Even South Asians, particularly educated urbanites, who do not believe in traditional ways have habits, remedies, food combinations, and day-to-day methods of preventing illness that are based on these traditional beliefs.

Traditional Treatment in South Asia

In South Asia traditional medical practitioners are readily available to almost everyone. Usually the first to be consulted, particularly in rural villages, is the Ayurvedic physician, sometimes a barber who also specializes in bonesetting or in treating snake-bites. Also to be found within walking distance are other religiously based practitioners and astrologers. An Ayurvedic doctor, often trained as an apprentice, will usually talk with a patient and his family together (Western-style "privacy" is usually not a concern), will sometimes take the patient's pulse or use a medical instrument such as a stethoscope to diagnose the illness, and then will prescribe herbal medicines or recommend bathing or soothing oils. The consultation time is usually short. Since fees or gifts are customary for traditional health services, many rural families try home remedies first. The tendency, particularly in rural villages and among the poor, is to wait until an illness is serious before professional care is sought from outside the village. The reason for this is to save money and time, not because people are fatalistic and believe nothing can be done.

Traditional medical services are available in urban areas as well, sometimes in more organized forms such as Ayurvedic hospitals and clinics. Although traditional healers are much more readily available than medical doctors, in many parts of South Asia this is not the only reason for choosing to use them. Many South Asians believe that traditional medicine is more natural, slower acting, and less strong, as well as having fewer side-effects than Western medicine. It is therefore preferred for chronic illnesses where a quick cure is neither important nor expected.

Some South Asians in Canada are likewise hesitant to use Western medicine. Many feel also that traditional treatments are more effective for certain diseases, such as rheumatism or asthma. Even urban, well-educated people may prefer traditional medicine for some symptoms.

Western Medicine in South Asia

India has one medical doctor for every 1,916 people, in contrast to Canada's one doctor per 550 people. Other South Asian countries are similar; Sri Lanka is an exception. There may sometimes be a physician in a larger village who serves surrounding villages as well. Some villages may have untrained "doctors" who give injections and supply Western-type drugs. More commonly, though, physicians practise in towns and cities. Since free public clinics are often absent or very crowded and health insurance is generally unavailable in South Asia, most people must pay for a physician's services and medicines, the latter usually being dispensed in the doctor's office. Thus a visit to a medical doctor can be expensive for village families and is avoided unless the disease is serious or the family can afford the fees, medicines, travel expenses, and time away from work.

Many South Asian villages, however, have trained and untrained midwives who deliver babies at home and provide pre- and postnatal care. Their services may include supervising delivery, giving advice about diet and behaviour, performing suitable rituals, and bathing and caring for mother and baby for some time after birth. Midwives are paid in cash or with gifts of food and clothing.

That hospitals are used only for more serious illnesses is suggested by the statistics: India in 1995 had only one hospital bed per 1,493 people, compared to one bed per 110 persons in Canada. Hospitals are usually located in towns and cities remote from many villages. When a village family does go to a hospital, no appointments are made and hospital staff are often very busy. Unless families know someone working at the hospital to whom they can appeal for help (a common way of dealing with such problems), patients and their families must take a number and wait in a queue, sometimes for several hours. When they finally see a physician there is little time for extensive taking of histories, physical examinations, or answering the patient's questions. Instead, the physician usually diagnoses quickly and decides immediately on treatment. Hospitals and physicians similar to those in Canada will have been experienced only by urban, middle-class immigrants from South Asia.

Disease in South Asia

While South Asia has a substantial urban middle class with satisfactory incomes and access to good health care, the great majority of South Asians are poor. Where incomes are low and uncertain, housing is crowded, water supply unprotected, sanitation inadequate, and nutrition poor. The relatively low standard of living is evident in the fact that a person born in 2002 could expect to live sixty-four years in India but seventy-nine years in Canada. In India in 2000, infant mortality during the first year of life was high, with sixty-five deaths for every thousand live births, compared to five in Canada.

Infections and parasitic diseases are the most prevalent in South Asia. South Asian immigrants to Canada may have experienced typhoid, dengue fever, cholera, tuberculosis, hepatitis, and amoebic dysentery. Of particular relevance is malaria. Although there have been relatively effective programs to eradicate this scourge, the incidence of malaria in India has increased recently, from a low of 100,000 cases and no deaths in 1965 to a high of six million cases in 1976. The area of greatest resurgence is Gujarat, where some

Canadian immigrants originate. Moreover, malaria is particularly common in many cities. The incidence of age-related illnesses, such as heart disease, cancer, stroke, and diabetes, is relatively low because of the low life expectancy. In 1999 India had the highest rate in South Asia for HIV/AIDS in young people aged fifteen to twenty-four: 7.1 per 1,000 for women compared to 1.8 in Canada and 3.4 for men compared to 2.8 in Canada.

Documented diseases among South Asian immigrants in the West are malaria, tuberculosis (including types other than pulmonary), several types of intestinal parasites, filaria, vitamin A deficiency, and rickets.

Seeking Health Care in South Asia and Canada

In cases of sickness in Indian villages, it is not simply the victim who decides on a suitable course of action. The whole family may be consulted (and sometimes neighbours) about the need to spend money on a visit to a doctor, and the final decision may rest with the head of the household. For example, when a child falls sick, the mother will often consult her mother-in-law about appropriate home remedies. The mother-in-law or household head will also decide if the child should be taken to a doctor or hospital. Many factors influence the decision besides cost and time. A wage-earner may be treated more promptly than others and a first-born son more quickly than a daughter.

Among South Asian villagers who have immigrated to Canada, the extended family often remains strong, so that the old ways of making health decisions persist, particularly in the early years of their residence. Elderly women often recommend home treatments, and elderly family members and the male household head are consulted about the need to see a doctor.

Especially in their early days in Canada, village families do not decide to use physicians on a regular basis but only for acute illnesses. In choosing a family physician, language familiarity is often important, but so are proximity and convenience, especially for the women. Today Canadian cities have large numbers of physicians of South Asian background who speak one of the Indian languages, though rural areas have few.

South Asian migrants of middle-class or urban background are much more familiar with regular medical care and more likely to leave treatment decisions to the patient or the immediate family.

Traditional Medicine in Canada

When South Asian villagers first come to Canada, they often continue to resort to traditional methods, even with health insurance and easy access to

Western medicine. Home remedies such as massage, bathing, and herbal medicines (either made at home or purchased from an Indian shop) may be used first, and a physician is sought out only for serious illnesses. Advertisements in some local South Asian newspapers reveal that traditional astrologers and palm readers also operate in Canada. Sometimes traditional treatments are used concomitantly with Western medicines or are even preferred for having fewer unpleasant side-effects and being less strong.

While greater variation exists among longer-term South Asian inhabitants of Canada, many still adhere to traditional tonics and ointments. Many more eat specific combinations of foods to prevent or treat illness, sometimes without knowing (or believing in) the theory behind the practice. Even South Asians who are well educated and think of themselves as modern or Westernized may be reluctant to discuss their use of traditional treatments.

Relationship between Doctor and Patient

In South Asia, patients and families often put great trust in doctors, whether traditional or modern. The patient expects the doctor to have all the answers and make all the decisions. The patient takes a passive role, answering but not asking questions, waiting for the physician to impart his diagnosis and recommendations. Medical advice is generally accepted without question. Moreover, the social distance between South Asian doctors and most patients is so great that the relationship tends to be formal, with patients typically using deferential forms of address.

It is also expected that the doctor will go beyond asking questions and should examine the patient by taking pulse and temperature and looking at the throat. Yet in many rural areas physical examinations as known in the West are very uncommon, so patients are not used to removing their clothing in the physician's office. However, the patient expects treatment in the form of medicine, injections, pills, or tonics. Failing such actions, the patient may be disappointed and lose confidence in the doctor.

These expectations can create dissatisfaction among South Asian patients in Canada when they consult physicians trained in the West. A doctor who says, "I do not know what is wrong. We need to do more tests," or "Come back the next time that symptom recurs so that we can investigate," may be perceived as incompetent. A doctor who asks the patient, "What would you like me to do about it?" may be regarded in the same light as the physician who says, "It is just a cold. There is no need for medicine." Doctors who behave and dress informally may also disappoint South Asians, who tend to prefer an active and commanding doctor who takes charge and writes prescriptions.

South Asian women tend to be hesitant and shy about being examined and treated by male physicians and may believe, along with their husbands, that a woman should have a female doctor. In South Asia, however, there is often no choice, while in Canada convenience of access is often a more important criterion than the doctor's gender except in the case of obstetricians, who should preferably be women. South Asian men may be embarrassed and reluctant to have a prostate examination, for example, if the physician is female.

Compared to non-Asian women, South Asian women in Canada are much less likely to receive Pap tests or mammograms. Many women do not know about these procedures since they are not readily available in South Asia, and those who do know may be reluctant to request or have them, especially if the Canadian physician is male. Women hesitate to have mammograms, even in screening centres entirely staffed by women, since the procedure involves removing clothing and being touched by a technician. South Asian women from rural areas have usually never had a pelvic examination, even those women who have had several children, and are thus reluctant to have one here. Women do not talk about "women's diseases" such as breast cancer with men, including their husbands. However, in the West, where many diseases are openly discussed in the media, it becomes easier for women to bring up these "taboo" illnesses with their spouses and doctors.

Hospitalization

Visiting

For many rural South Asians, hospitalization occurs only when illness is severe and often involves travelling to relatively distant towns. Family members may stay with the patient in hospital or visit daily to help with nursing tasks. Also, many families will bring food that they believe to be better than hospital fare. Relatives, friends, and neighbours, including children, make great efforts to express their concern for the patient and the family by making hospital visits.

These practices continue in Canada. Family, friends, and neighbours want to visit a hospitalized person, and the patient welcomes their attention. The patient will more likely feel happy than tired after a visit by a crowd of people, and may be dismayed if certain people do not appear. Visiting hours often take on the atmosphere of a family reunion with much food, talking, laughing, and eating. It is not enough to drop by briefly. Instead, visitors – both friends and family – are expected to sit and spend time with the patient.

Understandably, South Asian family members are sometimes disturbed when forbidden to visit the patient, as in an intensive care unit. In this case, it is not uncommon for family and friends to gather outside in a corridor, simply in order to be together near the patient. For many South Asians, hospital visits are a very important way to provide support for both the sick person and family. Hospital visits are believed to be right and proper by most South Asians, both in South Asia and in Canada.

Large numbers of visitors, lengthy visits, and gifts of food are often in breach of the rules of many Canadian hospitals. If limiting the number of visitors is desired, the hospital staff can most easily approach the patient's husband, father, or a male elder to explain the situation and to seek the cooperation of the others.

Hospital Food

Canadian hospital food can present problems for South Asians, particularly those with religious dietary restrictions. For example, a vegetarian may not accept a vegetarian meal prepared in a kitchen where meat was also cooked, or if the meat has simply been removed from the plate. Being told "Just don't eat the meat" on a plate is often not acceptable; the patient is likely to eat nothing.

Many South Asians, especially older persons, are more comfortable eating with their fingers and therefore need water to wash their hands before and after eating. Hospital food is too bland for most South Asians. In addition, since many South Asians believe that food and particular illnesses are related, they may be reluctant to eat some items and ready to suggest suitable substitutes.

Hospital Clothing

Some South Asian patients in Canada hesitate to wear clothing that others have worn before them, even where it has been washed and sterilized. They may worry that such clothing has been worn by an unclean person or by a patient who subsequently died. They prefer their own clothing where possible. South Asian women may prefer not to use hospital clothing for new babies since they may be particularly anxious about the harmful effects of used clothing.

Hospital Treatments and Surgery

Although many South Asians accept the doctor's authority to prescribe treatment, surgery is sometimes felt to be threatening. Only after detailed explanations about the surgical procedure and its necessity will the family agree. In some cases where surgery is refused, the decision is made not by the individual patient but by the whole family, and the patient will be taken home. In other instances the family may agree but will suggest an auspicious day for surgery on the basis of an astrologer's predictions. There is no religious or other belief that prevents blood transfusions or organ transplants.

However, hospital staff treating South Asian patients should know about some religious practices. High-caste Hindu men participate in a religious ceremony at adolescence in which a sacred thread (or string) is tied around the body; it goes over one shoulder and around the chest and is tied at waist-level. Because of its religious significance, this thread should not be cut or removed without the permission of the patient or his family. Strictly observant Sikh men do not cut their hair and do not shave their beards. If hair or beard must be cut, it is important to explain the need fully, both to the patient and the family. The Sikh man's bracelet and *kirpan* (small symbolic sword) must also not be removed. Muslims may wear thirty-three beads representing the names of God or small cylinders containing verses from the Koran around their necks or tied to their wrists. These should also not be removed unless absolutely necessary.

Most South Asians prefer that catheterization or enemas be performed by a staff member of the same gender as the patient.

Use of Medicines

The concern that Western medicines may be too strong or upset the body's balance leads many South Asian patients to avoid their use or prematurely stop taking them. This is true of all types of medicines, but especially of long-term psychiatric medicines. Once the person begins to feel better, the medicine is abandoned, since "If you're taking medicine you must still be sick."

Mental Illness

In South Asia, mental illness is sometimes believed to have supernatural causes, such as spells or curses cast by jealous relatives or acquaintances. These problems are resolved by visiting temples or shrines. Astrologers may also be consulted for a prognosis of the problem. Symptoms of mental illness are usually presented to a physician in somatic form, for example, as headaches, stomach aches, or burning bodily sensations, rather than as anxiety or depression. Depression, if acknowledged at all, is seen as being related to a specific life situation, such as a failed examination. Somatic complaints are more acceptable because mental illness is stigmatized and is generally hidden to safeguard the children's marriage prospects.

Such beliefs and practices persist in the South Asian community in Canada. Severely ill family members are not ignored or rejected but may be kept hidden and thus may remain untreated for long periods of time, only to arrive at hospital emergency rooms by ambulance or police car after uncontrollable outbreaks or suicide attempts. Less severe psychiatric symptoms like depression or neurosis are thought of as somatic complaints and presented to a doctor with a request for medicine. In some instances South Asian families will seek explanations from palm readers, astrologers, and other healers who practise in Canada. Such is the case of the parents who decided that their daughter-in-law had cast a chanting spell on their son, because he listened only to her. Where the problems are serious and the family has money, they may return to their home country for rituals and charms.

South Asian immigrant families experience a number of common problems related to leaving home and living in a new culture which seem to precipitate psychiatric symptoms. Because education is felt to be indispensable for upward mobility in Canada, failing a school examination may be devastating for a young person. Adolescents and young adults often face an insoluble dilemma in trying to balance traditional parental expectations against more liberal peer group pressures. A young South Asian girl may have two identities, one for home and another for school. The resulting stress and guilt may lead to depression, which if severe may bring suicide attempts, perhaps with household poisons. Psychiatric illness may be precipitated by a disturbance in family relations, such as the arrival of a mother-in-law from Asia or conflict between husband and wife over obligations to their respective families.

In other Western countries there is evidence that suicide rates are relatively high among young women immigrants from South Asia, particularly those recruited as brides by men already resident in the West. These young women usually have no family support of their own and must adapt to a new country and to a new extended family. Depression and anxiety, along with conflict with in-laws and domestic violence, may precipitate suicide.

While most South Asians treat these problems as somatic and prefer medicines, some patients in Canada do resort to psychiatric help. Western "talk" therapy is not usually compatible with traditional South Asian beliefs or expectations. The preference is for clear and authoritative advice about what the patient should do and how the family should help. The usual open-ended psychiatric interviewing method, with its assumption that the patient must be helped to find his or her own solutions, does not accord with South Asian expectations that the physician is in command. Attempts to elicit the family circumstances of the South Asian patient are not normally welcomed, since family harmony is usually more highly prized than individual well-being. The Western therapeutic value often attached to independence from the family is not usually acceptable to Indian psychiatric patients.

Kanwal, from India

Kanwal, now twenty-one, is in his second year at a community college. He lives with his parents, his sister, and two brothers in a suburb of Vancouver. His mother and father came to Canada nearly twenty years ago from a small town in northern India where his father was a school teacher. In Canada his father works as a parking garage attendant and his mother as a salesperson in a sari shop.

Three years ago, Kanwal's mother noticed that he seemed to be strangely fearful of one of the family's close friends, often retreating to the basement when the friend arrived. Also, she sometimes found him in his room, talking to someone who wasn't there. Then he announced that a professor at college had asked him to take charge of a huge project that could bring him and his family millions of dollars as well as instant fame back in India. These things mystified his parents. But one day they became very frightened when Kanwal began shouting at them and struck his mother in the face. At first they did not know what to do, but after several of these episodes they phoned a relative, a social worker, who advised them to take their son to the local emergency ward, which they did. Kanwal was hospitalized in the psychiatric ward for a week, given medications, and scheduled for clinic visits.

The psychiatrists who met him described multiple symptoms: delusions, grandiosity, hallucinations, poor insight, and aggressive behaviour. They believe that he has schizophrenia and that regular long-term treatment with anti-psychotic medication will control the symptoms.

Kanwal, on the other hand, believes that nothing is wrong with him.

Kanwal's parents do not believe in the medical diagnosis. Instead, they ask "Where in the family did this come from?" So they take him regularly to see a faith healer who is very well respected in the Indian community and who supplied Kanwal with an expensive talisman to wear around his neck. They also have costly holy water flown from India. Kanwal's parents note that his delusions moderate after a visit to the faith healer, but Kanwal says he doesn't believe in the faith healer: "I just go there out of respect for my parents." Instead, he argues, the reason for his improved behaviour after a visit is that the healer scares him. "She looks in my eyes for a long time and I come away feeling very scared for several hours." But the fact that Kanwal seems better after these visits confirms his parents' belief that their son is possessed and that the faith healer is driving out the evil in him. They say, "He must have been cursed" or "He is being punished for the sins of ancestors." Now they are considering some sort of sacrifice which they believe might solve the problem.

With permission of Dr. Kulbir Singh

Many South Asian families are more willing and able to use advice and help from community agencies and schools than from psychiatrists or the mental health system, especially when the sick person is an adolescent. Help provided in an informal and egalitarian way is generally more effective.

Pregnancy

In South Asia, pregnancy is considered a normal, healthy state. Consequently many women do not see the need to consult a doctor unless there is a problem. This is particularly true of women in rural areas, who usually plan on home deliveries. Help and advice are provided by the pregnant woman's mother or mother-in-law as well as by a midwife who visits periodically.

Life continues as usual throughout pregnancy. Couples continue sexual relations. Women who ordinarily work in the fields continue to do so, although they may avoid lifting heavy objects. In general the woman's diet remains the same, although she may avoid "hot" foods such as meat, eggs, and nuts, especially during the first trimester, because they are believed to encourage miscarriage or premature delivery. The emphasis is on "cooling" foods such as some fruit, coconut, yoghurt, butter, and milk, which may be eaten in increased quantities, particularly butter and milk.

There is a strong preference for male children among South Asian families, particularly as a first child. Consequently there has been in India a recent increase in requests for ultrasound by urban middle-class Indian women to determine the sex of the fetus. In India it is illegal to perform an abortion for reasons of gender preference, but abortion of females is sometimes illegally done all the same. Some South Asian women in Canada, concerned about the gender of their unborn children, have found physicians in the United States who are willing to do the testing and an abortion if the fetus is female.

In Canada, some South Asian women believe regular check-ups during pregnancy to be unimportant. Indeed, they may be avoided, or cause anxiety because visits to a doctor are associated with problems or abnormalities. Also, a young woman in Canada may be deterred from obtaining prenatal care by traditionalist relatives, in-laws, or mothers, who may discourage "new" practices, saying "I have the experience of giving birth to ten or twelve children and can advise my daughter. Is there anything new about childbirth here?" Ability to have regular check-ups is also influenced by the finances and family situation of the expectant mother. She may wish to have her sister or sister-in-law present at the birth but may be discouraged by the emphasis in Canada on her husband's presence.

South Asian women are encouraged to attend prenatal classes by physicians and public health nurses, but for a variety of reasons most prefer not to go. Language is often a problem, and many of the teachings offend the woman's idea of propriety. Sex is discussed openly with strangers, and movies of childbirth are shown, both of which make many South Asian women uncomfortable. Also, they are embarrassed about doing exercises in front of other people. Their husbands tend to feel even more embarrassed and uncomfortable in these classes and thus usually refuse to attend.

South Asian women who are recent immigrants may experience considerable stress during pregnancy, especially if they have married a man who is a relative stranger. While already making the typical adjustments to a new language, culture, in-law family, and husband, she may become pregnant immediately and suffer from morning sickness. Unable to confide in her husband or mother-in-law and with no family of her own, she may keep things to herself, lose weight, and receive little sympathy or help to deal with her emotional and physical stress.

An unmarried girl who becomes pregnant is often rejected by her family since virginity at marriage is highly valued, and lack of it greatly complicates marriage arrangements for all family members. In Canada, where financial aid is available to single mothers, it is possible for the rejected South Asian girl to live independently, but even so the loss of family and cultural support can be intolerable.

Childbirth

In South Asia the woman traditionally returned to her own parents' home for delivery of her first child, and sometimes for subsequent births. Although this is changing, most births still occur at home, supervised by midwives in the presence of the woman's mother, mother-in-law, or married sister. Childbirth is considered to be a woman's business, and husbands participate only insofar as they stay near the house in case of emergency. During labour the midwife often encourages the woman to be active, to walk around, and sometimes to drink herbal medicines to facilitate the process. Delivery is often in a squatting or sitting position. The baby remains with the mother after birth.

In Canada, where hospital deliveries are the norm, many practices will be unfamiliar to a woman who has previously had children in South Asia. However, she will of course have talked to her friends and have some idea about what will happen. Her husband usually accompanies her to the hospital but prefers to stay out of the delivery room. The woman's preference is usually for a natural delivery, and she will generally not request an anesthetic, leaving such decisions to the physician. Forceps and Caesarean section are usually accepted if clearly explained by the doctor. South Asian women not fluent in English experience additional stress during delivery and find reassuring the presence of an English-speaking married female relative or friend.

Asian babies born in the West are, on average, lower in weight than white Caucasian babies (2.96 kilograms versus 3.29 kilograms), but this difference is not usually the result of maternal malnutrition during pregnancy (Mason et al. 1982).

When a Muslim child is born, religious practice requires that a family member recite a prayer in the baby's ear as soon as possible. A male Muslim baby must be circumcised. For other religious groups circumcision is a matter of personal preference.

South Asian women, accustomed to keeping the baby with them at all times, may feel concerned at the Canadian practice of placing the baby in a nursery in certain instances.

The sex of the newborn child is of paramount importance to many Indian women and their husbands and relatives, especially newer migrants. For a South Asian woman the birth of a daughter may occasion crisis and fear of blame. Women who have had several girls and no sons may become stigmatized; people say, "She will only give you girls." If the baby is a girl, emotional outbreaks sometimes occur, and in extreme instances neither the woman's husband nor family members will visit the hospital.

After childbirth, particularly if the baby is a boy, visitors will come in large numbers to celebrate the event, bringing sweets for all.

Postpartum Period

The traditional practice in South Asia is for the mother and new baby to remain secluded in the home for a week to forty days, depending on region and caste. The belief is that the woman is at her weakest in this period, is most susceptible to chills and backaches, and requires rest. Failure of the mother to comply is believed to expose her to arthritis and other illnesses later on. Such periods of seclusion after childbirth are common among Indian women in Canada as well. Since the new mother is expected to be with the baby to the exclusion of all else, members of her extended family may help or a relative may come to stay for a month or so.

During the postpartum period, South Asian women are advised to eat "hot" foods and avoid "cold" ones. It is believed that heating foods strengthen the body, regulate the system, and encourage bleeding and discharge so that a flat stomach results. Cold foods are thought to cause weight gain. One snack commonly eaten by Punjabi women during this period is *panjiri,* a whole-wheat flour fried in butter with sugar, almonds, pistachios, raisins, and several kinds of seeds. All of these are heating ingredients. It is important to keep warm, avoid fans, and keep well covered even in hot weather.

Bathing is acceptable, but the water must be warm. Vigorous massages with oil are also used.

Visitors are welcome during this forty-day period and may bring gifts or cash. The new parents may also have a party to celebrate the birth. However, certain people do not visit, since they bring bad luck to the baby: widows, women who have lost children, and people in mourning. To avoid harm to the child, visitors are careful not to compliment or admire the baby to excess, lest parents worry about the effects of the evil eye. Parents may put black eyeliner behind the ear of the baby or tie a black thread to the baby to ward off the evil eye.

A woman is considered unclean in this postpartum period, and the couple abstains from sexual relations. At the conclusion of this seclusion she takes a special bath, and rituals are performed to mark her return to a clean state.

Breastfeeding

In South Asia, in both rural and urban areas, breastfeeding is preferred, although the baby of a middle-class mother who has to return to her job may be bottle-fed. Generally, though, women breastfeed for at least six months and sometimes up to two or three years. In Canada, some South Asian women prefer to bottle-feed, possibly believing it to be "modern" or simply to allow the mother-in-law the pleasure of feeding the new baby. Husbands, too, may influence the choice between breastfeeding or bottle-feeding. Some children are given a bottle up to ages three or four.

Family Planning and Sexuality

In South Asia, particularly in rural areas where children are needed to help with farm work, families are large; eight to ten children in a family is not unusual. Children are believed to be God's gift and are welcomed. There is no formal sex education for girls in South Asia, nor do most young unmarried girls know much about the menstrual cycle or methods of birth control. In contrast more young men are informed about birth control since they are allowed much greater freedom before marriage. While married couples have always known ways of preventing birth, abstinence and withdrawal being the most common, modern methods of birth control are still used by fewer than half the couples in India, and these are likely to be urban and middle-class, not villagers.

Families that come to Canada, or are started here, tend to be smaller because women have less help at home and often have jobs and because the cost of raising children is greater. Modern methods of controlling births are more acceptable and are used, but more often after the desired number of children have been born than to space births. The first child, usually born within the first year of marriage, is important because it demonstrates the wife's fertility to the husband and his family. Several closely spaced pregnancies may follow, but marital stress can occur where only daughters are born. Often it is the husband who makes decisions about family size. The favourite methods of contraception are the IUD and the contraceptive pill; diaphragms and condoms are seldom used. Breastfeeding is also understood to protect against conception.

A South Asian woman is not usually comfortable discussing family planning or sexuality with a nurse or doctor, especially if her husband or mother is present. Women usually talk more easily in private but even then may find discussion of sexuality difficult because they lack a vocabulary in any language for genitals or sexual functioning.

Abortion is thought of as killing the child and is thus not generally accepted by South Asians, either overseas or in Canada. However, illegal abortion is practised in South Asia and may be resorted to in desperate situations such as when an unmarried girl becomes pregnant or the baby is another girl. Legal abortion in Canada is somewhat more acceptable to South Asian couples, particularly if the woman is ill, if they cannot afford another child, or where pregnancies are very closely spaced. However, the decision is not just the woman's and her physician's but requires her husband's approval and perhaps his family's.

Disability and Rehabilitation

A South Asian family may find difficulty in accepting a disabled child or helping it in the ways that the Western health system expects. As with mental illness, some disabilities may be hidden because they reflect on the whole family, and some parents account for the situation in terms of karma. Some disabilities may be explained in either religious or supernatural terms, and the disabled person is taken to shrines and temples for ritual prayers. Disability may be understood in fatalistic terms, rather than being seen as a medical problem for which helpful treatments exist. A disability in a daughter is seen as a special problem by her parents because if she cannot marry she will remain a lifelong burden on them.

Many South Asian families are likely to accept and foster the dependence of disabled members, pitying them and helping them rather than encouraging them to greater independence, particularly if initial rehabilitation efforts produce little improvement. Exercises, independent social activities, and other rehabilitative measures advocated by the medical services may be disregarded simply because the South Asian family does not see independence as important or relevant.

Dental Health

In rural areas in South Asia dentists are rarely used. Instead, villagers may use home remedies (for example, a whole clove) for a toothache, pull out their own teeth, or go to traditional practitioners.

When rural South Asians come to Canada, most use toothbrushes but sometimes only irregularly. A dentist may be consulted for acute pain, but regular visits are not common, and yearly or six-month cleaning and check-ups are resisted mainly because many families cannot afford to pay for services that are not covered by medical insurance.

Bathing and Elimination

There is a general belief in South Asia that bathing in still water (as in a bathtub) is unclean, so South Asians generally bathe in running water, such as a stream, a shower, or clean water poured from a bucket. The same preference for showers is found in Canada but sometimes cannot be met in Canadian hospitals. South Asian patients would probably prefer a pitcher of water or a private area by a sink to the usual bathtub.

In South Asia many people do not use toilet paper but wash their bodies with clean water, using the left hand only (the right hand is traditionally used for eating). Most South Asians adapt to practices used in Canada. However, in South Asia and in some South Asian homes in Canada, a water tap or a bucket of clean water is available next to the toilet along with a pint-sized plastic pitcher or dipping bowl. In Canadian hospitals, some Indian patients, particularly elderly or new immigrants, may prefer to have a container of water and a bowl or pitcher provided in the toilet area or with the bedpan.

Food and Nutrition

Food has very important implications for religion and health in South Asia. Hot and cold foods, and the balance between them, can cause or cure illnesses. Certain foods are prohibited by the main religions, food preparation may be important, and there are times and situations when fasting is required.

Dietary restrictions and practices are of importance to many South Asians in Canada. They may refuse food because they do not know whether the food has been made with the acceptable ingredients. In a hospital, South Asians would find it helpful to be told whether dishes served to them contain beef, pork, shellfish, and so on.

Hindu Food Practices

Strict Hindus practise the doctrine of non-violence against living things and thus abstain from meat or fish. The more orthodox, especially women, do not even eat eggs. Because the cow is sacred, Hindus do not eat beef, veal, beef extract, or any other form of beef. However, dairy products are considered pure, although strict vegetarians do not eat Western cheese because it is made with animal rennet. Pork is forbidden as unclean. Strict vegetarians will be unhappy and may refuse to eat anything if served vegetarian items from the same plate that contains meat or if utensils used in cooking meat have been used to cook the vegetarian food. Alcohol is not prohibited but should be used in moderation only.

The Hindu caste system dictates that members of one caste cannot sit down to eat with members of another or eat food prepared or served by a member of a lower caste.

Fasting is used as a self-sacrifice to earn religious merit, to ward off evil, and to absolve sins. For example, a pregnant woman who has had two or three daughters might vow to fast for a certain number of days (for example, sixteen Mondays) if her next child is a son. Fasting may take many forms depending on individual interpretation, from total abstinence (no food or water for twenty-four hours) to one meal a day, or to eating only foods considered to be pure (for example, fruit, yoghurt, nuts, or potatoes). Once a year a Hindu woman may fast to give her husband a long life; she eats a meal before 5:30 a.m. and then not again until she sees the moon that night. Some fast in this way each month or week. Very few Hindus would insist on fasting when ill or in hospital, and even they would probably agree to take hot milk, fruit, tea, and salad without salt.

Hindus living in Canada vary a great deal in their adherence to these religious prescriptions.

Muslim Food Practices

Muslims follow dietary laws laid down in the Koran which forbid the eating of pork in any form or eating the blood of any animal. Special methods of slaughtering are used to produce meat that is *halal*. In Canada, such meat is purchased from a Muslim butcher. Foods containing non-*halal* meat products are forbidden, as are other foods cooked with utensils used in places where pork has been cooked. Only fish with fins or scales is allowed; shellfish is not permissible, although many Muslims eat it anyway. Alcohol is strictly forbidden. Some Muslims may not want to be in a place where alcohol is being consumed by others.

Each year all post-adolescent Muslims observe the month-long fast of Ramadan when no food or beverage is consumed from sunrise to sunset. Exemptions are made for young children, ill persons, travellers, and women who are menstruating, pregnant, or breastfeeding, but they are expected to make a compensatory fast at another time.

Just as with the Hindus, Muslims in Canada differ in their observance of religious rules.

Sikh Food Practices

Although there are no significant dietary restrictions in the Sikh religion, many Sikhs are vegetarians. Traditionally, beef and pork are not eaten, and smoking and alcohol consumption are prohibited. Some Sikhs also fast.

Diet and Eating Practices

Despite great regional variation, the commonest staple in South Asia is some sort of cereal, usually rice, or unleavened bread made of wheat flour. In the Punjab, from which many Canadian Asians come, many people are vegetarians who eat whole-wheat roti (unleavened bread), ghee (clarified butter), milk, buttermilk, brown sugar, lentils, seasonal vegetables, and fruit. Villagers usually have an early morning cup of tea followed by a large midmorning meal and another meal at the end of the day. Urban South Asians may have early tea, a larger breakfast at 9:00 a.m., a larger lunch at 1:00 p.m., tea with sweets or other snacks at 5:00 or 6:00 p.m., and a light supper at 9:00 p.m. Traditionally South Asians in both rural and urban areas eat with the fingers of the right hand, and water is provided to wash the hands before and after the meal.

Babies are not generally given special foods. Instead, solid foods such as soft rice, cream of wheat, mashed bananas, or potatoes will be given some time after the second month, followed, in the ninth or tenth month, by bread, rice, meat, or lentils cooked with some salt but no spices. By fifteen months, the baby is eating adult foods, including eggs, chapattis (unleavened bread), lentils, and rice.

After coming to Canada, South Asian families find it relatively easy to continue eating familiar foods since ingredients are readily available, at least in the larger cities. However, some junk foods are tempting, both because they are "modern" and because they are convenient for families where many people work on different schedules. The result can be poorer levels of nutrition than previously enjoyed by the family in Asia.

South Asian parents, especially newer immigrants, are likely to supply traditional school lunches such as roti or rice, in contrast to the usual Western sandwiches. If teased, the South Asian children may throw these lunches away and eat nothing. Some children prefer junk food because they see it as a way to be accepted by others.

Some South Asian mothers are confused about the relative food merits of various forms of milk (sweetened condensed milk, evaporated milk, yoghurt, and so on), to the detriment of their infant's nutrition. Mealtimes change in Canada as well, and the South Asian housewife may find herself cooking individual meals as each family member comes home from work. Most South Asians in Canada are relatively comfortable eating with cutlery in public even though they may eat with their fingers at home.

Food and the Prevention of Illness

Diseases are often held to result from an imbalance between hot and cold within the body. Hot or cold foods can therefore compensate to achieve balance. Whether a food is hot or cold is unrelated to temperature or spiciness, and the classification varies from region to region in South Asia.

Diseases thought of as cold, such as arthritis, rheumatism, respiratory infections, upset stomach, other gastrointestinal problems, and circulatory problems, are suitably treated with hot foods such as ginger and garlic. Cold foods are also avoided in cases of fever, when hot milk is offered instead. Following surgery, which is a cold state, cold foods are avoided because they may produce swelling in the affected area. On the other hand, hot foods accelerate healing. If these considerations are neglected, it is believed that the patient in old age may develop pain in the muscles or bones. Colds or other respiratory problems are also believed to be cold diseases, so the common Western home remedy, fruit juice, is not suitable. In fact it is believed that juices and cold milk will aggravate the condition. For hot states, such as pregnancy, cold foods are recommended, including yoghurt, milk, and fruit.

It is important for ill people to be given easily digested, soft food such as cream of wheat, lentils without spices, *khichari* (lentils and rice), and soup made of whole-wheat flour and milk. These are the foods a South Asian family might bring to a patient in hospital.

Beliefs about hot and cold foods are very strongly embedded in South Asian culture. Even South Asians who have lived in Canada for many years tend to follow these eating guidelines and modify their diets during illness and childbearing accordingly, taking care to eat the appropriate combination of foods each day.

Use of Alcohol

In South Asia there are some religious restrictions on alcohol consumption; the Muslim and Sikh religions prohibit alcohol. Many villagers are too poor to afford it, although homemade liquor is produced in many villages. Consequently, some South Asian men may drink, particularly middle-class urban men, but it is unusual for women to do so. When families come to Canada and achieve relative prosperity, alcohol, which is readily available, can become a problem for some men (but not women), particularly where men are feeling the stress of adapting to a new culture. Drinking alcohol and offering it to visitors is sometimes a symbol of economic success.

Excessive drinking among South Asian men in Canada has given rise to family conflict, misuse of family money, and in some cases extramarital affairs with non-Asian women. It is often associated with domestic abuse. This is not usually defined as a problem requiring outside help until it reaches a crisis. In that case religious or community services are more often acceptable and helpful than medical treatment.

The Elderly

Elderly South Asians who have lived in Canada for many years have less difficulty with aging than do those who have arrived late in their lives, sponsored by their children. The latter find themselves cut off from the support of friends and relatives at home, and they miss many religious activities that have been part of their daily lives. Many elderly South Asians in Canada feel lonely and saddened by the contrast between the social liveliness of the family compound or village and the isolation of the suburban single-family Canadian home. Often they lose dignity and respect because the knowledge gained through many years of experience at home is not useful in a new society. Most do not learn English, which further limits their ability to travel by bus to temples or friends' homes. Some elderly parents contribute to the family income by doing seasonal or irregular work like berry-picking or delivering flyers, but this is difficult for those who were well-educated professionals in their home country. Many elderly parents care for grandchildren left at home while the parents work, and conflict between the generations may occur over child-rearing practices. Some elderly parents are subject to psychological abuse by the family.

When South Asian parents grow old, they usually expect to be cared for by their children, particularly sons, and the sons recognize this obligation. Care is relatively easy in Asia where large families can share the day-to-day burdens. Residence in Canada does not often change the expectation, but it can alter the feasibility. If husband and wife must both work and there are no other relatives to share the responsibility for care of a sick or frail parent, the family will try leaving the old person at home, provided with lunch and other needs. So long as the old person can manage physically and mentally, this arrangement is usually satisfactory. At some point, especially if dementia sets in, the family may feel they have no choice but to place the old person in a nursing home. This will usually be done only as a last resort, after all other possibilities have been considered. The belief that old people should be cared for by their families is strong, and a certain stigma is attached to extended care homes. There are other reasons, as well, that deter use of long-term care, including the fact that many nursing homes are too expensive for most South Asian families to afford.

Some professionals in Canada have found that when families are considering nursing-home care for an elderly parent, the family benefits from visits to two or three nursing homes to see what they are like.

While there are a few nursing homes established by the South Asian community (for example, in the Vancouver area), they usually have long waiting lists. So most elderly persons must be cared for in a home that has a mixed ethnic population of residents and staff. Many elderly South Asians who have been sponsored by their children have never learned English. They can become very socially isolated in mainstream nursing homes even though staff sometimes use simple cue-cards and try to learn basic words of their language, for "pain," "toilet," and so on. If an elderly person is native-language literate, some families have helped with language problems by fastening to the elderly person's bed a list of common problems and questions written both in the native language and English, which allows the patient to point to the appropriate message.

As with other immigrant groups, elderly patients and their families can be confused by the choices offered by physicians in extended care. For example, a physician might ask a son whether he wants to have a "do not resuscitate" order on his elderly mother's chart or to allow tube-feeding. Such choices are not usually given in South Asian countries, where physicians decide. Children have therefore never discussed these issues with parents, nor have parents indicated their preferences by saying things like "I don't want to be kept alive by a machine," a statement common among elderly people in the West. Thus some family members are put on the spot by staff questions, not knowing what the issues are or what the parent might want.

For elderly nursing-home residents who wander, climb out of bed, and so on, staff are usually reluctant to use restraints unless there is real danger to the patient. They see physical and psychological benefits from allowing an elderly person to be independent and move around. In contrast, South Asian families are more likely to be concerned with safety and to request restraints, such as asking that a restraining belt be attached so an old person cannot leave a wheelchair. These issues are difficult to negotiate, especially if there are language problems.

Death and Dying

Religious and other cultural beliefs support the South Asian's acceptance of death as part of life. Death is not hidden. For Hindus, there will be another life after death, and death is openly discussed by all, including children. Associated with acceptance of death is the idea of fatalism, that death will come when it is time for the person to die. This time may either be preordained by God (among Muslims) or determined by one's karma (among Hindus and Sikhs).

While there are specific rituals and practices in each religious community, some beliefs are common to all South Asians. Death at home is preferred, because the dying person's family can care for him or her and because the appropriate actions can be taken both before and after death. A peaceful death at home, surrounded by family, is strongly preferred to death in hospital, especially as the family may perceive that the dying person is being unnecessarily "tortured" by medical procedures.

In South Asia it is generally not the practice for a physician to inform the patient that death is approaching. Though this practice is quite common in Canada, it is threatening to the South Asian patient and family. Instead, the family might wish to be informed and be allowed to discuss the impending death with a physician. It is unlikely that they would pass on such upsetting information to the patient. In some cases, of course, the elderly South Asian person may recognize that death is imminent and may talk about it openly and comfortably with relatives.

When death occurs, it is expected that surviving families and friends will express their grief openly, by moaning and crying. It is rare that a death is taken serenely, and a person who does so may become the subject of criticism or gossip.

Hindu Death Rituals and Practices

Relatives may bring clothing and money for the dying person to touch before distributing them to the needy. They may sit by the dying person and read from a holy book or chant prayers. Both rituals are believed to be helpful in the person's next life. The dying person may want to look at a picture of a god so that the god will be at the forefront of the mind at the time of death.

The eldest surviving son plays an important part in the rituals after death. Along with other relatives, he washes the body and dresses it in new clothing.

In the case of a married woman, red clothing and jewellery signify her married state. When a person dies in a Canadian hospital, the family prefers to wash and dress the body before it is removed from the hospital. Hindus are reluctant to agree to a postmortem on the body.

In India as well as Canada, bodies are cremated, usually on the same day as death, and ashes are kept until they can be thrown onto the surface of the sacred river, the Ganges. In Canada, however, the family may scatter the ashes in a local river or the sea. Traditionally, cremation ceremonies are attended only by men.

A mourning period of forty days follows. For the first eighteen days friends and relatives visit and care for the dead person's family, to help them bear their grief. On the eighteenth day the family provides food for high-caste Brahmins and the poor so that the soul of the dead person will rest in peace. Often a further remembrance ceremony occurs one year after the death.

Muslim Death Rituals and Practices

As a person nears death, family and friends recite verses from the Koran to give support and encouragement to him or her. At death, grief is shown by crying and lamenting.

Once death has occurred, the body is ritually washed before being buried with the face pointing towards Mecca. If death occurs in hospital, it is preferred that staff not wash the body but simply turn the head towards the right shoulder before wrapping the body in a plain sheet. During these procedures family members may wish to read passages of scripture or to make lamentation.

Religious rules stipulate that the body should be buried as soon as possible after death and that it be complete and whole. For these reasons, Muslims will agree to a postmortem only if it is legally necessary and will request that the organs be returned to the body for burial. In Canada there are now several Muslim cemeteries in areas with relatively large Muslim populations.

Sikh Death Rituals and Practices

When a Sikh dies, family members prefer to wash the body and prepare it for cremation. The body is viewed at the hospital if that is where death occurred. Sikh men and women go to the crematorium where the eldest son usually lights the funeral pyre. Open display of emotions is acceptable and even expected. After the cremation there is a memorial service at the Sikh temple, at which time prayers are said for the soul of the person. Often another ceremony is held on the yearly anniversary of the death. Like other South Asians, Sikhs do not readily agree to postmortems or organ donations.

Use of Health and Social Services

In South Asia, and in the many countries from which people of South Asian culture have emigrated, health services are privately run and must be sought out by the people who choose to use them. There are no government-sponsored social services as in Canada. Instead, families are expected to help relatives who are in need of money, household help, and other special care. There is little experience with social service agencies and sometimes a distrust of all government servants.

Thus, when South Asian families come to Canada, many find the activities of public health nurses and social workers unfamiliar and often threatening. In particular, home visits by such people are not always acceptable, and South Asian families are likely to use social service agencies only as a last resort, after seeking help from family, friends, the temple, or a physician. Financial help from social agencies is frowned upon and thus only reluctantly accepted.

Further Reading

Ananth, J. 1984. "Treatment of immigrant Indian patients." *Canadian Journal of Psychiatry* 29: 490-93.

Assanand, Shashi. 2001. "Cultural concerns of immigrant and visible minority women." In Rosemary Gaghlinger-Beaune, ed., *Modelling Equality: Support Groups for Abused Women: A Handbook for Facilitators*. Burnaby, BC: VINA (Violence Is Never Acceptable) Community Coordinating Committee. Sponsored by Burnaby Family Life Institute.

Bhandari Preisser, Amita. 1999. "Domestic violence in South Asian communities in America: Advocacy and intervention." *Violence against Women* 5: 684-99.

Bhattacharya, Gauri. 2000. "The school adjustment of South Asian immigrant children in the United States." *Adolescence* 35: 77-85.

Buchignani, Norman, and Doreen M. Indra. 1985. *Continuous Journey: A Social History of South Asians in Canada*. Toronto, ON: McClelland and Stewart.

Grewal, Manpreet. 2003. "Abused woman's mental scars will carry her in-laws' names." *Vancouver Sun,* 17 July, A13.

Jain, S. 1971. *East Indians in Canada*. The Hague: Klop Press.

Jiwani, Yasmin. 2001. *Intersecting Inequalities: Immigrant Women of Colour, Violence and Health Care*. Vancouver, BC: FREDA Centre for Research on Violence against Women and Children.

Kanungo, Rabindra N., ed. 1984. *South Asians in the Canadian Mosaic*. Montreal: Kala Bharati Foundation.

Mason, E.S., D.P. Davies, and W.A. Marshall. 1982. "Early post-natal weight gain: Comparison between Asian and white Caucasian infants." *Early Human Development* 6: 253-55.

Prathikanti, Sudha. 1997. "East Indian American families." In Evelyn Lee, ed., *Working with Asian Americans: A Guide for Clinicians,* 79-100. New York: Guilford.

Ramakrishnan, Jayashree, and Mitchell Weiss. 1992. "Health, illness and immigration: East Indians in the United States." In "Cross-Cultural Medicine. A Decade Later" (Special Issue). *Western Journal of Medicine* 157: 265-70.

Contributors to the first edition

Soma Ganesan, Physician, Vancouver General Hospital

Kuldip Gill, Anthropology, University of British Columbia
Guninder Mumick, Vancouver Health Department
Kanwal Inder Singh Neel, Richmond
Joseph Richardson, Ganges, BC
Reverend Vasant Saklikar, New Westminster

Contributors to the second edition
Mandy Channa, Penticton and District Multicultural Society
Habib Chaudhury, Gerontology, Simon Fraser University
D.P. Goel, Family Physician, Vancouver
Parm Grewal, South Asian Women's Centre, Vancouver
Mangula and Jagdish Kumar Jit, Vancouver
Truus Kotwal, Physiotherapist, Holy Family Hospital, Burnaby
Hardev Mann, Sunset Community Centre, Surrey
Kanwal Inder Singh Neel, Steveston Secondary School, Richmond
Penticton Focus Group: Six young female agricultural workers, recent immigrants
Shiraz Ramji, Gerontologist, Burnaby
Mary Regester, Nursing, University of British Columbia
The late Reverend Vasant Saklikar, New Westminster
Rob Sandhu, Transitions Program, University of British Columbia
Veena Sikka, MOSAIC, Vancouver
Kulbir Singh, Psychiatrist, Vancouver General Hospital
Sunera Thobani, Women's Studies, University of British Columbia

7
People of Vietnamese Descent

Dai-Kha Dinh, Soma Ganesan, and Nancy Waxler-Morrison

After the end of the Vietnam War, during the late 1970s and early 1980s, very large numbers of Vietnamese arrived as refugees in Canada – as many as 58,000 in one year alone. These were the "boat people" who escaped under devastating conditions and settled in refugee camps in neighbouring countries. Many of these refugee families have by now become well settled in Canada and in turn have sponsored relatives and spouses. These more recent immigrants from Vietnam make up two distinct groups, elderly parents and young wives. The new issues raised by these recent immigrants along with changes in established refugee families, such as the aging of the population, bring new challenges to professionals who work with Vietnamese.

Geography

Vietnam is about one-third the size of British Columbia, with an eastern coastline on the South China Sea and a common border with China to the north and Laos and Cambodia (Kampuchea) to the west. The country is geographically divided into three regions. The climate varies considerably from one region to another. Northern Vietnam, mainly mountainous with a small delta of the Red River, has four distinct seasons. Central Vietnam, which is mainly plateau, and Southern Vietnam, which is a large alluvial plain along the Mekong River, have a tropical climate with a wet season from May until November. In Hanoi, in the north, average temperatures can range from fifteen degrees Celsius in the winter to thirty degrees in the summer, while Ho Chi Minh City, in the south, is warmer, averaging between twenty-five and thirty degrees Celsius year-round. Adaptation to Canada's cold climate is therefore an initial problem for many Vietnamese immigrants.

Population

In 2000 the population of Vietnam was seventy-eight million, of which 80 percent were rural. Most Vietnamese work in agriculture, growing rice, maize, coconut, coffee, rubber, new varieties of fruit, and tea, or work as fishermen or on fish farms. The urban population is mainly in three large cities, Hanoi, Ho Chi Minh City (formerly Saigon), and Haiphong. One-third of the population is under fifteen years of age. Life expectancy in 1999 was seventy-one years for women and sixty-six for men.

Ethnic and Cultural Groups in Vietnam

While the large majority are ethnic Vietnamese, there are several minority ethnic groups: Thai, Muong, Tho, Cham, and Kha (Malay-Indonesians), East Indians, and, of most significance for migration to Canada, the Chinese, who constitute only 2 percent of Vietnam's population. All speak the Vietnamese language, which varies only slightly across the country.

The Chinese, most of whom descend from migrants from south China, have been in Vietnam for many generations. The majority speak either Cantonese or Trieu Chau, a dialect of Guangdong province, and most, particularly the Chinese in southern Vietnam, run urban businesses, ranging from one-person food stalls to large import-export enterprises. The Chinese community remains separate from the Vietnamese, each having its own residential communities, schools, and organizations. They hold negative stereotypes about one another, a pattern that lingers after migration to Canada.

History of Vietnam

Vietnam has for many centuries struggled against outside powers interested in its rich farmlands and its strategic position. Until the 1600s China sometimes occupied and controlled Vietnam.

French Dominance, 1883-1954

European expansion brought first the Portuguese and then the French. The latter penetrated Vietnam by means of Catholic missions, the French East India Company, and military force. French dominance continued until the 1950s, except for a brief time during the Second World War when the Japanese ruled and a short-lived period of Vietnamese independence in 1945-46. In 1954 the Vietnamese, led by Ho Chi Minh and the Communist Party, defeated the French at the famous battle of Dien Bien Phu.

French rule resulted in the introduction of French language and culture, the spread of Roman Catholicism, the building of cities, and a transformation of the rural class structure. Some peasants became rich landowners, while others lost their land and became labourers. Large extended families began to break up, leaving only the eldest son at home while younger children found homes elsewhere. More villagers moved to low-level jobs in towns where an urban middle class was growing. This "modernization" of many aspects of Vietnamese life was stimulated by French rule.

Division of the Country and the Vietnam War, 1954-76

After the 1954 defeat of the French, an international conference divided the country into North Vietnam, ruled by the Communists who were backed by Russia, and South Vietnam, ruled by the nationalists who were backed by the United States. The latter sent troops to Vietnam in 1965 to defend the South against the North. The Vietnam War (or the Anti-American War, as Vietnamese refer to it) ended in 1975 when the American forces withdrew in defeat, triggering the first wave of refugees: South Vietnamese government officials, members of the army, and their middle-class supporters, who rushed to leave the country.

Reunification of the Country, 1976

When the Communist government of North Vietnam took over the South, it began to carry out radical reforms there as it had done in the North after 1954. In the North, to achieve the goal of destroying all social classes, the government confiscated private property, collectivized land, and nationalized production. Two classes were recognized: public service workers (teachers, factory workers, traders) and peasants working on the land. Individual liberties were abolished. Polygamy and early marriage were prohibited, and men and women were pronounced equal. Many of these changes were replicated in the South, although with somewhat different economic policies.

These radical economic and social changes, along with a brief invasion by China in 1978 and a short-lived anti-Chinese policy in the North, led to a second wave of refugees – the "boat people" – in 1979, when many ethnic Vietnamese along with Vietnamese of Chinese background fled the country.

Vietnam since the Late 1980s

The government's radical social policies produced economic stagnation and international isolation and eventually forced Vietnam to introduce some free-market reforms in the late 1980s. Better relations were established with China, and in 1994-95 the United States lifted its nineteen-year economic embargo and re-established diplomatic relations. Today the Communist Party continues to control the government, and the economy is growing, but Vietnam still receives foreign aid. There is also some measure of government control of religious expression, of the press, and of opportunities such as university admission. In general, people's lives are improving, though many are still poor, particularly in rural areas.

Migration to Canada

Immigration before 1975

There were about 1,500 Vietnamese living in Canada prior to the end of the Vietnam War, mostly students or professionals who had come for training or economic advancement and had settled in Quebec where their knowledge of French was helpful.

The First Wave of Refugees, 1975-78

The early refugees, about 7,800 of whom came to Canada, sought safety abroad because they had been associated with the South Vietnamese government or the American forces. Many brought skills and language that facilitated their adaptation to Canada, since they were middle-class, urban, and relatively well educated. Many left behind most or all of their property and often some family members. Some chose Canada because they had relatives here. Most settled in Quebec.

The Second Wave of Refugees, 1978 to the Late 1980s

This second, very large group is generally referred to as the "boat people." As the Communist regime began to reorganize Vietnam's economy and society, an initial trickle of refugees began to appear in 1978 in places like Malaysia, Thailand, and Hong Kong. A year later that trickle had turned into a torrent; in one month, June 1979, an estimated 57,000 people left Vietnam by boat. This enormous exodus was at least in part encouraged and approved by the Vietnamese government. Almost all these migrants found themselves in refugee camps elsewhere in Asia, where they awaited admittance by Canada and other countries, a wait that sometimes lasted years. In 1979 and 1980, 58,000 refugees from Vietnam were admitted to Canada. By 1985 more Vietnamese refugees had come to Canada than to any other country.

The "boat people" represented a much broader segment of the population than those who left earlier. Of those reaching Canada, about 60 percent were ethnic Vietnamese. Some had previously migrated from North to South Vietnam when the Communists took over the North in 1954; others were Northerners who went south later.

About 40 percent of the refugees who came to Canada were ethnic Chinese who had lived in Vietnam for generations. They were forced out by government policies in which Chinese-owned businesses were expropriated by the state and the former owners were "relocated" to the countryside or to "new economic zones" (Dorais 2000). The loss of their livelihood and the traditional antagonism and distrust between themselves and the Vietnamese led them to fear for their future. Many fled by boat in semi-official voyages sanctioned by the authorities and costing them a good portion of their savings.

The experiences of this second wave of "boat people" were devastating. What property they were able to carry was often stolen or used to pay bribes before embarking. Pirates, many from Thailand, preyed on the boats, raping and murdering for the sake of what they could steal. One estimate is that 50 percent of those who left Vietnam's shores died or were murdered on the way. These trials were reflected, in the West, in the mental health problems experienced by refugees from Vietnam.

Those who did survive the exodus were held in refugee camps in Malaysia, Hong Kong, Thailand, and Indonesia. The United Nations and other international agencies gave financial support and instituted systems for screening and accepting refugees. But for the refugees themselves this arrangement resulted in delays of months and years before they were allowed to move on.

Family Reunification and Recent Immigration, 1982-2004

As soon as refugees began to establish themselves in Canada, they sought to sponsor family members for immigration. More than half of the 34,000 Vietnamese who entered Canada between 1983 and 1986 came to join their families. This pattern has continued, though the total number of Vietnamese immigrants dropped year by year, from 9,000 in 1990 to 2,707 in 1996.

At first, reunification usually involved close family members, children, spouses, and others who had become separated in the rush to leave or who had been left in Vietnam with the hope of joining up later. More recently, two distinct groups of immigrants have appeared. The first are elderly parents who are sponsored by their children, that is, by children who have become economically successful enough to meet the government's stringent requirements for sponsorship. The second group consists of newly wed young women chosen as wives by Vietnamese men on a trip to Vietnam. Most of these men had arrived in Canada as young, single refugees in the late 1970s and had not married in Canada because there were few Vietnamese women of a similar age. In contrast to the refugees, these sponsored immigrants do not have government help with settlement, such as finding jobs, but some do benefit from the support of the well-established Vietnamese community. In addition to these new immigrants, young people have begun to come on student visas for education.

Settlement of Refugees in Canada

Initial Settlement

Once they arrived in Canada, the Vietnamese "boat people" were aided by the federal government or by private sponsors, often church groups. Refugees settled where their sponsors or immigration offices were located and thus, at first, lived in many parts of the country. Some found themselves in small towns and even in the Arctic, isolated from other Vietnamese. This large group was less educated than earlier Vietnamese migrants, and few spoke English or French. Many were young, single men with no family. In their first year all received considerable help from sponsors and government with things like housing, schooling, work, language training, and health care. Their first few years were focused on the basics: establishing a home, finding any kind of work, learning enough English or French to survive, and dealing with the loss of home and the memories of escape from Vietnam.

Neither the ethnic Vietnamese nor the Chinese refugees had forerunners in Canada whose community they could join. The refugees distinguished themselves along lines of politics, class, and geography (northern or southern origin) and so could not easily join the earlier arrivals. Chinese from Vietnam, though they speak Cantonese, are thought of as Chinese-speaking Vietnamese by the Hong Kong Chinese community and were not usually included in Hong Kong community activities. Nor were they always included in Vietnamese activities. In contrast to many other immigrant groups, the refugees from Vietnam were faced with the task of constructing their own sense of community.

Becoming Established

By 2001 there were 148,000 persons born in Vietnam living in Canada, and the large majority had become Canadian citizens. Many had migrated within the country, mainly to live in Toronto, Montreal, Vancouver, or Calgary. Most had learned either English or French but spoke Vietnamese or Chinese at home. There were more men than women. Compared with people born in Canada, Vietnamese were somewhat less likely to be employed (66 percent of adult men had jobs compared with 76 percent of Canadian-born men) and had somewhat lower incomes. A positive sign for the community's future was the fact that a greater proportion of young immigrants from Vietnam aged fifteen to twenty-four were in school (69 percent) than of Canadian-born young people (61 percent).

Certainly a sense of community has been established. Large cities have Vietnamese newspapers and radio stations. There are many Vietnamese Buddhist temples and other religious organizations as well as associations of Vietnamese professionals of all kinds, social agencies such as seniors' drop-in centres, job-training centres, AIDS prevention services, and so on. Many refugee families have also become established, with good jobs, purchased houses, and well-educated children. And there are significant numbers of Vietnamese professionals, such as physicians, social workers, pharmacists, and nurses.

When Vietnamese refugees first arrived in the 1970s, they were divided according to their political allegiance in Vietnam. Most people were hesitant to trust someone known to have supported the "other side," whether Communists or nationalists. Vietnamese selecting a doctor often made inquiries in advance to determine the physician's politics. Social life also tended to divide along Vietnamese political lines. By the late 1990s this division seemed to be less important, in part because it appeared to be less important in Vietnam as well. However, whether the individual is originally from the north or the south continues to be an important factor, linked less to politics than to group stereotypes about the different life experiences in the once-divided country. Southerners sometimes believe that those raised in the north are less knowledgeable (for example, about Western medicine) because they have lived in poor conditions, while northerners may think of southerners as rude or culturally less refined. As a result these two groups still do not socialize more than superficially.

Reconnections with Vietnam

Many Vietnamese in Canada became well enough established to have time and money to visit Vietnam, often for several months. Money is important, because visitors are expected to bring gifts for relatives and friends – an expectation that prevents some from making the trip. Others send plane tickets to relatives so they can visit Canada. Vietnamese temples and other associations have organized and funded philanthropic projects in Vietnam, such as establishing clinics and orphanages, doing eye surgeries, and teaching English. Some young people have returned to work temporarily in Vietnam in order to learn about the country. While many retired persons consider returning permanently to Vietnam, very few do so, in part because regulations about property ownership are still unclear. The only permanent returnees are elderly parents who have been sponsored for residence in Canada by their children but who find it impossible to adapt to a new language and culture.

Jobs and Income in Canada

When the large wave of "boat people" arrived in Canada, government and private sponsors provided initial financial aid, expecting that the refugees would quickly find jobs. Sponsors sometimes paid little attention to the refugees' long-term employment goals or previous work experience. Getting work was just as important to the refugees themselves, who were keen to be financially independent. Yet most men were forced by necessity and lack of English to take low-level service and factory jobs that were often incompatible with their higher levels of education and previous work experience. Many men took on two jobs, working very long hours for little pay to meet living expenses and to buy clothing and medicines to send home. The economic burden was even greater because many felt strong obligations to help family members left at home or still living in refugee camps. The need to document savings in order to sponsor further family migration to Canada was an additional incentive to take two jobs, to search for work before learning adequate English, or to move to better-paying but perhaps dead-end jobs.

While it was not common for women to work outside the home in Vietnam, many immediately did so in Canada, where a second income was usually necessary to meet living expenses. As with the men, women were largely limited to poorly paid jobs in factories, hotels, hospitals, and restaurants. As a result, by 1981, 59 percent of adult Southeast Asian women in Canada were working, a fact that entailed considerable change in family responsibilities and roles.

By 1991 many who arrived as "boat people" had managed to obtain training, upgrade their skills, improve their English, and move into more stable and better-paid employment, even though incomes were lower and unemployment was higher, on average, than among Canadian-born persons. Many Vietnamese remained overqualified for their jobs, in part because they could not afford to take time from work to obtain Canadian qualifications. More than half of adult women, 54 percent, continued to work in 1991. Through the 1990s many continued to feel strong obligations to help relatives left at home or languishing in refugee camps by sending money or trying to qualify financially to sponsor them as landed immigrants.

At first the majority of Vietnamese workers were in manufacturing or service jobs, but soon many, particularly those of Chinese background, had opened small businesses such as restaurants and corner stores. In addition, by the end of the century there were more professionals and owners of mid-size and large businesses. However, in 2000 some of the "boat people" continued to have only minimum wage, hourly-paid employment, the kind of job they found on arrival in Canada in 1978-80. Some of those who were older when they arrived in Canada and who never learned much English or French have never been able to move from low-level jobs and therefore remain poor.

Religion

People in Vietnam have a rather pluralistic view of religion. A family might identify itself as Buddhist but might also worship at a variety of shrines and follow the precepts of Confucianism. Only the Christians, who make up 10-15 percent of Vietnam's population and are mostly Roman Catholic, see themselves as belonging to a specific religious organization with a distinctive set of practices. Even many Christians recognize the values associated with the traditional religions.

The majority of Vietnamese try to follow the central teachings of Confucius: to serve one's king or country, to respect one's teachers and father, to behave as a good and wise man. From Buddhism comes the idea of karma, which holds that one's destiny is set by one's moral behaviour in past lives. And pervasive throughout Vietnam is ancestor worship, whereby the souls of one's ancestors are believed to be the natural protectors of one's family. In Vietnamese homes in both Vietnam and Canada, there may be a small altar dedicated to Buddha and to family ancestors at which family members offer prayer and seek ancestral blessings.

In 1991, 43 percent of Vietnamese-born residents of Canada were Buddhists. When they arrived, there were few Vietnamese Buddhist temples, but over the years Buddhist monks have come from Vietnam and the number of temples has increased. By 1998, there were about thirty pagodas in Canada, the majority in Montreal, Toronto, and Vancouver but also some in smaller communities. Temples not only are places of worship but also tend to represent strong communities that provide mutual support and practical aid for persons in need. A smaller number of Vietnamese in Canada, 15 percent in 1991, were Roman Catholic, a group that has also initiated aid programs for social and medical needs in Vietnam. Some refugees were sponsored by Canadian Protestant groups, so about 5 percent of Vietnamese participate in or have organized their own Protestant churches. However, in 1991, a relatively large proportion of Vietnamese, 36 percent, reported no religious affiliation, compared with 15 percent of all immigrants and 12 percent of Canadian-born persons.

Language

In Vietnam, most people speak Vietnamese while the Chinese minority usually speaks both Cantonese and Vietnamese. Among Vietnamese speakers, differences in accents and colloquial expressions make it difficult for natives of the three main regions of the country to fully understand each other. Some older persons speak French, and a few know Russian, but

English is now the main second language among businessmen, academics, and government officials.

Most of the "boat people" who arrived after the Vietnam War refugees spoke neither English nor French. Some could not read or write their own spoken language. Thus, the largest proportion of people from Vietnam faced an acute language problem in Canada. Young children learned the new language quickly and became the go-betweens, thus threatening the traditional authority of father and mother. The adult's sense of isolation and lack of control over family life often continued until fluency was achieved in English or French.

By 1991, 85 percent of Vietnamese in Canada could conduct a conversation either in English or in French. Most still spoke Vietnamese or Chinese at home. As more and more children progressed through the Canadian school system, parents began to worry that the Vietnamese language would be lost; more recently these parents have begun to accept that the main language will be a Canadian one. In fact, by the late 1990s many young families of Vietnamese background communicated only in English or French. As a result some grandparents cannot communicate with their grandchildren, and the new English-speaking cohort of Vietnamese professionals such as doctors and social workers sometimes has difficulty communicating with older Vietnamese-speaking clients.

The more recent immigrants from Vietnam, young wives and the elderly who have come in the late 1990s, usually have little or no English when they arrive. Wives often do not attend language classes because they have family responsibilities and husbands are concerned about them leaving the home. Elderly grandparents who have come recently are also very unlikely to learn English.

Family Structure

For a person from Vietnam, the family is the main source of identity, and loyalty to family is primary. In Vietnam, the traditional family often included three generations, and this remains the ideal. However, nuclear families with husband, wife, and their children are now more common, given the socioeconomic changes in modern Vietnam. Even though large family networks may not actually live in the same home, the authority of elders, especially male elders, is still recognized, despite greater individual freedom on some issues, as in, for example, marriage "for love," which is the norm, not the exception.

Traditionally in Vietnam, women, had fewer rights than men, such as in access to education, but many women often worked, acquired professional training, or ran small businesses such as village rice mills. Indeed, women

Mrs. Nguyen, from Vietnam

Mrs. Nguyen, now seventy-four, came to Canada in 1992, sponsored by her two sons. She lives with her unmarried son in Richmond. She takes care of their apartment and has several Vietnamese friends from the temple but has learned only a few words of English. Two years after arriving she complained of pains in her stomach. Her son took her to a Vietnamese-speaking doctor, who prescribed pills for her to take as needed. But because the pills cost one dollar each, she was hesitant to use them. She tolerated the pain for two years, but then it worsened. After talking about it with a friend, she decided she must go back to the doctor.

Mrs. Nguyen was very reluctant to ask her unmarried son, who works as a labourer in a warehouse, or her other son, who lives about twenty miles away, to take time from work to accompany her to the doctor. Each son might lose a whole day's pay. She said, "I thought I knew where the doctor's office was so I decided to walk there. I tried to find the way. Well, the roads are like many flowers; I did not know which one to choose. I was lost. The roads here are wide and so long. Finally I had to ask for a taxi and it cost $9."

She continued, "When it was time for me to go home I walked out of the doctor's office and I did not know which way I should go, whether to go up or down the street. So I kept walking up the street; when I didn't see anything familiar, I walked back. I walked up then down and up again, then down again for a long time. Even if I had phoned my son at work I would have to tell him the name of the street, the corner where I am. But I could not say the name so even if I called my son he would not know where to find me. Often I tried to find my way around. Finally, I saw a white man reading a newspaper. I showed him my address and he showed me the way."

She then went on to say, "The doctor told me I should go for a test at the big hospital in Vancouver but I don't think I will go any time soon. I don't want to bother my children. I can't afford expensive taxis and I might get lost if I tried to go on the bus."

With permission of Tam Truong Donnelly

were considered "more rational and calculating in financial matters than men" (Van Esterisk 1980, 160). Thus, while elder men in the family were approached for major decisions, the wife or mother usually enjoyed considerable, if subtle, power.

The Refugee Families

Many families were separated when attempting to leave Vietnam. Some individuals left the country on their own, having been chosen to use family funds to go abroad in the hope that others might follow later. Others became separated during the exodus or in the refugee camps. In Canada many refugees initially created substitute "families" for economic and emotional reasons, by joining together to share housing. Some intact families took in others, creating extended families; few nuclear families could afford to live separately.

Obligations to family members outside Canada were very strong, often limiting the individual's or family's ability to become established by getting further training or buying a house.

The fact that most women found work more easily then men and therefore made important financial contributions to the family often undermined men's authority; additional stress occurred if a working wife sought in her own family the equality she saw in relationships between Canadian couples. The fact that Vietnamese women often continued to work even after their husbands found jobs meant that readjustments have continued far beyond the early years in Canada. In some of these families, permanent role changes have occurred, with husbands now taking pride in their cooking and often sharing child care with their wives.

After the initial problems were solved, other family issues become more important. Children adapted quickly to Canadian language and lifestyles and began to grow away from their families. Conflict, particularly at adolescence, left parents feeling that they were losing their hitherto unquestioned authority. Parents saw their children losing the Vietnamese or Chinese culture they wanted to preserve. This often coincided with parental realization that the family's future rested, not with themselves, but with their children. This realization led parents to strongly encourage and support their children's education. The children of these refugee families have become young adults, and most have become Canadian in choosing to live in their own nuclear families, not in extended families with their parents.

The refugee families lived through extremely stressful situations: escape from Vietnam, years in refugee camps, and then the challenge of starting anew in an unknown country with a very different culture and language. As a result they had to work hard and support each other, becoming what many professionals see as very strong and resilient families.

Family Reunification

Vietnamese who arrived as immigrants sponsored by family members already in Canada moved into a well-established Vietnamese community that provides support and services. However, many were totally unprepared for the reality of life in Canada, having heard sometimes inflated descriptions from Canadian Vietnamese visitors as well as having seen films and television programs that do not reflect the lives of average Westerners. Moreover, family members who have been separated for years find very large cultural gaps have opened and must be negotiated. Marital relationships may have suffered, and spouses may have had casual non-marital relationships during the separation. When reunited they must learn to live together again. Elderly parents sponsored by adult children also face difficulties since their knowledge and experience in Vietnam, the basis of their high status in the family, is not useful in Canada.

Men who came to Canada as refugees have recently been returning to Vietnam to find wives. Typically, these are men in their forties who choose a younger woman, sometimes as young as nineteen or twenty years of age. Because the sponsorship process takes time, some of these women arrive in Canada along with the couple's first child. Settlement tends to be difficult for these families. Women often expect, or have been led to expect, a higher standard of living than their husbands can provide. Husbands, in turn, worry that their new wives will leave them, as sometimes happens. As a result women may be discouraged from leaving the home for language classes or a job, and, lacking relatives in Canada, they become isolated. These women have left familiar surroundings to live in a foreign country, often with someone who is essentially also a stranger. There can be physical abuse if husbands lack the emotional or practical resources to deal with this situation. The task of establishing mutual trust is often difficult. The wife's first contact with formal support often occurs at pregnancy, when a public health nurse comes to visit. Relationships tend to improve when the wife makes contacts outside the home, particularly if she finds a job and learns some English.

Child-Rearing

Traditional Vietnamese child care seems unfamiliar to most Westerners, to whom much of it seems to consist of "spoiling" the baby. Instead of being allowed to cry, an infant would be held by the mother or an older sibling. Vietnamese children therefore did not start walking as early as Western children. When a new baby arrived, its predecessor would be abruptly weaned and handed over to the care of an older sibling.

Most child discipline and training was by example and thus was not usually a planned strategy. Toilet-training would occur only when small children decided to imitate their older siblings. In many families in Vietnam, toddlers did not wear underpants and urinated wherever they happened to be. The same learning-by-experience strategy was used for teaching other skills to young children: what to eat and wear, and how to speak. When parents did discipline children it might be by speaking, shouting, slapping, or asking the child to kneel facing the wall. While it did not happen often, parents were believed to be within their rights to beat a child, and outsiders were expected not to intervene. Yet Vietnamese parents expected their children to follow their guidance without discussion or question. One result was that children tended not to express anger openly but instead to be stubborn or passively uncooperative.

Many practical aspects of child-rearing changed over the years as families adapted to Canada. As well, new problems have arisen. For the first decade or so after they arrived as refugees, parents attempted to maintain control over their growing children. But parents have come to accept that, while they still provide some guidance, their children will be more independent in Canada as adolescents and young adults. The situation of adolescent girls has changed as parents recognize the advantages of the freedom to obtain a good education, notwithstanding the independence that goes with it. Parents see that education will not only improve their children's economic status but also give their daughters stronger positions in their marriages.

Most Vietnamese parents have learned through the media and elsewhere that physical abuse of a child is unacceptable and illegal in Canada. However, the Vietnamese professional community recognizes that child abuse and other family violence is a significant problem for some Vietnamese families.

The more recent arrival of Vietnamese wives who have been sponsored by men long resident in Canada has raised new issues for young children. Because many of these women are isolated, with no job, little English, and no relatives to help, they become depressed, a condition which then limits their interactions with their children. In some cases children's speech develops late, a problem not always noted until they begin school. Also, bottle-feeding may be prolonged and solid food not introduced if the mother has low energy or believes milk is the most nutritious food for the child.

Marriage

Marriages in Vietnam were traditionally arranged by both sets of parents, and couples rarely made independent choices. The new wife moved to her husband's father's home, thus joining a new family and learning to live and work with her mother-in-law. While most marriages were within an ethnic community, some Chinese men took Vietnamese wives. Neither husband nor wife expected a marriage to be close and personally fulfilling. They tended to socialize separately, and if the husband sometimes drank or visited prostitutes with his friends, his wife would shrug the matter off as typical male behaviour. The marriage itself was not usually threatened. Today in Vietnam some of these traditional marriage norms have changed, notably the shift from arranged marriages to marriages based on love.

When the largest waves of people arrived in Canada from Vietnam, there were many single men without families, fewer young unmarried women, and few intact families. The young men, once they had become economically established, at first often travelled long distances to find Vietnamese wives. Some of them married women from other Asian countries, such as the Philippines. Initially there were few intermarriages with Anglo-European Canadians, though in the new century these are becoming more common.

The single men who came to Canada as refugees and who return to Vietnam to meet prospective wives find women willing, and sometimes very eager, to migrate to Canada. Often these marriages are arranged in advance, with the bride coming from the man's home village or being related to a friend. These marriages, as described earlier, are sometimes dysfunctional and abusive and some break down. It is much less common for a young woman to return to Vietnam for a spouse, but when this occurs the outcome is generally much better for the couple.

Today the traditional separation of husband and wife roles is beginning to break down in Canada as those who arrived as children grow up here. It is more common to find spouses who have closer emotional relationships, who share household and child care tasks, and have mutual trust.

Divorce

Divorce was traditionally uncommon in Vietnam, as in other cultures in which marriages are arranged and thought of as family contracts. Women usually chose to endure the marriage rather than to suffer ostracism for having left their husbands. Today in Vietnam divorce has become more acceptable if living together has become physically or emotionally intolerable.

In Canada, divorce was not common among the couples who arrived as refugees. When it did occur, it often resulted from the stresses caused by the wife's becoming the breadwinner and the husband's central role being diminished; the stress would lead to abuse and then to divorce. As in Vietnam, divorce has now generally been accepted in Canada as better than staying in an untenable marriage.

Names

Names of both Vietnamese and Chinese people from Vietnam may confuse record keepers, though immigrants often adapt their names to Western conventions after they have lived in Canada for a while. However, family and given names are traditionally put in the opposite order from Western names. The family name comes first and the given name last, with one or sometimes two names in between. For example, a Vietnamese man might be Nguyen Trong Thiet (comparable to Smith George Jim).

Women in both Chinese and Vietnamese communities usually do not change their names after marriage. Thus married couples do not have family names in common. However, the children take their father's name, which means that mothers and their children have different names.

Common Chinese surnames from Vietnam are Chau, Ha, Luu, Ly, Luong, Ong, Pho, Tang, and Vuong. Common Vietnamese surnames are Cao, Dinh, Hoang, Le, Luu, Ly, Ngo, Nguyen, Phan, and Tran. Because at least two Vietnamese surnames are very common (Nguyen and Tran), Vietnamese people are commonly distinguished informally by use of their given name rather than their family name. For example, Nguyen Trong Thiet may be called "Mr. Thiet" in order to distinguish him from the many other people sharing the family name of Nguyen. Or a personal characteristic may be added (Vien map, or "fat Vien") to distinguish individuals.

Ages

In some instances confusion about a child's age may arise since, traditionally, a baby is one year old at birth, rather than at the end of the first year of life.

Values

Many people from Vietnam are preoccupied with maintaining face and avoiding open disagreement or confrontation. So long as relationships, particularly with one's superiors, are smooth, everyone knows how to behave, and everyone knows who has obligations to whom. Thus it is important to smile and to agree even when neither action really means consent or agreement. While a Canadian doctor may suspect that a Vietnamese patient has stopped taking prescribed medicines, the patient may deny the allegation, desiring to avoid embarrassing the physician by acknowledging that the instructions have been disregarded. Public health nurses may expect that a mother will bring her child to a well-baby appointment to which she has apparently agreed, only to find that the mother's so-called agreement was a polite "yes" meant to avoid disagreement. A "yes" during a conversation with a superior or stranger is a polite way to say "I am listening" but does not mean "I agree." To Westerners these actions may seem evasive, but to the Vietnamese they are honourable, and are meant to prevent mutual embarrassment.

Gestures

Facial expressions and body movements common to people from Vietnam have a high value in maintaining smooth and predictable relationships. Vietnamese prefer formal relationships with others, not the first-name or bantering mode of conversation adopted by Westerners. Politeness is important, resulting in smiles that do not necessarily mean agreement or even understanding. Impassive facial expressions and controlled body movements often make it difficult for Canadians to understand what a Vietnamese person is thinking. Yet, for the Vietnamese, the politeness and formality are entirely proper.

Vietnamese people are sometimes uncomfortable with steady and direct eye contact and would prefer fleeting glances, although eye contact during conversation is now the norm for middle-class persons. The person's head is believed to be sacred and therefore should not be touched without prior explanation. Patting a child on the head, a common gesture in the West, does not have the same meaning in Vietnam. Just as the head is sacred, the feet are profane and should not be pointed directly towards another person. A beckoning gesture with the index finger is considered rude.

Many Vietnamese who have lived in Canada for a time, especially those who have grown up here, tend to take on Western styles of day-to-day interaction.

Traditional Health Beliefs and Practices

In pre-colonial times, Vietnamese used a variety of strategies to deal with illness, such as herbal remedies, isolation of the sick person, and visits to shrines and temples. Even now, when Western medical treatment is available, traditional beliefs are common, and traditional methods of treatment are often the family's first choice. Many of these beliefs and methods have been brought to Canada and continue to be used alongside, or instead of, Western medicine.

There are four main notions about illness in traditional Vietnamese medical beliefs: hot and cold equilibrium, good and bad wind and water, supernatural causes of illness, and hereditary causes of illness.

Hot and Cold

The two opposing forces in the universe, yin and yang, as identified in philosophies across Asia, are represented in traditional Vietnamese medicine as "cold" and "hot" respectively. Heat and cold in the body must be in perfect equilibrium if illness is to be avoided. Where there is too much heat in the body, fever, colitis, or skin eruptions may result. Excess cold explains fainting, diarrhea, or paralysis, among others. The delicate balance of the body can be upset in many ways, for instance by strong emotions. But the most important disturbance is from the foods one chooses to eat. Some foods are hot, others cold, so careful choice is required to retain, or regain, equilibrium. Some herbal medicines, also classified as hot or cold, aid in balancing the body.

Thus, according to these beliefs, a woman is in a cold condition after childbirth because she has lost heating blood. She should therefore avoid drinking cold juice or water and should not shower or wash her hair. If a person has a fever, there is concern that heat is being lost. Consequently, the feverish patient should be warmly covered, should avoid foods classified as cold (many vegetables and fruits), and should eat heating foods such as eggs and rice. Western medicine is believed to be hot and sometimes is not taken, or the dosage is reduced, if the patient believes that the illness is a hot one.

Because many illnesses are believed to be the result of excess bodily heat or cold, a person from Vietnam sometimes describes them as such, thereby confusing Canadian health professionals. For example, if a Vietnamese complains of being "hot," he does not necessarily have a fever but may have symptoms believed to be caused by an excess of heat in the body, such as constipation, dark urine, or hoarseness. A "weak heart" may refer to fainting, dizziness, or feelings of panic; a "weak kidney" to sexual dysfunction; and "weak nerves" to headaches or an inability to concentrate.

Wind and Water

The Vietnamese classify wind (or air) and water as good or bad. A bad wind can quickly induce high fever, convulsion, and even sudden death. Bad water is believed to have a slower effect on health, causing chronic fever, anemia, or muscle-wasting.

An attack of a bad wind is believed to require emergency measures to dispel it quickly. For some manifestations of bad wind (such as headache, cough, or motion sickness), the bad wind can be released by creating small bruises on the body, commonly effected by rubbing the body with a coin or a spoon or by cupping, that is, by placing a hot cup on the body and letting it cool until the air contracts and draws the skin upward. When bruise lines appear, the bad wind has come to the surface and left the body. While many

Canadian professionals are now aware of this practice, health professionals have sometimes suspected abuse when they discover these bruises on a child's body. In fact, parents have simply used a traditional medical treatment that is believed to help cure.

Supernatural Beliefs

In Vietnam, supernatural forces are often used to explain mental illness and, in the past, epidemics. Epidemics that caused many deaths were formerly considered to be the way in which armies from the underworld recruited their troops. A person with a mental illness may have done something to offend a god who, in turn, punishes him with the illness, or his body may simply have been possessed by a ghost or demon that uses it to go about devilish work. Sorcerers may be called to the person's home, or the ill person might stay in a Buddhist temple where the ghost will flee in fear of Buddha.

These supernatural beliefs are of little importance to Vietnamese who have lived in Canada for some time.

Heredity

Traditionally in Vietnam, many communicable diseases were believed to be hereditary, a plausible belief since many members of the same family came down with the same illness, such as tuberculosis or leprosy. Parents carefully investigated the family into which their child might marry, in order to avoid such inherited diseases. Many diseases believed to be inherited became highly stigmatized, particularly leprosy. Lepers lived alone in small huts outside the village fence and had no contact with anyone. Food was left for them at the door.

More recently, with the advent of Western medicine, beliefs about hereditary illnesses accord much more closely with Western ones, although some of the traditional "hereditary" diseases are still stigmatized, notably leprosy and mental illness.

Traditional Medical Practitioners

As is true in most societies, Vietnamese usually try home remedies before going to a medical practitioner. But if homemade medicines or particular foods do not cure, the next step is a visit to the herbal practitioner, who may either subscribe to a theory taught by Chinese-trained "professors" (northern herbalists) or follow Vietnamese folk theory (southern herbalists). Each practitioner also owns a herb shop and may have inherited family formulas to treat specific conditions such as asthma, piles, or fractures.

While being treated by the herbalist, patients are normally less concerned with knowing the diagnosis than with obtaining medicines, usually in the form of dry ingredients that they can cook at home. Today in Vietnam traditional practitioners tend to be used for less severe sicknesses, although they do practise in hospitals where they care for chronic cases.

Traditional Medicine in Canada

The Vietnamese in Canada are very open to using Western medicine, particularly for serious acute illnesses, a choice made easy by medicare. However, many at the same time use traditional medicines even though they may be more expensive and labour-intensive than taking Western pills. Some obtain ingredients for traditional medicine from Chinese herbalists; others arrange for them to be brought in from Vietnam. Some people understand Western medicine in traditional terms, so that Western medicine is "hot" while traditional medicine is "cold." Thus, a person who uses a traditional remedy may wait at least six hours before using Western pills. Many believe that traditional medicines are safer and less strong then Western ones, and they sometimes use traditional herbs to counteract the stronger, fast-acting medicine the doctor has prescribed. Some use Chinese acupuncture, especially for chronic problems.

Western Medicine in Vietnam

The French brought Western medicine to Vietnam in the last century, but health services were slow in developing, particularly in rural areas. Some attempts were made to control epidemics through vaccination programs, but not until Vietnamese themselves began to be trained as physicians did ordinary people in the towns start to use Western methods. People in rural areas continued to depend on herbal doctors and home remedies for most health care.

By the end of the Vietnam War in 1975 there was only one doctor for every 10,000 people, but services began to improve as doctors were supplemented by "assistant doctors" who worked in village health stations and referred some patients to district hospitals. Hospital care, when it was available, was free except for the food, which families often brought from home. Rural health services were more developed in the north than the south.

By 1999 there was one physician for every 2,122 persons and a corresponding improvement in access to health care. Patients going to public clinics were required to pay for many services including doctors' examinations, laboratory fees, and medicines. After 1996 the government allowed private health services, which expanded rapidly, though access still depended in part on where one lived. Many private physicians in Vietnam are government doctors who divide their time between public and private clinics. Most city-dwellers and well-to-do rural residents seek Western medicine rather than traditional medicine for all important medical problems

Common Diseases in Vietnam

Before Western medicine became available for ordinary people in Vietnam, infectious diseases were common: malaria, tuberculosis, smallpox, cholera, typhoid fever, plague, meningitis, and polio. Parasites such as tapeworm and hookworm were endemic, and poverty explained high rates of malnutrition. Many young children died from gastrointestinal disease or pneumonia.

With the development of modern medicine and the expansion of preventive measures, many of these diseases have been eradicated, controlled, or effectively treated. In 2002 the recent improvements in health were evident in the average life expectancy of seventy years and an infant mortality rate of twenty infant deaths per thousand births (compared to Canada's five per thousand).

Malaria is still endemic, but with better treatment and prevention by 2002 only forty-two persons died from malaria in the whole country. Tuberculosis, usually in the lung, is less prevalent and more effectively treated; since 1990 all newborns receive BCG vaccinations. Diagnosis and prevention of leprosy have improved; there were 141 new cases in Saigon in 2002, contrasted to an average of 1,500 per year in the 1950s. Typhoid fever outbreaks sometimes occur, usually connected to floods, but a new vaccination program has shown some success. In the past trachoma was a scourge in the North, but by 2003 it was very much reduced. Malnutrition has been reduced by better transportation, more even food distribution among the population, and improved education and treatment. Since 2002, hepatitis B vaccinations are being given in all schools and hospitals.

HIV/AIDS was first diagnosed in Vietnam in 1990, and since that time it has spread to all parts of the country. WHO projects that there will be 200,000 new cases per year in the first five years of the new century. The large majority of those infected are injection drug users, who have access to cheap heroin produced in nearby countries, and sex workers, mostly young rural women. Since married couples tend to accept that infidelity on the part of the husband is a normal part of marriage, HIV is spreading to the general population through contact with prostitutes. Tuberculosis remains the most common opportunistic infection causing death of persons with AIDS. The government has begun public education programs as well as clinics for treatment of sexually transmitted diseases.

Western medicines are sold by drugstores without prescription, though the practice is illegal. Thus a family doctor practising in Vietnam often sees infections that are resistant to antibiotics because so many patients have used antibiotics at home in insufficient dosages for short durations and for inappropriate symptoms.

Diseases in Canada

Immigrants from Vietnam were and are relatively free of communicable diseases when they arrive in Canada because they have been medically screened abroad. Some arrive with health problems that can be treated fairly easily, such as intestinal parasites and anemia. Children are often incompletely immunized, and some people suffer from malnutrition. The standard Harvard height and weight chart is not always useful in assessing malnutrition in children since Vietnamese body sizes are often small; a well-nourished Vietnamese child may fall within the third percentile of the Harvard range. Because Vietnamese medical services are limited, there may be uncorrected genetic problems such as extra fingers and toes.

However, four major diseases are sometimes brought from Vietnam to Canada. Hepatitis B, mostly in sub-clinical form, may be apparent in a blood test. Hepatitis B vaccination is advisable for medical and dental staff working with people from Vietnam and for babies born of carrier mothers, since it is contagious through blood-to-blood contact. Vaccination is also advised for the spouse or sex partner of the infected person. The Canadian immunization program now includes hepatitis B.

In 2003 hepatitis C was found in many Vietnamese who arrived earlier as refugees. This disease may be acquired through either transfusions with contaminated blood or the use of non-disposable needles improperly sterilized.

Pulmonary tuberculosis is sometimes present in immigrants from Vietnam, usually in inactive form since tuberculosis screening is required for admission to Canada. Immigrants arriving with inactive tuberculosis are handed a form on arrival advising them to report to a clinic to receive information about preventive antibiotic treatment. However, many persons from Vietnam refuse the nine-month treatment program because of potential side-effects or beliefs that there is no need to take medicines when one has no symptoms. If reactivation occurs, it is usually during the first five years of the newcomer's stay in Canada. So it is important for all those with inactive tuberculosis to make regular visits to tuberculosis control clinics for examination and treatment for at least five years.

Leprosy, found only in tuberculoid form in Vietnam, can be easily missed by a medical officer conducting the immigration screening examination because its signs and symptoms may be so minor as to be mistaken for trivial skin diseases. Some cases were discovered in Canada among refugees from Vietnam. Tuberculoid leprosy, which does not spread by casual contact, is readily treated by dermatologists on an out-patient basis. It is important to refer patients who present long-lasting and hypoaesthetic skin lesions.

Malaria is sometimes brought from Vietnam but cannot spread in Canada because the anopheles mosquito carrier is absent. The disease is sometimes reactivated when the person has a low state of resistance, and it gives rise to inexplicably high and protracted fever.

After several years of residence in Canada, most immigrants from Vietnam generally present a good health picture. However, there is a tendency for them to develop certain specific diseases. Dental problems, both cavities and gum diseases, are common complaints. Constipation and hemorrhoids are fairly common and often linked. They are largely the result of a switch to softer foods with less dietary fibre but sometimes a consequence of people drinking insufficient fluid at work to avoid going to the bathroom during working hours.

Newcomers to Canada catch viral diseases very easily since they are not immune to the local viruses. For example, they are highly susceptible to respiratory infections during the influenza season.

Relationship between Doctor and Patient

As in the past, people in Vietnam still defer to health professionals. For the average person in Vietnam, the health professional is consequently rather remote and aloof. Doctors are special persons who are regarded as having a godsent gift to save people and help society. They are expected to be wise, to have good judgment, and to be dignified. Vietnamese patients entrust the doctor with almost total responsibility for medical decisions.

Like Vietnamese society, which has a hierarchical class structure, the medical professions in Vietnam are also organized hierarchically. Nurses are accessories to physicians whose role is to carry out the doctor's orders not to initiate activities; they apply bandages and give injections. Because public health nurses are government servants, they have special status and are respected and obeyed.

When people from Vietnam first go to a physician in Canada, they expect and prefer the doctor to behave like those at home. The doctor should be formal and unhurried, and patients assume that the physician in his wisdom will identify the illness without too many questions or an elaborate physical examination. Early in their stay in Canada, detailed questions about their lives or their families are particularly unwelcome, especially if the patient can discern no connection between the questions and the illness. Also, some fear that the very act of talking about an illness may induce or stimulate it. Patients do not expect detailed explanation of the diagnosis or the purpose of the recommended treatment. In fact, many people from Vietnam are unable to provide medical histories simply because their previous physicians did not inform them about such matters.

On the basis of past experience and customary preference, the Vietnamese patient may dislike removing more clothing than is absolutely necessary for a physical examination. In general, touching of the body should be kept to a minimum. For example, a man who has a respiratory problem might open only the top of his shirt to allow the physician to listen to his chest.

Physicians are expected to inform the patient's family, who often accompany the patient, about the illness and treatment, because other family members, particularly elders, often take responsibility for decisions and treatment. Vietnamese who were born in or grew up in Canada are more like Westerners in this regard.

Many Vietnamese prefer physicians from Vietnam, finding it easier to talk about personal things in a familiar language. Early refugees were reticent about their past lives until they had established where the physician stood in Vietnam's complex political world. This concern has diminished, in part because it is also less important in Vietnam. Many people choose Asian physicians where no Vietnamese doctors exist. While the ethnicity of the doctor is important, persons who have difficulty travelling independently because of cost or language are likely to select a doctor in the neighbourhood.

For gynecological examinations, women prefer female physicians and will accept a female nurse in the examining room, but not usually a family member. A Vietnamese male physician who senses the woman's reluctance and embarrassment may refer her to a female doctor.

In Vietnam, patients expect to be passive and dependent and expect physicians to take full command in accordance with their position and expertise. In Canada, health professionals may regard them as good patients because they ask few questions, make few complaints, and seem to comply with recommendations. To the Vietnamese this behaviour is felt to be polite, respectful to the professional, protective of one's self, and thus generally helpful in avoiding embarrassment. The Vietnamese person will show respect by consistently addressing the professional as "Doctor." However, this politeness can mask misunderstanding and disagreement, and a patient sometimes disregards treatment recommendations and subsequent appointments.

Because physicians are held responsible for treatment and cure, many patients from Vietnam find recommendations to change their own behaviour (stopping smoking or changing diet) unacceptable or difficult to follow. Since they expect doctors to prescribe medicines, other "natural" treatments that involve habit changes are less acceptable. For example, it would be very difficult to convince Miss Nguyen that she can use fluids and natural fibres in her diet to relieve constipation when she knows the physician can prescribe a laxative.

Vietnamese people also tend to be quite stoical in the face of illness and pain. Men, in particular, are reluctant to reveal symptoms, and sometimes delay treatment until pain or disability are great. This phenomenon is linked to beliefs about correct behaviour but also stems from the fact that many Vietnamese are paid by the hour and lose wages when attending appointments.

When first in Canada, people from Vietnam often find it difficult to adapt to the physician's appointment system and tend to arrive late. At home they were accustomed to an entirely different system, whereby they dropped in at the office and waited their turn, or appeared at the beginning of the physician's office hours, took a number, and returned at the appropriate time later on.

Gradually a person from Vietnam living in Canada learns that the physician will indeed keep confidences. The doctor can be trusted not to talk about the patient with officials or with other members of the Vietnamese community. Patients also come to expect the physician to take thorough histories, do physical examinations, and ask detailed questions; younger patients, in particular, learn to be assertive about their needs. In short, their expectations will increasingly conform to those of Westerners.

Hospitals

In the past in Vietnam, a decision to go to hospital was made only when there was no alternative, because it was believed that hospitals were places to die. Although modern Vietnam has a much more satisfactory hospital system, many of the old practices have not disappeared. Admission to hospital may be delayed beyond the optimal time for treatment; a patient may be taken home with the first appearance of improvement; elderly patients in particular may avoid hospitalization or return home early to avoid dying in hospital.

While the patient is in a Vietnamese hospital, a family member usually stays to provide personal care. The family sends food from home; in fact, in the Vietnamese language, to take care of a hospitalized patient is literally "to feed a patient." Family members can visit the patient at almost all times. The family has considerable control over what is done for the patient and even over treatment decisions.

When a person from Vietnam goes to a Canadian hospital, some of these experiences conflict with Western practices. During their first years in Canada some older people are reluctant to be admitted to hospital because of its association with death. To die away from home is believed to bring bad luck to one's children and to confuse one's soul, which may get lost on its journey to Nirvana. Nowadays the majority of Vietnamese consider the hospital a natural setting for dying under proper medical care.

Although Vietnamese willingly share hospital rooms with others, they prefer privacy and often want curtains pulled around the bed. Lack of privacy and fear of being overheard sometimes lead to evasive replies in answer to the doctor's questions. Problems of privacy are also posed by standard hospital gowns. Many people from Vietnam never reveal the body area between waist and knees, even to their closest relatives. They will wear hospital gowns if told to do so, but often with considerable embarrassment.

Because of traditional beliefs about the harmful effects of wind, many Vietnamese show great concern about drafts in hospital rooms. They fear that a wind may aggravate serious illness and thus prefer to have windows closed at all times.

A major worry of some Vietnamese is hospital food, not simply that the food is usually Western but that it is not easily classified in terms of "hot" and "cold." Jello is a prime example. Since it is unknown in Vietnam, patients do not know whether it is hot or cold, and some worry that they are being asked to eat something that may be bad for their particular illness. Others are simply unused to Western food and therefore do not eat what is offered. These problems are less common the longer the person has been resident in Canada.

Patients whose English is not strong worry that they cannot make themselves understood and will not understand what hospital staff tell them.

Unlike in Vietnam, in Canada the family can do very little for the hospitalized person. Food is provided by the hospital, and additional foods from home are discouraged or forbidden. Visiting hours are limited, and family nursing care is neither needed nor allowed. As a result, some families may feel that they have been forced to abandon the sick person.

Medicine and Other Treatment

In Vietnam most people try home remedies first, before seeking a physician. Common remedies are herbal drinks designed to rebalance the body by cooling or heating and a mentholatum-based ointment such as Tiger Balm which is rubbed on the affected part of the body, inhaled, or swallowed to prevent or treat a wind disease.

Western medicines are also used in Vietnam, many of them sold without prescription. Vietnamese families know antibiotics, penicillin, and psychoactive drugs, for example, but are not aware of possible toxic effects or interactions or problems of resistance. Chloramphenicol, which was introduced to treat typhoid fever, became popular for all feverish diseases with no awareness that its overuse could cause aplastic anemia. In rare cases, families from Vietnam have brought chloramphenicol to the West for use at home.

In Vietnam, it was expected that a good doctor would give medicine, and most physicians complied by prescribing not just one but several types of pills and perhaps one or more injections. It was unthinkable that no medicine would be given. In Canada, the same is expected of doctors at first. If the doctor says, "No medicine is really needed," a Vietnamese patient may feel cheated or misunderstood. Since patients expect rapid cures, a physician who repeats the same medication may find that the patient does not take it or fails to return; why should one continue with a medicine that does not work at once? Some may request certain drugs as they did in Vietnam, particularly "liver medicine" if there is digestive trouble or skin disease, or "heart tonic" for weakness or dizziness. Vietnamese persons in Canada learn only gradually to comply with the physician's recommendations and with medical prescriptions.

While most people in Vietnam have used Western medicines, in Canada there is still some resistance to their use. Western medicine is believed to be hot and is thus felt to be risky if applied to hot conditions. Also most people believe that Western medicines are too strong or inappropriate for Vietnamese. One way to avoid problems is to reduce the recommended dosage, a common practice among Vietnamese new to Canada. There is a tendency to stop taking medicines prematurely. It can be difficult to convince a Vietnamese patient that Western medical treatment is beneficial in the long term, particularly where there are no evident symptoms, such as with tuberculosis, high blood pressure, or diabetes.

Cultural beliefs and experiences with medical treatment in Vietnam lead Vietnamese to place a high value on some Canadian medical procedures while attempting to avoid others. There is enthusiasm for injections, which may derive in part from past experiences with quick cures from penicillin injections. People often insist on X-rays as well. Most laboratory tests are acceptable, such as urinalysis. However, many Vietnamese fear and resist tests that require even small samples of blood, in the belief that the body has a finite, irreplaceable amount of blood. Some may attribute symptoms such as headaches or weakness to the loss of blood during blood tests, even single tests done several years earlier. These beliefs change with longer stays in Canada and as people learn that blood tests may ensure better diagnosis and treatment. Anti-pain medication is seldom requested, probably because of the cultural value placed on stoicism. However, over time many Vietnamese living in Canada become willing to have laboratory tests and to use anti-pain medications.

Many women, particularly older women, are reluctant to have mammograms and Pap tests. Since these tests were not generally available in Vietnam, women do not know about them. In Canada, many avoid them because they are uncomfortable and embarrassing, especially if their physician is male. Young unmarried girls are extremely reluctant to have pelvic examinations and Pap tests unless they are absolutely necessary and clearly explained, in part because they fear the loss of virginity.

Many health professionals can attest to the reluctance of Vietnamese immigrants to agree to surgery. Only if they are convinced that there is no alternative will surgery be acceptable. Fear of surgery is partly a fear of hospitals as places to die and partly rooted in a cultural belief that the soul is attached to parts of the body and may be excised with those parts or escape from an incision, leading to death. Wandering souls are problematic for both the dead and the bereaved family. Vietnamese may be especially reluctant to consent in cases of minor surgery, such as to correct strabismus or remove extra fingers and toes. If a biopsy or Pap test is described as "cutting tissue," it may be refused. If Vietnamese do consent to surgery they may want to consult a horoscope to select an auspicious day. These cultural beliefs begin to fade with longer residence in Canada.

Contraception

Traditionally in Vietnam contraception was neither highly valued nor legal. The family was a source of happiness, and children were highly appreciated. Furthermore, the French colonial authorities followed dominant Roman Catholic policy and discouraged modern birth control. In the 1960s urban physicians found that there was a demand for contraceptive pills. Some herbal decoctions were used to prevent contraception or to induce abortion, but until after the Vietnam War most rural Vietnamese did not know about modern contraceptives.

However, as a result of social changes and government family planning programs in the 1990s, the government of Vietnam has reported, some form of modern contraception was being used by 75 percent of married women, and the number of births per woman dropped from 5 in 1980 to 2.3 in 1999. Women recently arriving from urban areas of Vietnam are likely to know of and use modern methods, but women from rural areas less so.

Vietnamese refugees to Canada were introduced to modern contraception in many refugee camps, usually in the form of Depo-Provera, a long-term contraceptive injection. Some Vietnamese women in Canada subsequently requested Depo-Provera, while others, repelled by its serious side-effects, grew reluctant to use any contraceptive at all.

However, having moved to Canada, where there may be no extended family to help and where rearing children is expensive, most women are willing to discuss modern contraception, particularly if the physician or nurse is a woman, and to accept some form of it. The IUD is most commonly accepted. Birth control pills are not popular. Women find taking a daily birth control pill is difficult, and many believe that the pills will cause obesity, mood changes, and skin problems. Vietnamese women will choose sterilization if they have had more children than the family can afford to raise, even though some worry that, if sterilized, they will become masculine and lose their libido. Professionals will find that it is important to explain clearly that contraceptive methods will not change one's personality or gender. Some men use condoms (though often without spermicide) but are unwilling to have vasectomies. Younger Vietnamese who were educated in Canada have learned about contraception in the school system and are well informed. Finally, professionals should be aware that some Vietnamese families are large, not because of failure to use contraception effectively, but because they have chosen to have many children.

Pregnancy

Pregnancy is traditionally believed to be a normal condition, but one in which care should be taken to maintain the body's equilibrium. Thus pregnant women should avoid too much hot food (meat, alcohol, coffee) as well as cold food (bananas). They may, however, crave foods that are astringent such as green mangoes. Tonics of various kinds are often taken to strengthen the mother and to shrink the fetus so as to ease delivery. There is a strong belief that continued physical activity is important right up to the time of birth. For this reason pregnant women often avoid naps or rest.

Many Vietnamese women believe that behaviour during pregnancy can affect not only the delivery and physical health of the mother and child but also the child's moral development. Pregnant women should avoid contact with people who are dishonest for fear of contaminating the unborn child. Moreover, the mother should behave impeccably herself by giving food to the poor, not complaining, not being jealous, and so on. For similar reasons, sexual intercourse is ended at the third month of pregnancy.

Recently in Vietnam, formal prenatal care is being used by many more women, especially city dwellers. Thus some newer immigrants to Canada have had experience of regular check-ups and health education. Once in Canada, most women are willing to make regular prenatal visits to the physician and even attend prenatal classes, particularly classes conducted in Vietnamese or Cantonese. Some husbands are willing to attend, especially if they know other men who are going. Husbands who are drawn into these classes often learn how to share interests and concerns with their wives, something that they did not do before. Some professionals see these classes as an important way to strengthen the family.

Childbirth

The birth of a baby is a normal process. As the Vietnamese say, "The bud opens and the flower blooms." While many women from urban Vietnam have had hospital deliveries by a physician, those from rural areas are more likely to have had babies at home with the help of a midwife. In both cases, the women endured the pain of childbirth with stoicism and seldom with the benefit of an anesthetic. Once women arrive in Canada, some of these practices begin to change, including the use of anesthetics. If pain relief methods are made available, Vietnamese women use them and even request them, although the maintenance of self-control and stoicism during labour is still evident.

There is a tendency for Vietnamese infants to weigh less at birth than Caucasian infants; in one part of the United States the median weight for Vietnamese babies was 3,260 grams as compared to 3,459 grams for Caucasians. Some physicians see this as a genetic effect that is likely to continue.

All babies, whether male or female, are treated with tenderness. However, sons are preferred, as suggested by a common saying, "A single boy, that is positive; ten girls, that is still negative." Sons are important because they perpetuate the family name and allow the family to fulfil its responsibilities to the ancestors. Traditional methods were thought to guarantee the sex of the child, such as planning conception on an odd-numbered day of the week in order to produce a son. Preference for boys is important to many families in Canada; for instance, a woman who gives birth to a third daughter and no sons may get depressed.

Traditional beliefs classify the woman's body after childbirth as cold because she has suffered stress and loss of blood during delivery. In rural Vietnam, therefore, many women followed the practices of "mother-roasting" common in Southeast Asia; that is, placing a small charcoal fire under the mother's bed to keep her warm. This practice has disappeared among urban women, but there are other ways of countering the cold imbalance, many of which have been brought to Canada.

After giving birth, women are reluctant to bathe or wash their hair, for fear of cooling the body further. Sponge baths with very warm water are much more acceptable. It is important, too, to avoid cold foods such as water, fruit juices, raw vegetables, and fruit. Hot, spicy, and salty foods are preferred, along with rice, eggs, tea, sweets, chicken broth, and a special "stew" made of rice, pork, and fish sauce. Even though Vietnamese women do not normally consume alcohol, many drink red wine or wine with ginseng after childbirth in the belief that these will cleanse their system. Avoiding drafts, air conditioning, and open windows is important. After birth the new mother expects and hopes to rest for at least one month. Elderly women who experience weakness in their bodies, such as in their arms and legs, often attribute these problems to not taking the right precautions after childbirth.

In Canada, the one-month period of rest after childbirth remains the norm. Many women who have hourly-paid factory work stay home for a month even with no assurance that their job will be available at month's end. If possible the new mother's own mother or her mother-in-law will come to help. The end of the baby's first month is celebrated by as large a party as the family can afford, such as a backyard barbecue for as many as 150 guests.

In Vietnam's villages women commonly breastfeed for one year and a half and usually let the child wean itself. Urban women, especially those who work, are more likely to bottle-feed. Babies are not usually offered solid food until six months. In Canada, despite the advocacy of breastfeeding by physicians and public health nurses, most women bottle-feed, even women who have lived in Canada many years. Some prefer bottle-feeding because it is more "modern." Others stop breastfeeding early due to conflict with jobs. Many women are conscious of their breasts and prefer firm breasts rather than the sometimes droopy breasts they fear will result from breastfeeding.

Mental Health

To people in Vietnam, mental illness usually means severe disorders, not the relatively minor problems such as anxiety that Westerners often include in that category. Once a person is diagnosed with a mental illness, hope of a cure is lost. Persons with mental illness are feared and rejected, and their family members feel shame. It becomes the collective responsibility of the family to care for the sick person as long as this can be managed at home.

Traditionally, mental illness is often explained in astrological terms, such as being born under an unlucky star. Sometimes the suffering is attributed to misdeeds in previous lives or malevolent spirits. Treatments consist of exorcism ceremonies, rituals by Buddhist priests, and sometimes a stay at the Buddhist temple. Meanwhile, family members devote themselves to good behaviour and religious piety.

After Western medicine came to Vietnam, psychiatric hospitals became available, but only patients who were unmanageable and profoundly disturbed were taken there. One large hospital, with 1,900 beds, provided little therapeutic activity for patients, few professional staff, and offered only electric shock and, later, drug therapy. Few expected the patient to return home. With the advent of psychotropic drugs, some families began to seek medical treatment at earlier stages of mental illness, but most people adhered to traditional beliefs about causes and cures.

Mental Illness among Refugees

The experience of leaving Vietnam and eventually settling in Canada certainly increased the risk of mental illness among refugees. Almost all refugees left Vietnam with very little preparation and often no choice. Many suffered terribly in the escape by sea. This was followed by prolonged stays in overcrowded and unsanitary refugee camps. Upon arrival in Canada, some were settled in areas with no ethnic support groups and where the climate was harsh. All lost their homeland, and often their property, business, and customary social networks. Many lost their sense of security, identity, and self-esteem. Separation from family was a major factor causing depression and anxiety. Some of these problems were later eased by subsequent reunion with family members and by regrouping within Canada by moving to large metropolitan areas.

Some were not able to adjust to loss and change and developed mental disturbances six months to three years after arrival in Canada. In the early years of residence in Canada, refugees who did develop psychiatric problems were often kept at home without treatment because their families were ashamed. Delayed reactions to loss and trauma were precipitated by job loss, an automobile accident, or family conflict, which then led to psychiatric illness. First contact with formal treatment was often in hospital emergency rooms, the sick person generally having arrived by police car or ambulance.

Professionals found that after a first contact with a psychiatrist, the person often resisted all treatment until becoming ill again. Only then was the person willing to accept treatment, especially if the professional had established a supportive mood and sense of trust in the first encounter.

Families were reluctant to agree that minor psychiatric problems, such as adolescent problems in school, should be treated by a physician, particularly a psychiatrist. Consulting a psychiatrist seemed equivalent to declaring a family member insane.

Many Vietnamese refugees managed to adjust to their new situations within three years or so. However, even after decades of settlement, some who came to Canada as refugees in the 1970s are still dealing with the memories of traumatic experiences in the past. Post-traumatic stress disorder tends to resurface when individuals achieve more stability or get older.

Family physicians have noticed that problems of mental illness have generally diminished over the years since the refugees arrived, though the refugees are quick to say that memories of these experiences never disappear.

Mrs. Tranh, from Vietnam

About six years ago, Mrs. Tranh's son sponsored her immigration to Canada. She is a widow who lives with her son and daughter-in-law in a Montreal suburb. At first she was able to help the family by walking to and from school with their youngest child and doing some of the cooking, but for the last year or so she has spent her days in her own room not talking to anyone. She eats the meals the family brings to her and takes care of her room, but otherwise she just sits and gazes out of the window. When her son asks her what is wrong she simply says, "I am quite all right. I need nothing more."

Finally, Mrs. Tranh's son asked a Vietnamese mental health professional to come to their home to see what was wrong with her and suggest something the family could do to help. At first Mrs. Tranh refused to talk or answer questions. Then the mental health worker began to describe the common plight of elderly parents uprooted from their familiar community and transferred to Canada where they have no friends of their own, no English or French, and little knowledge that is useful to the family. He suggested that this often leads to feelings of sadness and depression. As he talked, Mrs. Tranh began to nod in agreement and finally, tentatively, began to say that this is how she feels.

Mental Illness among Immigrants

Vietnamese who came to Canada under the family reunification program in the 1990s and early 2000s often find settlement emotionally difficult because they were not prepared for the challenges. In particular, mental health problems are sometimes apparent among the new wives of Canadian Vietnamese men, among the men themselves, and among older parents of refugee couples.

Though there are many community supports for seniors, some elderly people are very isolated, especially if they have not learned English and cannot easily travel or if they are kept at home for child care and household tasks. Often they cannot communicate with grandchildren who do not speak Vietnamese. As a result, depression is fairly common, perhaps first signalled by a retreat to a private room and a refusal to talk or to be touched. Such persons tend to refuse treatment unless professionals visit their homes and find ways to engage them in conversation about their situation.

Wives who have been sponsored by older husbands from Canada often suffer from depression. These women are usually young and have high expectations but soon find they are without family support, have no job, no skills, little English, and little money. After childbirth, when lack of sleep adds to stress, they may suffer from postpartum depression. Their husbands may also be depressed, because they have financial worries, fear their young wives will leave them, and have few coping skills to draw on.

Mental Health Treatment

The culture of Buddhism says that one should learn to deal with the stresses of daily life without burdening others with one's problems. The Confucian code teaches people to respect and obey their seniors such as parents and teachers. With this heritage, psychiatric patients with a Vietnamese background are not willing to discuss personal feelings about their family or older relatives and will tend to describe their childhood as satisfactory. They will generally not accept "talk therapy" that investigates family relationships as their central psychiatric treatment.

Instead, the Vietnamese patient and family expect the mental health professional to act promptly: take a brief history, make a diagnosis, and provide medical treatment. A physical examination is expected, because without it the psychiatrist is not a "doctor." Patients and their families are unfamiliar with, and threatened by, intrusive, open-ended questions such as "Tell me about yourself" or "I wonder what you think of your illness." Moreover, a doctor who says, "I hope that we can work together in finding a solution" is not respected. Vietnamese expect the mental health professional to be authoritative and direct; in return, they will accept and follow recommendations faithfully, especially those that come from a Vietnamese professional.

Thus, discussion of past experiences or current problems is more acceptable if it is combined with medical treatment, such as drug therapy, or with some kind of social intervention. Once the Vietnamese patient feels comfortable talking, it is useful to focus on psychosocial factors that may have contributed to the illness. For example, when working with refugees, professionals have found it helpful to discuss: (1) life, problems, and stresses in the home country; (2) escape or departure, who came, who stayed, the experience; (3) refugee camp experience; (4) attitudes towards and problems of living in Canada; (5) current worries and outlook for the future. These topics provide a framework for linking past experiences to current symptoms in ways the patient can understand and may not have recognized.

Today, with education from the mass media, available Vietnamese-speaking mental health professionals, and very good Vietnamese community networks and referral systems, at least in the larger cities, most mental health problems are being dealt with sooner and more effectively.

Nutrition and Food

In Vietnam most people prefer a diet in which boiled white rice is the staple. In fact, the literal translation of the word for "meal" is "time to eat rice." In addition to rice, fresh green vegetables and fresh or dried fish are commonly served, along with fermented fish sauce. If the family can afford it, chicken or pork in small quantities is also eaten. Noodles are sometimes substituted for rice, especially in soups. Water and tea are common beverages, and fruit is often eaten as a snack. The fat content of the traditional diet is low, and normal caloric intake is about two-thirds of the Western norm.

Foods are classified as hot, cold, or neutral, and it is important to balance these qualities to prevent illness. Hot foods such as meat, fish sauce, sweets, coffee, spices, garlic, ginger, and onion should be offset by cold foods such as most vegetables, fruit, potatoes, fish, and duck. When an illness results from heat loss, one should avoid cold foods. Common foods for people who are ill are a rice gruel to which sugar or sweetened condensed milk has been added or a dish made from pieces of salty pork with fish sauce. Over the years in Canada, overt concern with hot and cold foods begins to diminish.

In Vietnam, the same kinds of foods are generally served at all three meals. Rice along with vegetables and perhaps some meat in very small amounts are set out in bowls from which each person, including the young child, chooses what he wants. The family meal in which everyone sits together and where one course follows another is not common, nor are meals occasions for conversation.

When people from Vietnam settle in Canada they generally prefer the foods they ate at home, such as *cha gio* (deep-fried rice paper rolls filled with meat, egg, or chopped vegetables), *pho* (a soup made of noodles and meat), and *nuoc man* (fermented fish sauce). In urban areas many of these ingredients are available in Chinese markets.

However, over the years some changes have occurred, in part because women who are employed do not have time to cook and also because many Vietnamese, particularly children, have developed a taste for Western foods. Quick and relatively inexpensive fast foods have become popular, leading to a significantly increased consumption of soft drinks, peanut butter, ice cream, and pastries. Many now eat significantly more milk, beef, butter, margarine, eggs, and potatoes. Because meat is much cheaper in Canada than in Vietnam, it is no longer a special treat for celebrations. One woman said, "In Canada, we eat party food every day!" The increase in carbohydrates, sugar, and fat has meant that some Vietnamese, including children, have gained weight, and a few have become obese. There is some evidence, too, that the nutritious, well-balanced Vietnamese diet has been replaced by a poorly balanced one.

A large proportion of Vietnamese, like many Asians, are intolerant of lactose, the sugar in milk. Using too much milk produces diarrhea and stomach aches, mainly in those over age six.

Alcohol and Drug Use

While rice wine is available in Vietnam, men traditionally do not consume large quantities of it. Their drinking is almost always confined to group celebrations; men never drink alone. Drunkenness is unacceptable, because of the value placed on formality, politeness, and face. Also, like many Asians, Vietnamese men after consuming alcohol often suffer uncomfortable symptoms, such as flushed faces, trembling, palpitations, and rapid breathing. Women do not drink alcohol except for "medicinal" wine after childbirth.

In Canada the situation is different. There has been an increased use of alcohol among men, especially those who arrived very young and those born here. Vietnamese men here tend to consume more alcohol than the Canadian norm. Men tend to drink in social groups, such as at evening parties where wives do the cooking. Some drink heavily, and alcoholism has become a problem. In some cases alcohol is used to manage depression. The majority of women do not drink except after pregnancy.

In Canada, illegal drug use is found in some teenaged and young adult men who are involved in the illegal production and sale of drugs, especially marijuana. They are seen by professionals when they have acute psychotic symptoms such as delusions and hallucinations, but they are often unwilling to accept any treatment. Few young women use illegal drugs.

Bathing and Elimination

Daily bathing is important to people from Vietnam, except for certain times when it is thought to be risky for the reason that bathing may cool the body and create illness. Therefore, a woman usually does not bathe or wash her hair when menstruating or after childbirth. If bathing is unavoidable during these vulnerable times, a sponge bath with very hot water is thought to be safest. After living in Canada for some time, many adopt the Western norm of daily bathing.

In rural Vietnam flush toilets are rare, and toilets are designed so that the individual can squat rather than sit. New immigrants to the West initially have some difficulty adapting to the Western style of elimination.

Dental Health

Vietnam has many fewer dentists than Canada, and only the very rich and privileged have had access to dental care. This lack of care and the malnutrition and unbalanced diets caused by protracted war have fostered serious dental problems among immigrants from Vietnam. Adults and children often have decayed or missing teeth. Periodontal disease, indicated by spongy and bleeding gums, is also common.

In Canada cavities and gum diseases are common complaints, especially if immigrants ingest less calcium because they live in soft-water areas and eat softer foods than traditionally found in the Vietnamese diet.

Even though great value is placed on healthy white teeth and most Vietnamese are eager to receive dental care, a visit to a dentist in Canada is often postponed if money is needed for other more important priorities.

Rehabilitation

In Vietnam, very few medical resources were available for rehabilitation, such as for correction of birth defects or for treatment of chronic diseases like epilepsy. Immigrants to Canada do not have experience or knowledge of such measures and tend to ignore local rehabilitation programs. For example, braces for child victims of polio epidemics in Vietnam may not be accepted because the family feels that further suffering will result from additional medical attention. The need for long-term medication for a condition like high blood pressure with no symptoms and little discomfort may not be understood by the family, so the medication may be abandoned. In instances where surgery is recommended for corrective purposes,

Vietnamese families may feel that the dangers of surgery far outweigh the benefits and decide that it is better to live with strabismus, say, or a cleft palate.

Sexuality and Sexually Transmitted Disease

In Vietnam, married couples do not talk about sex, nor do they educate their children about it, and married women accept that their husbands will have other sex partners. This is especially true in rural areas but is common in cities as well.

In Canada many of the same norms apply. Among those who arrived as refugees as well as among more recent arrivals from Vietnam, couples do not discuss sexual relations and so cannot easily make joint decisions about contraception. Parents rarely teach children about sexuality or disease prevention; some say, "Let the school do that," while others are opposed to schools being involved at all. Many young women are unable to talk about sex, in part because they are expected to be "pure" and not know about it; often they do not have the necessary vocabulary.

Vietnamese in Canada know how HIV/AIDS is transmitted. However, some young women believe, or allow themselves to be persuaded, that if partners love each other there is no chance of infection. Many men continue to have sexual partners outside marriage. Now that everyone knows how quickly HIV/AIDS is spreading in Vietnam, some wives worry that their husbands will become infected on visits there.

The Canadian-born, younger Vietnamese are more likely to be well informed about sexuality and more ready to talk about it with their partners and their children. These younger people are quite willing to ask physicians about disease prevention.

Aging

Traditionally, old people in Vietnam were respected and privileged. Their long lives gave them wisdom to advise the young, and they were called upon when important decisions had to be made. After death they were worshipped. All their children were expected to return the parental concern and love they had received, but it was usually the eldest son who cared for parents in his home until their death.

In Canada in 1991 only 4 percent of the Vietnamese-born population was over sixty-five years of age. The majority were female, and following traditional expectations almost all lived with immediate family or other relatives.

Since 1991 some of the initial refugees have become elderly, while older parents have arrived from Vietnam sponsored by their children through the family reunification program. These two groups of seniors have some things in common. With many husbands and wives at work, elderly parents often become babysitters and housekeepers and are isolated from the rest of the Vietnamese community. Isolation is especially likely if they have not learned English, have no money of their own, and feel unable to use public transportation. Some seniors "don't want to bother their children" with requests for transport or other extra help. Some grandparents with little English are even isolated in their own homes because they are not able to communicate with their English-speaking grandchildren. Depression is common among seniors and is most often reported in somatic terms, perhaps as headaches or fatigue. In the United States, abuse of Vietnamese seniors has also been reported. This is almost always in the form of a psychological tactic such as "the silent treatment," that is, treating the elderly person as not there; if it occurs it is most often found where both parents work, there are small children, and financial pressures are great.

By now the seniors who arrived as refugees and grew old in Canada usually have some form of pension, and thus some economic independence, and if they have learned English they do very well. Many return for visits to Vietnam; some spend six months there each year, and many have participated in philanthropic projects in Vietnam. But others experience inner conflict over the issue of a return to the site of their suffering. Many elders continue to relive the traumas of the past and fear that a visit to Vietnam will traumatize them once again.

Seniors sponsored under the family reunification program are much less able to adapt to Canada than those who grew old here. Perhaps as many as half of these seniors return to Vietnam permanently, in part because life is now better there but also because in Canada they are "mute and deaf," being unable to speak or understand the language, and because they tend to be extremely isolated in their children's homes. The life experience and wisdom they bring from Vietnam is of little use to their children here. Those who remain in Canada are often depressed. They have no friends in Canada, are very unlikely to learn English, have left behind everything familiar, and have to get along with children whom they had not lived with or even seen for many years and who have made many changes in their own lives.

Some elderly parents living in Vietnam visit families in Canada, but many families are reluctant to extend invitations because they cannot afford private health insurance to cover possible illness here.

Almost all Vietnamese children make great efforts to care for elderly parents in their own homes. They find it heartbreaking to have to put a parent in a nursing home. But the economic pressures that force both husband and wife to work long hours may make impossible the proper care of an ill or disabled parent at home, so the only choice is admission to a nursing home. It is estimated that the majority of Vietnamese elderly persons needing regular nursing care in Canada today are living in nursing homes, not with family. This is usually a very distressing experience for the old person, especially one who does not speak English. Families visit regularly, daily or at least weekly, and often bring familiar food, but other meaningful social contact may be minimal.

Community support for elderly Vietnamese is strong, particularly in the larger cities, where there are Vietnamese seniors' centres, Buddhist temples, Catholic churches, and other service organizations.

Death and Dying

Traditionally, among the Vietnamese there is a strong feeling that death should occur at home, not in hospital. At home one's family can provide comfort, and one can die in peace. For some Vietnamese, death away from home means that the soul will wander, having no place to rest. The family will often make every effort to take a dying person home. If death does occur in a hospital, it becomes important to move the body home as soon as possible.

These beliefs gradually change with longer residence in Canada. Families come to accept that the hospital is where the best care can be given for critically ill or dying patients. If the person who dies in hospital has been given the appropriate last rites, the spiritual needs of the family are fulfilled, and the body can then be sent to the funeral home without any further concern.

Generally, the dying person's family wishes to be informed that death is imminent, but prefers that the patient not be told. After death, families seldom, if ever, give permission for an autopsy unless it is required by law. They do not wish to cause more suffering to the dead person.

Traditional mourning practices require that family members wear white clothing for fourteen days, followed by the wearing of black armbands. On the forty-ninth day after death, the surviving family members organize a ceremony where food is provided for the entire family and for close friends and neighbours. A smaller ceremonial gathering may occur after one hundred days. Then, the person's eldest son organizes a ceremony each year on the anniversary of the death. The child or wife of a deceased person must wait three years to marry, and the husband must wait one year.

Further Reading

Bong, Nguyen Quy. 1985. "The Vietnamese in Canada: Some settlement problems." In K.V. Ujimoto and Gordon Hirabayeshi, eds., *Visible Minorities and Multiculturalism: Asians in Canada*. Toronto, ON: Butterworth.

Chan, Kwok B., and Doreen M. Indra, eds. 1987. *Uprooting, Loss and Adaptation: The Resettlement of Indochinese Refugees in Canada*. Ottawa, ON: Canadian Public Health Association.

Donnelly, Tam Truong. 2004. "Vietnamese women living in Canada: Contextual factors affecting Vietnamese women's breast cancer and cervical cancer screening practices." PhD diss., Faculty of Graduate Studies, Individual Interdisciplinary Graduate Studies, University of British Columbia, Vancouver, BC.

Dorais, Louis-Jacques. 2000. *The Cambodians, Laotians and Vietnamese in Canada*. Canada's Ethnic Group Series, Booklet No. 28. Ottawa, ON: Canadian Historical Association.

Government of Canada. 1996. *Profiles Vietnam: Immigrants from Vietnam in Canada*. Ottawa: Statistics Canada, Immigration Research Series.

Indra, Doreen. 1985. "Khmer, Lao, Vietnamese and Vietnamese-Chinese in Alberta." In Howard Palmer and Tamara Palmer, eds., *Peoples of Alberta: Portraits of Cultural Diversity,* 437-63. Saskatoon, SK: Western Producer Prairie Books.

Le, Quyen Kim. 1997. "Mistreatment of Vietnamese elderly by their families in the United States." *Journal of Elder Abuse and Neglect* 9: 51-62.

Muecke, Marjorie A. 1983. "In search of healers: Southeast Asian refugees in the American health care system." *Western Journal of Medicine* 139: 835-40.

Nguyen, San Duy. 1982. "Psychiatric and psychosomatic problems among Southeast Asian refugees." *Psychiatric Journal of the University of Ottawa* 7: 163-72.

Rekart, Michael L. 2002. "HIV/AIDS in Vietnam." Paper presented at UBC Institute of Asian Research, University of British Columbia, 9 October.

Stephenson, Peter H. 1995. "Vietnamese refugees in Victoria, BC: An overview of immigrant and refugee health care in a medium-sized Canadian urban centre." *Social Science and Medicine* 40: 1631-42.

Tepper, Elliot, ed. 1980. *Southeast Asian Exodus: From Tradition to Resettlement*. Ottawa: Canadian Asian Studies Association.

Tung, Tranh Minh. 1980. *Indochinese Patients: Cultural Aspects of the Medical and Psychiatric Care of Indochinese Refugees*. Washington, DC: Action for South East Asians.

Van Esterisk, P. 1980. "Cultural factors affecting the adjustment of Southeast Asian refugees." In Elliot Tepper, ed., *Southeast Asian Exodus: From Tradition to Resettlement,* 151-72. Ottawa: Canadian Asian Studies Association.

Zhou, Min, and Carl L. Bankston III. 1998. *Growing Up American: How Vietnamese Children Adapt to Life in the United States*. New York, NY: Russell Sage Foundation.

Contributors to the first edition

Donna Shareski, Vancouver City Health Department
Vien Thien, MOSAIC, Vancouver
Tammy Thiet, Vancouver City Health Department

Contributors to the second edition

Tam Truong Donnelly, School of Nursing, University of Calgary
Tina Huyen, Multicultural Family Support Services, Vancouver
Cho Van Le, Kitsilano Mental Health Team, Vancouver
Nghia Nguyen, Evergreen Community Health Centre, Vancouver
Mary Regester, School of Nursing, University of British Columbia
Donna Shareski, Bridge Health Clinic, Vancouver

8
Refugees in Canada

Natalie A. Chambers and Soma Ganesan

> A refugee is: "Any person who ... owing to a well-founded fear of persecution for reasons of race, religion, nationality, membership of a particular social group or political opinion, is outside the country of his nationality and is unable or, owing to such fear, is unwilling to avail himself of the protection of that country; or who, not having a nationality and being outside the country of his former habitual residence as a result of such events, is unable or, owing to such fear, is unwilling to return to it."
>
> – Convention Relating to the Status of Refugees, United Nations, 1951

By 2000 about 30,000 refugees were arriving in Canada every year. Unlike most of the immigrants described in this book, refugees did not choose to leave their home country and come to Canada. They fled persecution and often violence at home and feared for their safety if they should return. Many arrive in Canada after long and difficult journeys; others have waited in a refugee camp in a second country, often for years, before boarding a flight to Canada.

Becoming a refugee inevitably entails poverty and loss of social status through being forced to abandon property and even family members. Refugees may already suffer from a variety of physical and mental health problems on their arrival, and on settling in Canada they are typically confronted with profound culture shock. They have had little or no time to learn English or French or to become familiar with Canadian culture, and many have no family or friends here to support them.

Natalie Chambers interviewed professionals and refugees, reviewed the literature, and wrote this chapter. Soma Ganesan provided introductions to professionals and acted as consultant on chapter content.

Not only are the social problems and health concerns (particularly mental health concerns) of refugees different from those of ordinary immigrants, but also government policy drastically limits refugees' access to health services, work, and social benefits. This is particularly true of asylum seekers, the larger of the two groups of refugees to be described.

A professional can respond effectively to the physical, mental, and social concerns of a refugee only by understanding the overall refugee experience and the difficult processes that refugees must go through to become settled in Canada. Knowledge of the refugee process allows a professional to anticipate and deal with the inevitable stress, sometimes very prolonged, that the refugee may experience as a result of leaving home, coming to Canada, and struggling to survive on the margins of Canadian society. It is therefore critical for professionals to identify (1) whether their clients are refugees rather than immigrants, (2) which category of refugee status they belong to, and (3) where they are in the very complex stages of the refugee acceptance process. In the course of working with refugees, moreover, professionals should learn to work with the refugee services available to help their clients.

Despite the variety of cultures and experiences among refugees who come to Canada, it has been noted that there are "certain consistencies in the refugee experience and refugee behavior" that may assist professionals in their work with refugees (Stein 1986, 5). To identify some of these common problems, we talked with health providers, family doctors, psychiatrists, nurses, and other knowledgeable persons, as well as with immigration and refugee-serving agencies. These individuals included both immigrants and Canadian-born persons who work daily with refugees. Everyone emphasized that the professional must use the information presented here as a guide only and must go on to learn about what refugees face from personal contact with refugees themselves.

This chapter briefly outlines the formal definitions of refugees and the services available to them and presents some of the social, physical, and mental health issues that challenge them. To contrast the unique experiences of refugees from different countries, we include two case studies of refugees from Somalia and Afghanistan.

Reasons for Leaving

Refugees flee their home countries to escape conditions they feel to be threatening or unbearable. Most fear violence or persecution, and most have suffered deprivation at home and during their escape.

Elsewhere in this book are detailed accounts of the experiences of refugees from Central America, Iran, China, Vietnam, Cambodia, and Laos which demonstrate the importance of knowing something about refugees' home countries. Refugees everywhere tell similar stories. In the 1990s the Canadian government and private sponsors focused on the urgency of protecting Albanians from the genocide in Kosovo in the former Yugoslavia. Five decades of armed conflict in Colombia have created more than two million refugees who flee in the face of being kidnapped and suffering torture and death at the hands of the Colombian security, their paramilitary allies, and opposition guerrilla groups. As in many other countries that are engaged in armed conflict, defenders of human rights, trade unionists, and journalists are targeted for "disappearances," torture, or outright murder. Since intertribal fighting first broke out in 1999 in the Darfur region of western Sudan, 110,000 refugees have fled into neighbouring Chad. In Somalia, clan divisions continue to force families to flee into Ethiopia, where they may wait several years before being resettled in countries like Canada. In Sierra Leone, fighting between government forces and revolutionary groups since 1991 has created a constant flow of refugees. Around the world at any given time, according to refugee-serving agencies, armed conflict is under way in about thirty countries.

Refugees from each country, and even individual refugees from the same country, may have had very different experiences. But all share the fear of staying at home and have made the courageous and life-altering decision to leave.

Refugee Camps

There were an estimated twenty million displaced persons around the world in 2003, many of them in refugee camps in adjacent countries. For example, most refugees from Somalia have spent years in camps in Kenya and Ethiopia before being admitted to Canada as refugees. Many refugees from Afghanistan lived in camps in Pakistan or Iran; Somalis fled to Ethiopia and Kenya; Sudanese stayed in camps in Chad; and in the past Vietnamese, Cambodians, and Laotians were sheltered in camps just inside the border of Thailand, as well as in Malaysia, Indonesia, and Hong Kong.

Refugee camps usually begin as makeshift shelters providing minimal services. Many of the countries where refugee camps emerge are poor, and their governments usually want to discourage further refugees from arriving. For these reasons refugee services are often left to aid agencies such as Doctors Without Borders or the Red Cross. The largest camps in Asia and Africa have become permanent places of sanctuary as a result of long-standing conflicts in neighbouring countries. For example, over time the camps in Pakistan for Afghanis became permanent settlements and are now suburbs.

Most refugees in camps plan on returning to their home countries when stability is restored. But after years of waiting for this to happen, many refuges resign themselves to lives in exile and apply to be resettled in Western countries, including Canada.

The camp experience is often an integral part of the trauma of being a refugee. For example, a camp in Maro, Chad, in Africa, had no essential services such as water, medicine, and sanitation until outside agencies arrived. For nine months the only source of food was mangoes grown on local farms, followed for months by a diet of cereal and little else (Denes 2003). This situation is not unusual. Refugee camps are usually overcrowded and have poor sanitation, a high risk of fire, and a short supply of food and other necessities. Inhabitants of refugee camps are usually the poorest of those who flee, since persons with money tend to find alternative paths of departure. Some refugees may manage to start small businesses inside camps, such as market stalls or selling cooked food. Some men may find temporary work in nearby towns or agricultural areas, though working outside the camp sometimes involves the risk of being arrested and returned to the home country.

Camps generally do not provide adequate support for the most vulnerable persons, notably the elderly, children, and pregnant women. Pregnant women are at risk of infection with tuberculosis, hepatitis, or malaria, and they have to give birth in unsanitary conditions if suitable clinics are not available. Refugee children are extremely vulnerable to malnutrition, which, if they survive, can have consequences for them in later years. A physician may see a well-nourished ten-year-old in Canada but will not have the medical records that would show this child once lived in a refugee camp, suffering severe malnourishment and probable brain damage at ages one or two, which may explain learning difficulties in Canada now (Galler, Shumsky, and Morgane 1996, 230).

Camps are not always benign and protected environments. Some Afghanis waiting in camps in Pakistan became addicted to heroin, which was readily available for sale inside the camps, and upon their return to Afghanistan have overwhelmed the meagre addiction treatment services. Refugee camps in Africa have been invaded by armed men who murdered those who belonged to different ethnic or political groups. Sometimes a camp replicates the social, political, and ethnic conflicts of the home country, confronting refugees with the same problems in a new form. Refugees also suffer if some camp workers become corrupt and demand bribes for essential services, such as routine health checks or support for refugee applications.

Refugee-service professionals have noticed that refugees who live in camps tend to block their memories of the past or thoughts of the future and focus on the day-to-day camp routines. This is a survival technique for enduring the trauma. Many refugees after arriving in Canada continue to use this strategy of "splitting time to handle stress" (Beiser 1999, 124-45) sometimes for years until they are fully settled in their new home.

Origins and Destinations

The events and conflicts that force individuals to flee their home countries occur in places all over the world. The countries from which refugees come to Canada change continually. By 2001 the numbers of persons arriving from the former Yugoslavia, mainly from Kosovo, Bosnia-Herzegovina, and Croatia, had greatly diminished only to be replaced by refugees from Afghanistan, Colombia, and the Congo. In 2001 the top source countries for persons admitted as refugees into Canada were Afghanistan, Sri Lanka, Pakistan, Yugoslavia, Iran, Colombia, Iraq, Sudan, and the Congo. In all, 27,899 refugees arrived that year.

In 2002 the largest proportion of refugees, 61 percent, settled in the major metropolitan areas of Ontario, 27 percent went to Quebec, and 8 percent settled in British Columbia. Each metropolitan area receives refugees from somewhat different countries, depending on such things as ease of travel and where others from the country have settled earlier.

The Two Refugee Categories

When a person asks Canada for protection as a refugee, the government must consider the request and decide if the claim is valid. Under Canada's Immigration and Refugee Protection Act of 2002, there are two main pathways through which individuals can apply to become accepted as refugees in Canada: (1) the Refugee and Humanitarian Resettlement Program, for people applying from outside Canada as "convention refugees," and (2) the In-Canada Refugee Protection Process, for persons applying from within Canada as "asylum seekers." These two types of claim for refugee status will be explained below and discussed separately. Convention refugees and asylum seekers have had dissimilar social and psychological experiences. Convention refugees, who arrive sponsored by the resettlement program, have far better support from government services than asylum seekers, who appear in Canada with no status beyond their statements of claim. Moreover, unlike applicants for convention refugee status, who endure the stresses of evaluation and possible refusal in a distant land, asylum seekers are present in Canada throughout the arduous evaluation period and aware that more than half such applications are refused.

Resettled Refugees from Abroad

Every year the Canadian government relies on the Office of the United Nations High Commissioner for Refugees (UNHCR) and private sponsoring groups, such as Canadian church groups, to identify approximately 10,300 refugees abroad for resettlement in Canada. These refugees are called "resettled" or "convention" refugees, the latter referring to the UN Convention on refugees, which defines refugees as having "a well-founded fear of persecution for reasons of race, religion, nationality, membership of a particular social group or political opinion." The sponsoring groups have local representatives who visit most refugee camps, and almost all these refugees apply for sponsorship to Canada from a refugee camp.

Persons applying from outside Canada to become refugees must pass a medical examination, and criminal and security screening procedures must prove that they are of no risk to Canadian security. They must also demonstrate the ability to become self-sufficient in Canada within three to five years, and they must be financially sponsored by the government, a recognized group, or a private organization.

Most refugees who are accepted into Canada from overseas arrive as permanent residents. Others, whose applications were expedited, perhaps to give urgent protection, may arrive as "protected persons," and they may have to wait several months before receiving permanent resident status.

A major problem in the refugee process is associated with the hurried departure of most refugees from their home country. Many have left behind everything they could not carry and during the trip to the camp have spent any money they carried. They may not have brought with them their birth certificates, passports, documents showing their education and training, or other papers. And now it may be difficult or even dangerous to attempt to obtain such papers from home.

Applicants from outside Canada must meet the UN definition of refugee stated above and their situation must be one of the following:

Country of Asylum Class

They are outside the country of origin – for instance in a refugee camp – and "seriously and personally affected by civil war, armed conflict or massive violation of human rights."

Source Country Class

They meet the definition of convention refugees, but they still live in their home country, perhaps detained or imprisoned. They are suffering serious deprivations of the right of freedom of expression or dissent and the right to engage in trade union activity. Only individuals from the following countries have been identified by the Canadian government to be eligible for this class: Colombia, Democratic Republic of Congo, El Salvador, Guatemala, Sierra Leone, and Sudan (Canadian Council for Refugees 2002).

Other Refugee Application Streams

Urgent Protection

In some cases UNHCR requests that Canada provide urgent protection for people subject to "immediate threats to their life, liberty or physical safety" in their home country. These are priority cases to which Canada usually responds in twenty-four hours, and attempts are made to move the refugee to Canada within three to five days. These urgent refugees are not usually required to attend an interview with an immigration officer. They may have experienced recent, intense trauma, and their swift move to Canada adds to that stress. Refugees from Sudan and Colombia, for example, have been processed within three days. One man arrived in Canada with bullets still in his leg. Their trauma is often so recent that considerable cultural competency is required to help them.

Women at Risk

Women who are living outside Canada and need urgent protection because they are "in a dangerous situation without family protection or the protection of local authorities" must still pass medical examinations and security checks. But they "do not have to show that they have settlement potential" (Citizenship and Immigration Canada 2003).

Family Reunification of Resettled, or Convention, Refugees

Family members often become separated during their departure or later on journeys or in refugee camps. Once a convention refugee has arrived in Canada, there is a one-year window of opportunity to apply for reunification with others in the family, provided these family members' names were included in the refugee's initial application.

Services for Resettled, or Convention, Refugees in Canada

Resettled, or convention, refugees are eligible upon their arrival in Canada to receive certain services to aid their settlement experience. They are met at the airport and given temporary accommodation, assistance with finding permanent housing, and a supply of basic household items. They receive financial orientation, assistance in locating work or other continued financial support, and in some cases an income supplement for up to one year. They are also eligible for provincial medical services upon arrival. In provinces where health insurance premiums are required, such as British Columbia, these payments are waived for the first year.

Convention refugees are also eligible to apply to the Immigration Loans Program to cover the costs of medical examinations, travel documents, transportation to Canada, and the Right of Permanent Residence Fee (costing $950 in 2004). Refugees who accept immigration loans are expected to repay the amount, and interest may apply after a period of one to three years. Individuals who wish to return to their country of origin within two years of arrival in Canada may also be eligible for loans from the Canadian government to cover their transportation back.

Refugees arriving in Canada usually do not know about the services for which they qualify. An organization called Community Airport Newcomers Network (CANN) sends representatives to meet refugees at Vancouver International Airport. Written material is of little use if arriving refugees cannot read it. Professionals can be especially helpful by providing accurate information about these services in person.

Asylum Seekers in Canada

Individuals who arrive in Canada and then claim asylum must apply to become refugees through a different process. In 2001, 44,726 individuals made refugee claims from within Canada. Also that year, "of 28,418 refugee claims finalized by the Immigration and Refugee Board, 13,383 (47 percent) were found to be *bona fide* refugees" (Canadian Council for Refugees 2002).

Fleeing the Home Country

Asylum seekers have often made long and dangerous journeys to come to Canada. Many have spent years in refugee camps, some have come straight from conflict in their home country, and others have lived illegally in other countries while saving money to travel to Canada. Some have been forced to travel through many other countries in order to arrive finally at a place where they can board a plane. For example, asylum seekers from Afghanistan have been known to walk across Iran into Turkey before being able to board a plane to a Western country such as Canada. The risks of such a journey include mountainous terrain, hypothermia, and being shot or captured by border patrols. Many asylum seekers have no option but to pay most of their money to illegal smugglers who arrange false identification documents and transport to enter Canada. Refugees who lack the money for the full journey often work illegally in intervening countries, in restaurant kitchens, or on farms and construction sites, to pay for the next stage of their trek to Canada.

The In-Canada Refugee Protection Process

Asylum seekers are expected to make a claim for protection as soon as they arrive within Canadian territory, at the border or airport. Under international law, Canada is required to protect anyone in Canada who claims to be unable to return to his or her own country because of being "seriously and personally affected by civil war, armed conflict and massive violations of human rights" (Citizenship and Immigration Canada 2003). That is why Canada has a system for fairly evaluating such a claim originating within this country.

An exception to Canada's responsibility to accept all asylum seekers reaching its borders came into effect in late December 2004. Since that time the Safe Third Country Agreement between the United States and Canada requires asylum seekers to make refugee claims in the first of the two countries, Canada or the United States, in which they land. In practical terms, this means that most asylum seekers from Central or South America and many from other countries must make their claim in the United States, whose border they encounter first. They will be turned back by Canadian border officials if they have previously been allowed into the United States. This new agreement will affect an estimated 40 percent of those who would seek asylum in Canada.

After a claim for protection has been made, the eligibility of the claim to receive evaluation is supposed to be determined within three days, although this is rarely the case (Canadian Council for Refugees 2002). Once a claim is deemed eligible, it is up to the Immigration and Refugee Board (IRB), an independent tribunal, to determine if the person meets the criteria of the UN Convention and qualifies for protection. If the claim is unsuccessful, the person must leave the country in thirty days. The board's decision can be appealed, on procedural grounds, to the Federal Court for judicial review or to the Minister of Immigration and Citizenship, on compassionate grounds. It is estimated that just over half (50-55 percent) of asylum seekers' applications are denied, so that nearly half are in fact genuine refugees. Those applicants whose claims are successful become "protected persons" and are eligible to apply for permanent resident status in Canada.

This brief description of the formal process that asylum seekers go through to become, they hope, first "protected persons" and later permanent residents in Canada does not do justice to the actual experience. The bureaucratic process is long, usually more than a year and often much longer. Some of the procedures require applicants to recall very traumatic events they have tried to forget, and during this extended period without refugee status they must survive on very little money and little formal support. It is important for professionals working with asylum seekers to understand these bureaucratic steps, when they are likely to occur, and the implications they have for the refugee's physical and mental health. We list them here and then describe the experience of these events in some detail.

1 To begin the process, individuals present themselves to an immigration officer, generally at an airport or border crossing, and make their initial claim for asylum in Canada.
2 They are required to complete a refugee claim form describing their experiences and the reasons why they left their home country. Their refugee claim is assessed for eligibility, and if approved their case is referred to the Immigration and Refugee Board.
3 Individuals and families must find their own accommodation in Canada when they arrive. Many may attempt to locate distant relatives, friends, or simply other individuals from their home country for assistance in orienting themselves to Canada.
4 Before they can receive financial aid, asylum seekers are required to take an employment orientation session in English or French.
5 Following this, asylum seekers are eligible to receive minimal financial aid.
6 Upon receiving "hardship benefits," asylum seekers are finally eligible to seek the services of a lawyer through Legal Aid. They require a lawyer to help them prepare for their hearing with the Immigration and Refugee Board.
7 Asylum seekers must prove their identity; this may involve obtaining documentation, such as birth certificates or passports, from their home country.
8 With the assistance of a lawyer, asylum seekers are required to fill out a Personal Information Form (PIF) that for a second time, after their initial claim, describes the reasons why they have come to Canada and explains their claim for protection.
9 A hearing with the Immigration and Refugee Board is often scheduled many months later. If the application is approved by the board, the claimant becomes a "protected person" and may apply for permanent residence in Canada.

Making a Statement upon Entering Canada

To make a refugee claim from within Canada involves having entered Canada illegally since the individual does not have an entry visa and probably lacks identifying documents. Many refugees from war-torn countries have had their documents confiscated or destroyed at home. Those who do have passports must destroy them before approaching an immigration officer or risk being sent back immediately to their home country. Most asylum seekers have learned this on their journeys and find ways to dispose of passports on the plane.

Such "paperless" refugees presenting themselves at an airport or border crossing must fill out a refugee claim form describing in detail their experiences at home and their reasons for claiming asylum in Canada. This process of telling their story can be extremely challenging for genuine refugees traumatized from their home experience and stressed by the journey to Canada. Moreover, the combination of so much at stake, the environment of a busy immigration office, and a likely lack of fluency in French or English makes it especially difficult to present, on the spot, a coherent statement of all relevant facts.

Asylum seekers, having been persecuted by government officials in their home country, are understandably fearful for their safety in this new country. They may be suspicious of authority figures and afraid to tell their story to an immigration officer, especially one in a position to turn them away. These difficulties can be exacerbated by the lack of awareness and sensitivity of authorities. For example, one asylum seeker having difficulty filling out the refugee claim form asked for help. The immigration officer responded by handing over the completed statement of another refugee. Seeing this, the man became afraid to record his own story because it might be revealed to others. He knew that if he had revealed his story in his own country, his life would be in danger. Women who have fled their home country after being raped by government officials or the military will almost certainly still be too traumatized, afraid, and ashamed to record these facts on the claim form.

Despite these obstacles, asylum seekers may be accused later of making a false claim if omissions are found in the account in their initial claim form. A story found later to be incomplete may lead to their claim being rejected by the Immigration and Refugee Board. What's more, asylum seekers generally do not know this when they fill out the initial claim form and discover it only later.

Employment Orientation and Financial Aid

Many asylum seekers have little or no usable English or French and find difficulty following the complex bureaucratic steps. For example, asylum seekers who have no other means of supporting themselves in Canada may be eligible to apply for employment authorization. However, first they must attend an Employment Orientation course. Only after completing this course can they apply for financial help. Then they find that, in 2004 in British Columbia for example, this "hardship benefit" amounted to only $25 a week.

Obtaining a Lawyer and Filling Out the Personal Information Form

Once asylum claimants have retained a lawyer through Legal Aid, they must tell their entire story again in detail to their lawyer. This second telling of their story may occur up to twelve months after they first set it down in the claim form on arrival in Canada. In the meantime, many refugees have put a great deal of emotional energy into trying to forget their traumatic experiences. The result can be discrepancies with details recorded in the original claim. These inconsistencies sometimes complicate and jeopardize their refugee hearing.

With the help of a lawyer, asylum seekers prepare a Personal Information Form (PIF) that must include details of the traumatic events that caused them to leave their country, including dates, names, and so on. Some refugees forced to rehearse events they have been struggling to forget become very confused and distressed. Professionals report that at this stage some of them begin to have nightmares and insomnia.

Obtaining Identity Documents

To make a refugee claim it is necessary to prove one's identity. Identity is judged by Canadian standards, which demand a passport, birth certificate, driver's licence, high school certificate, or other precise record. In many cases asylum seekers do not have these documents. Efforts to obtain them from the home country can sometimes be extremely dangerous for family members who have stayed behind. Individuals from Afghanistan, Somalia, Iran, Burundi, and Sri Lanka consistently face serious problems in obtaining identity documents from their home countries. Some governments have never even issued identity documents to their citizens. Women and young people, particularly from rural areas, are most likely to lack identity documents, having never possessed driver's licences or school certificates (Canadian Council for Refugees 2002).

While a refugee claim may be processed without satisfactory identity documents, only individuals from Somalia and Afghanistan are able to gain permanent resident status in Canada if they still lack identity documents five years after they are deemed "protected persons." "Protected persons" from other countries remain in limbo until they can meet the standard for proof of identity for application for permanent residence.

The Hearing with the Immigration and Refugee Board (IRB)

A year or so after coming to Canada, refugees receive notice of their IRB

Hearing. This is their opportunity to prove their story. For many, the hearing represents a critical and often terrifying ordeal, because the system does not allow for an appeal on the merits of the case but only if there are serious procedural errors on points of law. Due to the lack of legal aid in some places, many claimants find they must represent themselves or accept minimal or poor legal assistance.

During the time leading up to the hearing, professionals working with asylum seekers notice that refugees' mental health often deteriorates. They may experience depression, anxiety, nightmares, insomnia, loss of appetite, panic attacks, and so on. For this reason health and social service professionals should be aware of the date of a person's IRB Hearing in order to be sensitive to changes in physical and mental health, and in order to offer reassurance that these disturbances are normal and experienced by most asylum seekers.

Many refugees expect the IRB Hearing to be like a criminal court. In some ways it is, since it involves "a high degree of examination of small details and re-telling of the facts. Consistency plays a huge role" (VAST 2002, 6). Confusion or incoherence about dates and events may lead to more aggressive questioning by board members, and mistakes or the inability to recall details accurately can be devastating in weakening the refugee claim and leading to its rejection. Survivors of torture, in particular, often are unable to remember aspects of their abuse or may feel too vulnerable to share shameful memories. Experts have commented that this results in a contradictory situation in which those who are most vulnerable and most in need of protection are usually the "least able to articulate the reasons why" (ibid., 14).

Many refugees have blocked out memories of their traumatic experiences, and such blocking out may actually have been critical to their survival. The process of preparing for and participating in the hearing, that is, re-telling details of events, brings all of these events to the surface. The Vancouver Association for the Survivors of Torture (VAST), an organization that assists asylum seekers in their applications, suggests that "the first and most important tool is to acknowledge the existence of stress and then get direction from the person" about what can help them reduce their anxiety. VAST advises professionals, when possible, to provide some concrete information to their clients about what to expect in the hearing, including mundane details such as the setting of the room, who will be there, and the procedures that are followed. They reassure refugees that the IRB is familiar with and sensitive to the emotional and psychological strain of the hearing and that refugees can request breaks during the hearing if they find it too difficult. Because many people find that recounting their story triggers crying, they can also be reassured that "none of this behavior will negatively impact their Hearing outcome" (ibid., 3). They suggest that deep breathing is often useful to manage stress during the hearing.

Refugee children and teenagers may experience an intense crisis as they approach the hearing date. Some may have been asked to attend and tell their story, but even those who do not attend are undoubtedly affected by the distress of their families in the months leading up to the hearing. They will likely experience the same physical and mental health challenges as do adults. Regular attendance at school may provide them with some stability and a welcome distraction from their home situations, but refugee children and youth may find it difficult to interact with others or to concentrate on school work. Suzie, a refugee mother, described the effect on her daughter of the upcoming hearing. "My daughter had a panic attack. Her high school took her to the hospital in an ambulance ... I had a counselling session with my daughter ... my daughter said, 'I am afraid about the future, about what is going to happen to us.'" She concluded, "It's not just killing me, it is killing my kids" (ibid., 10). This family was unfortunate enough not to be given an immediate assessment of their case following the hearing. They were forced to wait three agonizingly long months before being informed that they had indeed been accepted to Canada as "protected persons" and could now apply for permanent residence.

Medical Examination

Upon the completion of the hearing and on becoming "protected persons" in Canada, individuals must arrange an appointment with a Designated Medical Practitioner (DMP) who conducts medical examinations on behalf of Citizenship and Immigration Canada. (Asylum seekers who had medical examinations done prior to this in order to obtain work and student authorizations do not have to be examined again.)

Medical examinations involve the following: a chest X-ray for individuals eleven years and older, testing for syphilis and HIV for individuals fifteen years and older, and urinalysis for those over the age of five. Individuals are also screened for hepatitis, parasites, sexually transmitted diseases, and tuberculosis.

Applying for Permanent Residence

Once asylum seekers have been accepted as "protected persons" by the Immigration and Refugee Board they can apply for permanent residence in Canada, a status considered by the government to be a privilege and not guaranteed. Like all other applicants for permanent residence, protected persons must satisfy a points system that considers education, language ability, work experience, and potential to adapt to Canadian society. The

Nasiri, refugee from Afghanistan

When Nasiri and her twenty-year-old daughter arrived in Toronto in 2001 they were exhausted – but also exhilarated at having finally reached a safe place far from the chaos of Afghanistan.

Nasiri had lived through twenty-six years of war at home. Many times she had been threatened by Taliban troops for her attempts to teach school-age girls in her own home. Girls were forbidden to attend school, and women who worked risked being punished by death. In 2001 her husband and sons were killed and their home destroyed by an American bomb. Deeply saddened by their loss and fearing for their own lives now that their men could no longer protect them, Nasiri told her daughter that they must leave Afghanistan. Her husband had money hidden away that would pay for the journey, and he had instructed her on how to leave if it became necessary to do so. They paid smugglers to guide them to the Pakistani border and provide them with false identification. Once in that country they continuously dodged officials until they could fly out several months later.

After about six months in Toronto, Nasiri felt more and more pain under one arm; she could barely lift her arm to reach things and could not carry heavy shopping bags. But she was too nervous to go to a doctor, fearing the expense of medicines and bus fares. She was also worried about having a stranger look at her body, especially a male doctor. Eventually her worried daughter heard of a walk-in clinic that had a woman doctor, and she accompanied her mother to interpret in her basic English. The physician insisted on doing a physical examination and then told them that she would need to see a doctor at the cancer clinic. The clinic would call to arrange an appointment.

The following day Nasiri received a call notifying her that she and her daughter were required to attend their refugee hearing in four weeks. Since that time she has spent most of her time in their bedroom, praying. Her silence is occasionally broken by sobbing. "I can't go to the clinic," she told her daughter. "They won't let us stay in Canada if I have this awful disease. They will send me back to Afghanistan. If I'm going to die, I want to be with you here." She feared that this disease would kill her, and that would leave her daughter to fend for herself in a strange country. Eventually her daughter begged Nasiri to return with her to the female physician, in the hope of receiving some reassurance to put her mother's mind at rest.

processing of the claim and the final acceptance documents can take up to four years to be issued, and sometimes as long as ten years, as in the case of some Somali refugees who were unable to obtain identity documents from officials in their country.

Asylum seekers whose claims are not accepted are ordered to leave Canada. But many remain. In 2003 it was estimated that there were 36,000 such persons in the country, many working illegally in construction and service jobs for low pay. Many have "settled" and established families, but of course they do not have the security of Medicare or the other protections available to permanent residents and citizens (Jimenez 2003).

Community Agencies Providing Support

A number of non-government organizations and church groups, mainly in urban areas, offer services for asylum seekers. However, these groups are usually non-profit and limited in resources. Since non-governmental organizations are not allowed to set up desks inside airports, asylum seekers may have difficulty identifying agencies for assistance. Refugee-serving organizations usually have multilingual workers and offer translation services and advocacy for asylum seekers. Other services they may provide include financial and employment orientations, temporary accommodation and assistance in locating permanent housing, access to a food bank, assistance with completing application forms, support for refugees in detention, information for parents about the Canadian education system and assistance identifying schooling, introductions to Canadian host families, and referrals to other agencies.

Working in Canada

Convention refugees are eligible to work upon their arrival. They receive assistance in finding work and other support and, in some cases, an income supplement during the first year. By contrast, asylum seekers are eligible only to apply for a one-year work authorization. First they must prove that no other form of public assistance is available to them. Then they must apply for the work authorization and undergo a medical examination. Applications can sometimes take as long as six months because the results from medical examinations are often delayed in Ottawa. A delay leaves the person with no way to obtain work legally, and out of desperation some individuals may accept illegal employment.

Changes to the law in 2004 mean that non-permanent residents of Canada are no longer able to obtain a social insurance number (SIN) without proof of an offer of employment – in spite of the fact that it is difficult to impossible for individuals with poor language skills to obtain written offers of employment for temporary, low-skilled jobs. Furthermore, SINs for non-permanent residents are now issued with an expiry date. Both asylum seekers and convention refugees are therefore assigned a social insurance number that begins with "9," indicating temporary residence in Canada. Many employers infer from this that the individual will not be here permanently, cannot be relied upon, or is an illegal worker. As a result, refugees may be the "last to be hired and first to be fired." Only if they obtain permanent residence status will the "9" in their SIN be replaced by another number. The stress of being unemployed, combined with other pressures connected to refugee status, has been linked to higher rates of suicide and mental disorders (Report 1988).

Once they receive work permits, many refugees have difficulty finding work. Given that many of them, especially asylum seekers, do not have usable English or French, opportunities for employment are usually limited to low-level, poorly paid jobs, often in roles that do not use their skills or training. One refugee from Vietnam, an engineer, worked for several years as a church janitor before he could move into a position as a technician at a large hydroelectric facility. A public health physician from Cambodia started work as a dishwasher in a small restaurant before she could obtain a more suitable job as an aide in a nursing home.

Health of Refugees upon Arrival in Canada

Convention refugees are required to have a medical examination before being admitted into Canada. This process screens out some applicants and leads to treatment for others before they arrive. Convention refugees are vaccinated before leaving the refugee camp unless their applications were expedited, as with Kosovo refugees in the 1990s. However, the medical exams are usually conducted shortly after the application for refugee status is made, which can be months to a year before their arrival in Canada. Since they may have been exposed to disease and parasites during this intervening period, they may require another medical exam shortly after coming to Canada.

Asylum seekers who have come to a port of entry on their own will not have had any formal medical screening before their arrival. However, health organizations across Canada are set up to do medical examinations for asylum seekers who self-refer or who are referred to them by refugee-serving agencies or other non-governmental organizations. Individuals who do not go independently to have a medical screening, such as for work authorization, will not receive an exam until after their IRB Hearing, which could be several years after their arrival.

For individuals who request medical screening shortly after arriving, health care professionals may be the first Canadian professionals they meet. For this reason, some health organizations, such as the Bridge Community Health Clinic in St. Joseph's Hospital in Vancouver, have health care workers who specialize in working with refugees and who are fluent in a number of different languages. Community health clinics generally screen asylum seekers for parasites, hepatitis B if from endemic areas, hepatitis C, STDs, and HIV if the individual is considered at risk, as well as doing Pap tests and mammograms. Asylum seekers can also request to have immunizations. Health care workers who have experience working with refugees may also provide referrals to other refugee-serving agencies for advocacy, counselling, legal aid, and for information on other settlement issues.

HIV/AIDS

Beginning in 2003 the Canadian government required that all immigrants be tested for HIV/AIDS. In the case of refugees, however, a positive test does not bar their admission to Canada. As a result of this policy some refugees recently diagnosed with HIV/AIDS will not have had any pre- or post-test counselling or support. As yet, few services have been set up to link these refugees to appropriate professional help.

Refugee Health Benefits in Canada

Even though refugees may have received some information about their health benefits at the airport or elsewhere, the stress of arrival and settlement, lack of English or French, illiteracy in their own language, and many other factors contribute to their unawareness of services available to them. Health professionals can be very helpful by ensuring that they have accurate information.

As of 2004, convention refugees arrive in Canada eligible for provincial health insurance. In addition, they receive Extended Interim Federal Health Insurance, which covers the cost of eyeglasses and basic dental care, including cleaning, pulling, and filling teeth but not cosmetic or restorative work. Extended Interim Health is valid only for one year following their arrival in Canada. In provinces where premiums are required, convention refugees do not have to pay them during their first year of residence in Canada.

By contrast, asylum seekers are not eligible for provincial health insurance. After they submit their claim to an immigration officer and their claim is approved for referral to the IRB (in principle within three days), they become eligible for Interim Federal Health Insurance (IFH), which provides coverage until their hearing and then, if their refugee claim is successful and they become "protected persons," for up to three months after that. At this point they can become covered by provincial health insurance.

Interim Federal Health Insurance covers essential services and emergency care, so they are eligible for hospital care, but there are limits. If the amount billed to IFH is greater than the insurance allows, the resulting debts in the refugee's name are forwarded to collection agencies (Anderson 2002). The IFH program provides only low-cost generic medicine, and many asylum seekers are unable to pay for more expensive medications if these are prescribed by doctors unaware of this financial constraint. Furthermore, IFH does not pay for counselling sessions with physicians, which is a limitation and disadvantage for asylum seekers who may prefer to use their family doctor instead of the special counselling services offered by refugee agencies. A disincentive for health professionals is that they must send their bill for IFH services to the federal government and then wait for reimbursement, sometimes for long periods of time.

All children born in Canada, including children of asylum seekers, are Canadian citizens at birth. A child born to parents not eligible for provincial health insurance becomes eligible for this coverage after a three-month waiting period if the family intends to remain in the province.

Barriers and Challenges to Good Health Care for Refugees

Refugees face enormous challenges in obtaining good health services in Canada, problems often much greater than those of other immigrants. Health professionals working with refugees are challenged as well, since little information is readily available about refugees with their diverse cultures and experiences. The population of refugees changes very quickly, and health professionals may not be prepared for persons with unexpected languages and cultural backgrounds. Moreover, the few professionals experienced in working with refugees have difficulty meeting their varied and pressing needs. In large cities, but often not in rural areas, community resources exist to assist health professionals, but many of these agencies find themselves overburdened and underqualified, especially when it comes to identifying refugees' mental health concerns (Charlton et al. 2002).

Refugees are three times less likely to speak either English or French when they arrive in Canada than are immigrants who arrive through the independent, family, and business class processes (Report 1988). The language problem has been dealt with in different ways, to which we now turn.

Physicians from Refugees' Home Countries

Family doctors who share the language and culture of their patients are an extremely valuable resource for refugees. However, refugees settling outside the major metropolitan areas may have to bear the cost of long-distance travel and lost wages just to find a physician they can talk to. Then, too, refugees may be understandably reluctant to use a physician from their home country until they are certain of the doctor's politics and social position in their culture. Most Vietnamese refugees had little or no English when they arrived in Canada (a few had French), so they asked for Vietnamese-speaking doctors. But before making an appointment they would first inquire among other Vietnamese whether during the Vietnam War the doctor had sided with the Americans or with Ho Chi Minh's revolutionary army. These and other indications would help them judge whether the physician could be trusted to protect their privacy and understand their trauma. Indigenous peoples from Central and South America sometimes discovered on arriving in Canada that they were expected to confide in Spanish-speaking health professionals. Many were understandably traumatized at having to answer questions from these Spanish-speaking authority figures who belonged, or were perceived to belong, to the groups who had persecuted them.

Use of Interpreters

Many health professionals have found it helpful to use the services of interpreters. Especially when refugees are involved, it is important to identify, if possible, professional translators who not only have an adequate medical and mental health vocabulary but also are aware of ethical issues such as assuring confidentiality. Unfortunately there are not many professional interpreters working in the physicians' private offices. Hospitals may have access to AT&T telephone translation services, but this process is impersonal, time-consuming, and often disruptive to a trusting relationship between professional and patient. The use of interpreters remains a barrier to effective communication, especially in counselling.

Both trained interpreter services and telephone translation are expensive, so many hospitals rely on ad hoc translation by untrained staff, from nurses to kitchen aides and janitors who speak the required language. Other patients, relatives, and children may also be asked to interpret, thus creating problems of confidentiality, censorship, and incorrect translation. In some settings, as in nursing homes, commonly used terms such as "pain" and "toilet" are written in the patient's language side by side with English so that both patient and staff can point to the message they want to convey.

Discrimination and Racism in Canada

Asylum seekers face unusual challenges in dealing with the stigma of their uncertain status in Canada. Popular stereotypes see them as "bogus refugees" and as a drain on resources in Canada. Public perceptions of asylum seekers are compounded by negative coverage in the media of selected individuals who do seek to abuse the system. Not only persons born in Canada but also landed immigrants and even convention refugees may regard asylum seekers as "jumping the queue" by coming to Canada before applying for refugee status. However, as shown by the decisions by the Refugee Board, nearly half of asylum seekers have documented, legitimate reasons for fleeing to Canada for protection.

In addition, asylum seekers as members of visible minority groups may be stigmatized or face discrimination by members of mainstream society, including health professionals, for their skin colour, clothing, accent, or poor English. They frequently encounter verbal or physical abuse, discriminatory hiring practices, and difficulty in finding housing. These experiences can cause profound confusion and low self-esteem.

Families and the Refugee Experience

Professionals working with refugees in Canada have found it very important to know whether families have been separated. Many refugees arriving in Canada have been removed from their families through death or travel. Families sometimes lose each other in their flight and end up in different camps. Families may split between members who stay, often the elderly, and those who leave, whether voluntarily or by family decision. Many refugees suffer the daily anxiety of not knowing the whereabouts of other family members or even whether they are alive. Difficulties of communication compound this anxiety, because mail or telephone contact may be perilous for family members still at home. Some refugees suffer profound guilt at having survived when other family members and friends lost their lives.

Aisha and Hussein, refugees from Somalia

In 1999 twenty-eight-year-old Aisha, her husband, Hussein, and their five children finally were "settled" in Canada as convention refugees. Although the family was originally from Somalia, the ongoing civil war had forced them to flee their home, and they had spent six years living in a refugee camp in Kenya.

Life was very hard in the camp. There was no running water, and sanitation was very poor. At the camp they met people who had already been waiting nine years to be resettled in a safe country. Aisha and Hussein did not discuss their happier memories of the past in Somalia before violence and chaos began to shape their lives, and they soon began to find it almost impossible to think about what each new day might bring.

From their very first night in the camp, Aisha struggled to care for and feed her two children, and she battled with malnutrition constantly during each of her subsequent four pregnancies. One of her babies was born so small and weak that he died shortly after delivery, but Aisha had no time to mourn their loss. The family constantly fought hunger and worked hard to comfort their children in their flimsy canvas shelter.

Hussein went missing in their final year in the camp. He had decided to seek work outside the camp in a nearby village. After several months he was caught and arrested by Kenyan officials. Aisha had not known if she would ever see her husband again and feared he had been killed. When the family's application to be resettled in Canada was finally approved, Aisha had little choice but to board a flight to Toronto without him. She informed friends in the camp that she would find Hussein's cousin in Toronto when they arrived in Canada.

Aisha and her five children arrived in Toronto in the middle of November wearing sandals and thin cotton garments. It was winter, and they were completely unprepared for the cold. They had never even seen snow before. How could they survive in such a harsh climate?

In broken English and with a heavy accent, Aisha successfully communicated to an immigration official that she was looking for a relative in Toronto. In an attempt to help, the officer looked up the name in the phone book and gave her the number for someone with a similar-sounding last name. After being instructed on how to make a call, Aisha dialled the number and spoke rapidly in Somali to the person who answered. It was not her husband's cousin, but the Somali woman was helpful. She offered to pick Aisha up from the airport and invited her and her children to stay with them a few days, or longer, while they located her husband's relatives. Within a week Aisha and her children were staying in the cramped house of her husband's cousin. She was relieved to have found some family support while she began rebuilding her life in Canada.

Within a month the Somali community had helped Aisha to find a job as a seamstress in an industrial estate where many other Somali women worked. It was an enormous adjustment for Aisha and her children to live in Canada alone without Hussein. Suddenly Aisha was the head of the household, and the family was completely dependent upon her meagre income.

Aisha had learned some English in Somalia, and, as she had hoped, her English improved quickly once she was in Canada. She was thankful for their safety, but she was constantly overwhelmed and depressed by the responsibilities of single parenthood. She seldom allowed herself to think of her husband or her life in Somalia because these thoughts seemed to tear at her soul.

After two years Aisha finally gained news of her husband; Kenyan officials had sent him back to Somalia, from where he made his way to Ethiopia and finally arrived in Toronto exhausted and traumatized. He found the adjustment to Canadian life very challenging. He discovered that his wife had become more independent than when they lived in Somalia, and it made him very angry when his children paid attention to their mother but not to him. A year after his arrival, Hussein was still unemployed and spending his days socializing in Somali cafes with other unemployed Somali men. He and Aisha have to start their lives over again. They try not to think of the past and the old way of life in Somalia that they miss so much.

Families of refugees become extremely vulnerable to breakdown through a combination of long periods of separation, the conflict between the values of Canadian society and their own values, and the pressures of integration and economic survival.

Refugee Children

Leaving Home

Refugee children may experience settlement and mental health problems that are not shared by immigrant children who entered Canada through normal immigration. They may have been separated for long periods from their parents, siblings, and extended family members. They may have learned that information was withheld from them for a variety of reasons. They might have been told they were going on a short trip or to visit a relative only to discover, months after arriving in Canada, that they would never be returning home. Parents caught up in the refugee process may not have kept their children fully informed, or may have chosen to shield their children from anxieties, or may have wished to avoid dealing with their children's desires to return home. Young children, and of course infants, will not be fully aware of what is happening, but they will perceive and suffer from the tension and trauma affecting their parents.

Health

Refugee children may have health problems that were not diagnosed or treated prior to their arrival in Canada. Professionals have noted malnutrition, incomplete immunization, parasites and worms, and delays in growth and development. Some refugee children may have been sexually abused in refugee camps. In 2002 some school administrators and teachers noted an increasing number of refugee children with special needs, including Down's syndrome and post-traumatic stress syndrome (ESL Consortium 2002, 2).

Many refugee children arrive in Canada with no birth certificate or other official documents to establish their age. Sometimes parents do not know their children's precise ages, and in some situations bone testing may be done to determine a more accurate age. A date of birth of 1 January and then the year may have been arbitrarily assigned.

School Experiences in Canada

Many refugee children enter school fairly soon after arrival while their families are still in "survival mode." The central family issues are the basic worries about jobs, money, and future status in Canada. Recent years have seen the arrival of increasing numbers of refugee families from places such as Afghanistan and Somalia with multigenerational illiteracy and poor or no spoken English or French. Their children may be extremely frustrated to arrive at a Canadian school and be completely unable to understand what is happening. Some older children feel infantilized by the education system. And yet, school may also seem to refugee children a safe place where there is consistency and stability.

Professionals have noted that children whose parents are uneducated or illiterate tend to have low levels of conceptual and language development. With these disadvantages, illiteracy in a native language can make literacy in English or French difficult to achieve and in the long run may hamper a child's integration into Canadian society (ESL Consortium 2002, 2). Recent adult refugees from Afghanistan, for example, may have little or no education, particularly the women, and after twenty years of war and repression their children often arrive in Canada with almost no schooling. As was true of some Cambodian refugees, these parents would not themselves know how to support their children's schooling – by reading aloud, encouraging homework, and so on – even if they did have the time to do so despite being preoccupied with economic survival. Refugee children may perform poorly, lose interest in school, and drop out early and then face a lifetime of low-paid jobs or welfare.

In some refugee families the father has been separated from his wife and children, leaving his family without its traditional head. These situations may "create long-term negative changes in responsiveness to legitimate authority. In some cases, this problem is compounded at school when children respond poorly to female teachers who, of course, form the majority of the teaching population" (ESL Consortium 2002, 4).

Counselling Refugee Children

All refugee children have lost their home. Many have been faced with long periods of separation from one or both parents and siblings. Some may have seen loved ones killed or brutalized. As with adult refugees, it is important to allow refugee children to tell their stories when they are ready. But some children may never be ready, and they should not be asked about such information if they do not volunteer it.

Many professionals say that in counselling a refugee child, it is very important to involve the family rather than to isolate the child from the social and cultural reality of daily life. Families may join in the counselling sessions, or family members' points of view may be discussed with the child. Also, focusing on a behavioural problem, such as not wanting to go to school, rather than on the child as a "problem person," may help to minimize blaming in the family and encourage the formation of family alliances to solve the problem.

Refugee children are exposed to Canadian values in the schools, and, like other immigrant children, may feel conflict between the values of their home society and cultural practices here. Parents feel the same conflicts and often attempt to protect their children from mainstream Canadian life by isolating them or using strict disciplinary methods. Other challenges for older children may be exposure to drugs, gang recruitment, and sexual exploitation. Professionals can be more supportive and effective in counselling if they learn about and respect the family's own cultural beliefs concerning childhood and child-rearing (Olness 1998, 234).

Survivors of Torture

Persons working with refugees are unlikely to know whether their clients have been tortured, since specialists recommend that this topic not be raised until the client does. Some never do. If disclosure does occur it is usually in the context of the refugee's story of loss, not simply a raw description of things that were suffered.

Torture continues to be practised in more than half of the world. It is often crude, including punching, beating, and burning with cigarettes. In some countries, such as Sri Lanka, Turkey, and India, where the army and the police are commonly known to use torture, tormenters are careful to use methods that do not to leave scars, such as suspension or electric shocks. Even where torturers leave permanent visible damage, the lesions heal and may not be recognized by Canadian professionals (Hargreaves 2002).

If a refugee does talk about having been tortured, it is helpful to learn about the survivor's cultural perceptions of it. For example, "Cambodian refugees who had been tortured believed this was done to them because of their karma. They felt responsible for their own suffering" (Olness 1998, 230). Some have suggested that, when the home culture of the refugee has influenced how the torture was both conducted and experienced, the survivor may benefit from indigenous cultural practices, such as might involve elders, senior family members, and traditional healers (Mollica and McDonald 2002, 30).

Persons who have been tortured "often suffer from chronic fatigue and mental exhaustion" (ibid., 29). Some problems are long-lasting, such as feelings of incompetence and powerlessness. Professionals have reported that "intellectual performance, especially deterioration in memory and the ability to learn new tasks and ideas, is associated with head injury (beatings to the head), starvation and the secondary cognitive sequelae of PTSD [post-traumatic stress disorder] and depression" (ibid.). Sometimes psychological pain is expressed as somatic symptoms which prevent the person from working and which thus prolong helplessness and poverty.

Some professionals stress the importance of helping torture survivors reconceptualize their recent past to recapture a sense of their identity prior to and independent of the troubles that led to their torment and flight. This approach seeks to help survivors frame the torture experience as a phase in their lives, a phase now over, rather than as a permanently defining factor. The strategy is not meant to minimize the long-term effects of the experience but to focus instead on providing "the opportunities to work, take part in religious and spiritual activities and participate in education or training programmes" (ibid., 30), in other words to take charge once again of building their lives.

The Vancouver Association for the Survivors of Torture offers a variety of services to refugees, including some based on the idea that the "effects of torture are clearly on the body. The body has a memory and so the body also needs to be addressed. People carry tremendous stress in their bodies" (VAST 2001a, 12). Some techniques used by their bodywork therapists include acupuncture, craniosacral therapy, shiatsu, and reiki, which are offered by therapists selected with care and attention to their compatibility with the needs of the client.

Health professionals who work with victims of torture hear some very shocking stories. In certain circumstances, such as during the official medical assessments for the refugee's application, it is necessary to inquire about the details of the torture. In these circumstances it is especially important for health professionals themselves to have a support team of their own with whom they can share their concerns. Professionals who do this work stress that it should not be done in isolation.

Mental Health

Almost all refugees experience some mental health problems. Common among these are sleeping problems of all kinds, depression, obsessive thoughts, alcohol and drug use, anxiety, suicidal thoughts and behaviour, and post-traumatic stress symptoms. Emotional distress is often expressed physically as headaches, body pains, loss of appetite and weight, and so on. In addition, many refugees experience acute loneliness and social isolation, which exacerbate depression and low self-esteem.

Despite common mental health problems, many asylum seekers will not mention their mental health concerns or symptoms to a medical doctor, in the mistaken fear of compromising their application to remain in Canada. In the case of asylum seekers, mental health problems may fluctuate in relation to the stages in the refugee application process. We have noted earlier that an impending hearing before the Immigration and Refugee Board may trigger acute anxiety. If the board delays its decision, asylum seekers often experience an increase in anxiety around the time they expect to hear the result. Health professionals also find that refugees, even when they receive a positive decision by the board, do not always experience elation or mental relief. In fact, on finally being accepted into Canada, many asylum seekers experience a sinking feeling and a new anxiety. At this time their relief becomes the occasion for grief for the home that has been lost, grief and guilt about family and friends left behind, and a sense of emptiness about the future challenges that await them. For some, this time of transition is as difficult as the earlier wait.

Psychological Symptoms

Common symptoms among refugees are depression, insomnia, frequent waking, nightmares, loss of appetite, weight loss, intrusive memories (often of past traumatic experiences), as well as associated physical symptoms such as headaches and general aches and pains.

Focus on the Present

For the first few years after refugees have been in Canada, many tend to "split time," that is, they separate out the present, on which they focus their energies and thoughts, and disregard the past and the future. "Under normal circumstances, most people have an integrated time perspective. Time-splitting helps people adapt to extraordinary circumstance" – in this case, having lost their home and coming to a new country with all the demands of adapting to a new culture, learning a new language, finding work, and establishing a new social network (Beiser 1999, 135). Professionals see this focus on the present as a survival technique that helps individuals avoid depression, and it may explain why refugees often want to avoid re-telling their "refugee story." During the ten years or so after they come to Canada, refugees tend to abandon time-splitting, although most remain more focused on their present and future lives than on the past (Beiser 1999).

Distraction and Forgetfulness

A common complaint among refugees is not being able to concentrate. Many refugees describe being in an ESL class, hearing what is being said, but just not taking it in because their minds are distracted. They try to listen but cannot help being preoccupied with other thoughts, about the challenges they face or the events of daily life. Asylum seekers, for example, may be obsessively rehearsing the details of their Personal Information Form, a crucial stage in the application process when they must tell their whole refugee story. The struggle with a new culture and a new language can overwhelm the mind with immediate details and displace careful plans.

To deal with at least some forgetfulness, professionals often suggest that refugees obtain a diary in which to write where they are supposed to be each day. Physicians can help by writing down the most important information they want to convey, such as the diagnosis, how and when to take the medicine, possible serious side-effects, when to return, and a phone number for an appointment.

Issues of Trust

Many refugees have understandable difficulty trusting people they do not know well. They are likely to disclose psychological problems only when they have developed personal relationships with individual settlement workers or health professionals. Some fear to disclose mental health problems at all, believing that this will adversely affect their application for protected person or permanent resident status in Canada. Experiences in their home country may serve to make refugees suspicious that professionals here will disclose confidential information to others. It is therefore vital that health professionals should reassure refugee clients that there will be no bad consequences of candour, that patient confidentiality is guaranteed, especially in relation to government authorities. Many refugees are afraid, or suspicious, of authority figures such as immigration officials and are understandably reluctant to talk to the police because in their home country the police were not their protectors.

Some refugees feel intimidated and frightened about going to new places or even about going outdoors at all. They feel safer at home, and may stay inside for days and weeks on end. This makes it difficult for them to visit service agencies, and they may be particularly reluctant to join group meetings with others from their home country for fear of encountering supporters of the people they feared at home.

Sleeping Problems

Sleeping problems are common among refugees, and many suffer from insomnia and nightmares about their past traumas or their present situation. Sleeping problems are exacerbated by the strain and uncertainty of their present circumstances, by not knowing the whereabouts or safety of family members, by health and relationship problems, and by post-traumatic stress disorder.

For asylum seekers disrupted sleep can become more severe during certain high-anxiety stages of the refugee process, such as just before the IRB Hearing. Health professionals can help by understanding the refugee process and their client's stage within it, which will enable sleep disorders to be prepared for and quickly identified.

Sleeping problems impair refugees' physical and mental health and their ability to function effectively. Many refugees find it difficult to wake up early in the morning and be ready to face the day at an early hour. They may miss important appointments with doctors or lawyers if an eight o'clock meeting requires getting up at six in the morning. Professionals who work regularly with refugees are aware of this reality and try to accommodate it. An understanding of the causes and consequences of sleeping disorders among refugees helps dispel the stereotype that refugees are "lazy."

Suicide

A number of refugees become depressed and suicidal. Thoughts of suicide may be entertained when a refugee feels that there are few options available through which to participate in society and lead a normal life. In these circumstances it is particularly important for professionals to normalize the process by explaining the sequence of emotional ups and downs routinely encountered by claimants going through the steps of gaining refugee status.

Some suicidal persons may need to be hospitalized for protection and treatment, but professionals need to put a great deal of effort into making sure that hospital care is necessary and, if so, that it is not stressful. Persons who have been traumatized in their home countries or during their escape may be re-traumatized by being confined to a ward or a room in a situation that mimics earlier experiences.

Drug and Alcohol Abuse

Refugees may abuse drugs and alcohol for several reasons: as a temporary escape from challenges and traumas, to combat depression, and as a means by which a socially isolated person can socialize with others and gain a sense of inclusion.

Counselling Refugees

Health professionals can be much more effective in counselling refugees if they are aware of how easily their clients can be re-traumatized. It is not necessary for a professional to know exactly what happened to the client; refugees can be spared having to tell their "refugee story" yet again. Refugees who have been tortured may have scars, but specialists in this line of work advise the professional to wait for a time (which may never come) when the patient is comfortable enough to volunteer an explanation for them. When professionals need to learn the story to assemble any medical evidence in support of the claim for the IRB Hearing, it is preferable to review the person's Personal Information Form (PIF) in which that story is recorded rather than to ask the person to talk about it. The role of the health professional is to provide support while allowing the refugee to set the agenda.

The Vancouver Association for the Survivors of Torture has developed some general guidelines for work with people who have survived political violence (VAST 2001a, 3). These recommendations may also be useful more broadly for working with any refugee, because they have all experienced the trauma of exile. The guidelines suggest that refugees find it helpful to maintain a steady routine, so that meals, going to bed, and getting up occur at the same times every day. Upsetting memories can be stimulated by exposure to noisy, busy, and confusing environments, as well as by violence on television. The recommendations also stress the importance to the refugee of maintaining contact with other people outside the home.

Delivering Sensitive Health Care to Refugees

There are probably as many "refugee experiences" as there are refugees. The information in this chapter is intended only as a general introduction. It cannot substitute for the knowledge of each refugee's situation that comes from sympathetic, supportive personal contact.

This chapter explains why it is crucial for a professional to learn whether the client is an immigrant or a refugee and, if the latter, whether a convention refugee or an asylum seeker. The services available to the two types of refugees vary radically. Moreover, while convention refugees are fairly certain that they will have a future in Canada, asylum seekers have a long period of insecurity before discovering whether they can put down roots. As a result, the physical, emotional, and social problems experienced by the two types of refugees may be quite different.

The majority of refugees arrive in Canada with little or no usable English or French. This means that contact with health professionals is often stressful and unrewarding for both parties. Professionals need to be aware of the formal translation services available to them, through trained interpreters and telephone translation, and should be cautious about using untrained persons such as hospital staff and family members. Some physicians have found that writing brief notes for the patient to take home, such as the diagnosis, how to take the medicine, side-effects, and so on, is helpful since it allows the patient to find a family member or friend who can read the note and help explain it.

Persons working with refugees can be very helpful if they are aware that most refugees are living on very meagre and often insufficient budgets. The cost of transportation, for example, can severely limit the person's ability to return to the physician for follow-up, or to attend ESL or support group meetings. Some organizations who serve refugees recognize this problem and provide their clients with free bus tickets.

Further Reading

Beiser, Morton. 1999. *Strangers at the Gate: The "Boat People's" First Ten Years in Canada.* Toronto: University of Toronto Press.

Buckland, Robin. 1997. "The everyday experience of Somali women in Canada: Implications for health." Master's thesis, Faculty of Nursing, University of Ottawa, Ottawa, ON.

Canadian Council for Refugees. 2002. "Role of NGOs." State of Refugees in Canada: http://www.web.ca/~ccr/state.html.

Charlton, A., D. Damstrom-Albach, C. Friesen, Dr. S. Ganesan, K. Nesbitt, R. Peters, and J. Smythe. 2002. "Refugee Mental Health: Moving Forward." Survey and Symposium Report. Coordinated by Chris Friesen, Immigrant Services Society, and Soma Ganesan, Psychiatry, University of British Columbia, Vancouver.

Citizenship and Immigration Canada. 2003. "Humanitarian Component." *Facts and Figures 2002: Statistical Overview of the Temporary Resident and Refugee Claimant Population.* http://www.cic.gc.ca/english/pub/facts2002-temp/facts-temp-6.html.

Denes, Melissa. 2003. "Refugee camps: A kind of home." *Guardian Unlimited.* 13 December. http://www.guardian.co.uk/, Archive search: "Melissa Denes, 13 December 2003."

ESL Consortium. 2002. *Growing Diversity: Settlement and Integration Services for Immigrant Children in a New Century.* Vancouver: School Districts of Burnaby, Coquitlam, North Vancouver, Richmond, and Surrey and Vancouver School Board.

Galler, J.R., J.S. Shumsky, and P.J. Morgane. 1996. "Malnutrition and brain development." In W.A. Walker and J.B. Watkins, eds., *Nutrition in Pediatrics: Basic Science and Clinical Applications,* 2nd ed., 194-210. Neuilly-sur-Seine, France: Decker Europe.

Hargreaves, Sally. 2002. "A body of evidence: Torture among asylum seekers to the West." *The Lancet* 359: 793-94.

Jean, François, ed. 1993. "Somalia: Humanitarian aid outgunned." *Life and Death and Aid: The Médecins Sans Frontières Report on World Crisis Intervention.* Médecins Sans Frontières. London and New York: Routledge.

Jimenez, Marina. 2003. "Under the radar." *Globe and Mail,* 15 November, A1.

Mollica, Richard, and Laura McDonald. 2002. "Old stereotypes, new realities: Refugees and mental health." *United Nations Chronicle* 2: 29-30.

Olness, Karen N. 1998. "Refugee health." In Sama Loue, ed., *Handbook of Immigrant Health,* 227-41. New York: Plenum Press.

Report. 1988. *After the Door Has Been Opened: Mental Health Issues Affecting Immigrants and Refugees in Canada.* Report of the Canadian Task Force on Mental Health Issues Affecting Immigrants and Refugees. Ottawa: Health and Welfare Canada.

Stein, Barry. 1986. "The experience of being a refugee: Insights from the research literature." In C. Williams and J. Westermeyer, eds., *Refugee Mental Health in Resettlement Countries,* 5-23. Washington DC: Hemisphere Publishing Corporation.

UNHCR. 1979. *Collection of International Instruments Concerning Refugees.* Geneva: Office of the United Nations High Commissioner for Refugees.

VAST. 2001a. *VAST Quarterly* 2, 3 (June). Vancouver: Vancouver Association for the Survivors of Torture.

VAST. 2001b. *VAST Quarterly* 3, 1 (December). Vancouver: Vancouver Association for the Survivors of Torture.

VAST. 2002. *VAST Quarterly* 3, 2 (March). Vancouver: Vancouver Association for the Survivors of Torture.

Contributors to the second edition

Dr. Cheryl Anderson, Ravensong Community Centre, Vancouver
Alexandra Charlton, Centre Coordinator for Storefront Orientation Services, Vancouver
Catherine Eddy, Manager, Multicultural Liaison Program, Vancouver School Board

Chris Friesen, Immigrant Services Society of BC, Vancouver
Hana Hussein, Cultural Studies and Health Research Unit, University of British Columbia
Fowzia Isse, Cultural Studies and Health Research Unit, University of British Columbia
Rosmin Kamani, Family Physician, Vancouver
Scott Laurence, School Counsellor of Refugees, Vancouver School Board
Francis Macqueen, Coordinator, Vancouver Association for the Survivors of Torture
Deega Mohammad, MOSAIC, Vancouver
Firouzeh Peyvandi, Afghani Settlement Worker, Immigrant Services Society of BC, Vancouver
Sherry Shaghaghi, Afghani Settlement Worker, Immigrant Services Society of BC, Vancouver
Donna Sharesky, Community Health Nurse, Bridge Health Clinic, Vancouver
Dawit Shawel, Somali Settlement Worker, Immigrant Services Society of BC, Vancouver
Victoria Stafford, Head Nurse, Bridge Health Clinic, Vancouver
Lynn Wells, Penticton and District Multicultural Society, BC
Elaine Wynne, Family Physician, Vancouver Association for the Survivors of Torture, BC
Fahima Yusuf Ali, Somali Settlement Worker, MOSAIC, Vancouver

Conclusion
Delivering Culturally Responsive Health Care

Joan M. Anderson, Sheryl Reimer Kirkham, Nancy Waxler-Morrison, Carol Herbert, Maureen Murphy, and Elizabeth Richardson

This concluding chapter highlights the issues and trends most likely to have an impact on the care of immigrants whatever their ethno-cultural background. These common themes are important not only for the groups described in the book but also for other groups not mentioned, because newcomers to Canada share many similar experiences. Health professionals caring for patients from a particular ethnic group will also want to consult the appropriate chapter. But in the end a better understanding of cultural background is only a gateway through which a professional can proceed to build a sympathetic and productive relationship with each client as a person.

The Context of Care

Since 1990, when the first edition of this book was published, Canada has become even more culturally diverse, with immigrants and refugees coming from many parts of the world. The chapter on refugees, for example, noted that by 2001 the top source countries for refugees to Canada were Afghanistan, Sri Lanka, Pakistan, the former Yugoslavia, Iran, Colombia, Iraq, Sudan, and the Congo. In all, 27,899 refugees arrived in Canada that year. In 1998 mainland China overtook Hong Kong to become the major source of immigrants to Canada of Chinese background. In 2002 the top source countries of immigrants to Canada were China, India, Pakistan, the Philippines, Iran, Republic of Korea, Romania, United States, Sri Lanka, the United Kingdom, and the former Yugoslavia. In 2002 a total of 203,947 immigrants and 25,111 refugees entered Canada.

In fifteen years there have been major changes in the Canadian health care system. The escalating cost of health care has increased pressures for cost effectiveness and efficiency in hospital administration and for more home care. Restraints in health care spending in the 1990s reduced the number of staff who now care for an ever more acute and complex patient population across both hospital and community settings. Increasingly the realities are shortages of hospital beds, rapid patient turnovers, and little ongoing in-service education for staff on issues such as intercultural care.

Shorter hospital stays have meant that patients are now going home while they still require a significant amount of care, making the transition from hospital to home a critical time for them and their families. With a new emphasis on a seamless transition from hospital to home, some patients are given home care services, which relieve the stress on the family. But others are not and must manage on their own. These changes have affected all patients, but newcomers to Canada may experience special difficulties. An inability to communicate effectively with health professionals and not knowing what questions to ask even when they do speak English or French impair their ability to navigate the health care system and tap into community resources. Hospitalization and the transition to home are no easier now than they were fifteen years ago for immigrant patients and their families.

The last fifteen years have also seen an increase in the complexity of health care. New medical technologies have made treatments more intricate and therefore more difficult to explain in discussing the pros and cons of treatment. Informed consent must be obtained, which means that clinicians must be assured that patients and their families understand the procedures that are to be undertaken and their risks. Ethical and moral issues must be negotiated across cultural and linguistic differences. Health problems such as HIV/AIDS cut across populations but have to be dealt with differently depending on cultural backgrounds and socioeconomic class. Such changes have made more challenging the task of health care professionals.

The last fifteen years have also brought opportunities. Researchers and hospital personnel are working more closely to address health care issues, and there is a growing awareness of the importance of translating knowledge from research into practice. We have had opportunities to conduct research projects with patients from different ethno-cultural backgrounds and to work closely with health care professionals – who are themselves becoming more culturally diverse. Sometimes it is the health care professional from an ethno-cultural minority group who experiences discrimination. Many have related incidents in which they were demeaned, or their care was refused, by Anglo-European patients. Administrators are now challenged to balance the need for a harassment-free workplace with the need to care for all patients. They must find ways of dealing with sensitive issues of racism and of talking about them openly.

Health care professionals from different ethno-cultural groups who are fluent in languages other than English have told us about the pressures on them to interpret for the patients of their colleagues. These requests have added stress to their own heavy workloads. Other issues are also surfacing.

For example, attempting to provide culturally responsive care by matching a health professional with a patient of the same ethnicity can lead to unexpected tensions. Patient and health care provider may be from contrasting socioeconomic backgrounds and share little except language. In some cultures more than others, dynamics of age and gender can enter into health care interactions. Professionals report being sometimes pressured by patients or families unused to universal health care to provide extra or "special" care. Yet, having a health care provider who can speak the same language provides tremendous comfort to a patient and can improve the level of care, especially with assessments, pain management, and patient teaching. There is no easy set of guidelines in these situations. Administrators and health care providers can only evaluate each case with the aim of providing culturally responsive care in a safe working environment.

Our research projects have studied the issues and best practices of providing culturally responsive health care in this changing environment. While many professionals have a sound knowledge base and are aware of what ideally ought to be done in intercultural care, they are increasingly forced by patient numbers and the severity of illnesses to set priorities. They must focus on ensuring the safety of the most critically ill patients – and are distressed at being unable to give the kind of care that they know other patients deserve. However, the barrier most often mentioned by health professionals in our studies is language, a recurrent theme throughout this book. Inability to communicate, explain, and understand is the leading source of frustration for professionals, patients, and their families alike.

Despite these challenges, practitioners have devised ways of "connecting" with patients from different language groups and cultural backgrounds, even when time runs short. Some of these methods are described in the practical guidelines as a way of helping practitioners learn from one another in their day-to-day work.

Emerging Ideas about Intercultural Care

When the first edition of this book was published, many practitioners found daunting the idea that they might be expected to know about the cultures of an ever-increasing number of new immigrants to Canada. Some of them may have misunderstood how this book is meant to be used. The various chapters discuss the countries from which people come, their histories, and some of the things that influence how people use health care and manage health and illness. This information can help health professionals interpret what patients and their families tell them. But it is by no means a recipe for practice. In the fifteen years since the first edition, professionals have become quite aware of the dangers of stereotyping people, that is, of seeing a particular person as merely a representative example of a culture. Information about cultural practices and beliefs does not add up to a prevailing image of an individual from that culture, a stereotype. Cultural information has an entirely different purpose.

To provide culturally responsive care, the professional needs to focus on the context of each person's life and experiences – with an immigrant even more than with a mainstream Canadian. What is different with immigrant patients is that the practitioner risks making assumptions about the patient based on mainstream Canadian culture and ethnic stereotypes. If this happens, the professional's judgment becomes clouded with incorrect inferences: the situation is not what the practitioner thinks. It is to avoid this mistake that this edition stresses the assessment process: making an effort to learn about an immigrant patient and family is even more important than with a patient who shares the practitioner's culture and from whom the practitioner can effortlessly and accurately pick up nuances. Only by being alert to possible cultural misunderstandings can the professional gain an adequate sense of what the patient is saying and what the family situation really is.

This approach to intercultural care is in keeping with perspectives such as "culturally responsive care" and "cultural safety," concepts developed by Maori nurses in New Zealand, and now widely drawn on in the Canadian context (Ramsden and Whakaruruhau 1993). Culturally safe practice includes not only recognizing and respecting the cultural identity of others and taking into account their needs and rights, but also recognizing our own personal and cultural history and the ways in which it influences our interactions with patients and their families (Anderson et al. 2003). So the strategy recommended here, far from memorizing facts about different ethnic groups, is to engage with people as individuals to find out about their particular situation, which can only be done adequately with the help of cultural background knowledge to ask insightful questions and understand the answers.

A patient's culture is important as background; the practitioner must learn also about the circumstances that make up the foreground. Not being able to find a job in Canada, downward mobility in the workforce, living in poverty, how health care services in Canada are organized, and how this differs from the home country – all these events and conditions interact with culture to determine newcomers' experiences, how they seek help, and how they manage health and illness. What the professional must also do is learn about the experiences that may be evoking cultural responses: the life opportunities, the day-to-day living situation, instances of discrimination and stereotyping, and other circumstances that may be involved.

These emerging ideas about intercultural care, along with the current trends in Canadian demography and health care, help in understanding the significance of the common themes identified in the preceding chapters.

Common Themes from the Cultural Overviews

Understanding Diversity and Avoiding Stereotypes

People from a given ethnic group share beliefs, values, and experiences but are quite diverse among themselves. They differ greatly in their combination of social class, religion, level of education, rural or urban origin in the home country, and length of time in Canada. These factors make patients differ in their beliefs about health, illness, and help-seeking, in their expectations of health professionals, and in their practices regarding health and illness. South Asians, for example, come not only from a variety of regions with different languages and dialects but also from several distinct religious groups. The Chinese living in Canada also come from different regions and countries with different languages and dialects and great variations in experience. There are differences between people from mainland China and those from Hong Kong, but there are also major differences among people from the mainland, while there are similarities among Chinese from all source countries. Confucianism and Buddhism, for instance, are unifying philosophies for people from many backgrounds, fostering similarities in their responses to health and illness.

In some countries a small urban elite enjoys a high standard of living while most people in all areas live at a subsistence level. This contrast makes for major differences in health beliefs and practices, expectations of health professionals, and patterns of use of health care services. Ideas about the use of Western medicine, the place of preventive health care, and the concept of rehabilitation are likely to vary among people from the same ethnic group according to social class. An upper-class urban Iranian family is most likely familiar with Western medicine and health care and able to afford excellent care on a par with European and North American standards, unlike a poorer Iranian family with access only to relatively rudimentary health care.

Ethnic factors operate in varying degrees in the lives of people. Some people closely follow traditional practices. Among Vietnamese in their home country, traditional beliefs are still common, and traditional methods of treatment are often the family's first choice. Many of these beliefs have been brought to Canada, and traditional methods continue to be used, alongside or instead of, Western medicine. An example is the belief about "hot" and "cold." Many Vietnamese think that a woman is in a cold condition after childbirth because she has lost heating blood, and that she should therefore avoid drinking cold juice or water and should not shower or wash her hair.

Sometimes components of traditional culture are built into an otherwise modern lifestyle. Conversely, persons who appear traditional may be familiar with many aspects of the Western way of life. It should not be assumed that if an Indian woman wears a sari she will use traditional health care practices or is unfamiliar with English. It is often assumed quite incorrectly that persons dressed differently do not understand English and are somehow "different." Nor should it be assumed that a patient dressed in Western clothes and fluent in English will therefore understand the Canadian way of doing things. Cultural differences create misleading or misunderstood cultural signals and therefore make it especially important to find out what someone from a different culture is really like.

Problems of Resettlement in a New Country

Despite their ethnic diversity, immigrants share many experiences. Most of these relate to everyday life issues: filling out a job application, going to a job interview, getting and keeping a job, finding adequate housing (often a huge problem for refugees), managing child care, struggling with a new language, shopping in a supermarket, banking, navigating on public transportation. Of course not only immigrants find difficulties with these things from time to time. But in combination they can cause anxiety and distress with a major impact on health. Quite likely these will be among the issues when immigrants seek help from health professionals. Downward job mobility is an ever-increasing problem for professionally trained immigrants. Many enjoyed prestige and a reasonable standard of living in the home country and came to Canada assuming that their skills were needed, indeed hoping to improve their standard of living. Upon arrival, many professional people have had to take menial jobs to make a living. Lacking fluency in English or French and without Canadian qualifications, they cannot practise their professions. To survive, they have to take whatever jobs they can find; a doctor might work as a taxi driver or janitor. Many have been deeply disappointed by the realities of life in Canada.

Some immigrants are from the lower socioeconomic groups in their countries of origin and therefore do not have much education. They may have difficulty learning English even after several years' domicile in Canada, particularly if they could not read or write their own home language. Illiteracy can be a source of difficulty in hospitals, especially among older immigrants, even those who have lived here for a long time. Health care professionals might assume that a patient can read and therefore provide written materials in the patient's language. But many people are too embarrassed to say they cannot read, so it should never be assumed that people will be able to read pamphlets that are given to them.

With access only to low-paying jobs, many immigrants are faced with a life of poverty and despair. The stresses are often heightened when there is an illness. Many who work in menial jobs do not have the benefits other Canadians take for granted, such as sick time and time off work to see a doctor or go to a clinic. Many work in non-unionized jobs and get paid only for the hours they are actually on the job. Hospitalization and illness may mean a loss of job. A lengthy illness might also mean a loss of job for the family member who has to look after the sick person. These factors add to the stresses of illness, and may contribute to depression or to psychosomatic illnesses, especially when there are few sources of support. Failure to keep clinic appointments or to buy medicines could be the result of not being able to take time off from work and accept the loss of pay, or even of a lack of money to buy a bus ticket, rather than ethno-cultural factors. This means that health professionals have to be constantly aware of people's life situations, and the hardships that come from the process of uprooting and resettlement. For visible, dark-skinned, non-English speaking minority groups, the problem of racism in neighbourhoods, schools, workplaces, and health care institutions may be real, and also a source of depression and despair.

Some people did not choose to migrate. They fled political strife in search of refuge here. Others saw Canada as the "promised land" where they could start over and make a better life for themselves and their children. Health professionals need to keep in mind that people who voluntarily migrated to Canada bring different sets of experiences from those of refugees who were compelled to leave their countries for their own safety.

The experiences of refugees have been described in the chapters on various ethnic groups, while issues that cut across all refugee groups are the focus of Chapter 8. Many left their possessions and loved ones behind, not knowing if their relatives were dead or alive. Many want to go back "sometime" in the hope that they will find and be reunited with their loved ones. Many have suffered great hardships in the refugee camps, which contributed to the trauma of being a refugee. Some have been in camps such as in Maro, Chad, in Africa, which had no essential services, no water, medicine, or sanitation, until outside services arrived. Food is scarce in most camps, and many refugees arrive in Canada malnourished. A large number of refugees have been the victims of torture, such as those coming from Central America. The pain of the refugee experience goes far beyond the physical wounds. Children are haunted by nightmares of murders they have witnessed, adults are plagued by sleeplessness, and families mourn for those who have been killed, imprisoned, or "disappeared." Asylum seekers face particular challenges; many are made to feel that they are not welcome in Canada and have an uncertain status until their refugee claim is processed.

The difficulties experienced by refugees may not easily be shared with others outside the immediate family. Language barriers, a feeling of marginality in Canadian society, and unfamiliarity with the way of life here, all add to the sense of isolation. While immigrants may have been pulled to Canada for a variety of reasons, and can return to their home country if they wish, refugees are pushed out of their countries, and "returning home" is usually not an option.

Gender-Related Issues and Family Adjustment

Issues surrounding gender and family life are central to this book and are relevant to the delivery of health care services. One issue is the role of women in some societies and the changes that occur on migration to Canada. Often the man is traditionally the breadwinner while the woman takes care of the home. In Canada, however, many immigrant women out of economic necessity must find employment outside the home. The family as a unit benefits economically from the woman's income, and some women find that they gain the respect of their husbands by making a financial contribution to the family. Nevertheless, role changes within the family sometimes lead to family conflict. As women become more aware of their rights in Western society, and as they become more independent, their husbands may grow to resent the Westernization of their wives.

Men also face difficulties. A man may feel that he has lost status within the family if he is unable to fulfil the role of breadwinner; he may "lose face." Many men do not quickly find a job they regard as suitable, and their wives are usually able to find a job first. As their wives earn money and get ideas about freedom in the new country, husbands lose status in the eyes of their children and feel that they are no longer head of the family. This can lead to depression in men, as noted in Chapter 4 on Iranians, and to problems of family violence, as noted in Chapter 6 on South Asians.

Both men and women therefore go through a process of readjustment in order to cope with their lives in Canada. Women may find this process especially difficult when they are part of their husbands' households and their own families have not immigrated to Canada. They may have few sources of support in their community. Many women fear that airing family problems outside the home will provoke gossip in the community and may eventually get back to the family. So, even a woman with a large extended family may feel socially isolated if she has no one to turn to for help with personal problems.

In some groups, divorce is not usually an acceptable option for women, who are brought up to believe that keeping a marriage together is their responsibility. For example, among the Laotians and Cambodians, Iranians, and traditional South Asians, divorce is rare and disapproved of strongly. In many communities divorce and separation may stigmatize a woman and lead to her rejection by the community. She may therefore choose to remain with her husband even though the marriage is unsatisfactory, since facing life on her own without social support would be even more difficult.

Many women face another problem. Those who lack English and professional qualifications become trapped in low-paying jobs with no hope of mobility. As with men, highly educated women may find that their qualifications are not recognized and they have to start over in Canada (Mojab

1999). Deterrents to acquiring English include lack of time because the woman has to work outside the home, difficulty in following language instruction, and lack of adequate child care. Although many aspire to fluency in English and better jobs, few are able to achieve either. The sources of distress for many women, then, lie in the socioeconomic circumstances of their lives and should not be ascribed solely to their cultural or ethnic backgrounds.

Women who are not in the labour force can also have difficulties in Canada, especially after they have raised their children. Some feel a loss of purpose after the children have left home. Furthermore, they have found that housework is not valued in Canadian society. Many feel socially isolated, especially if they lack English or French.

Another issue facing both men and women is the break-up of the family unit as a result of moves to Canada. It is not unusual for one family member to gain entry to Canada and for relatives and children to follow later. Not only does this pattern of migration disrupt social support networks but family members must also readjust to one another and redefine their family relationships once they are reunited in Canada. In some families, business matters dictate living arrangements. For example, some families from Hong Kong, mainland China, and Taiwan are referred to as "astronaut families" – the father commutes between his business in Asia and his North American home. This puts extra strains on family relationships and may be very difficult for his wife and children.

Understanding the dynamics of family life and the importance accorded the family is essential if culturally responsive care is to be provided. Physicians, nurses, social workers, and other health care professionals need to recognize that solutions acceptable to Canadian-born women may be unacceptable to some immigrant women. For instance, an immigrant woman may flatly refuse to leave an abusive family for fear of being shunned by the community she depends on. Western feminist approaches to the care of a woman which focus mainly on issues of patriarchy may be unhelpful or aggravate her situation. Many immigrant women live in a complex situation, having to deal with the triple discrimination of skin colour, gender, and social class. Encouraging Western-style "assertiveness" and "division of labour" in the home without an awareness of the family's expectations may inflame family feuds and isolate the woman. A woman who loses the support of her family and her community may have no one else to turn to because she is part of a non-Western, non-English-speaking immigrant group that is marginalized in Canadian society. Health professionals also need to be acutely aware that some of the stereotypes about "third world women" as passive and lacking in assertiveness can be harmful and undermine women's competencies. As stressed elsewhere, understanding the woman's particular situation is indispensable to helping her.

Influence of the Extended Family on Health Care Decisions

In many immigrant families, the family unit is not only a source of emotional support but also an economic unit. Even if family members do not all live in the same household in Canada, many aspects of extended family life may be carried over. Family members may be consulted on important decisions. They may help one another with child care or with other activities intended to make life in Canada smoother. For many families from developing countries, obligations and expectations within the family unit are unaltered by geographical separation. The extended family plays an important part in decision making about help-seeking and illness management.

Even though older family members (such as grandparents) may have a weaker position in Canada than in the home country, they may still have a say in health care. Usually, there is deep respect for elders (notably among the Chinese, South Asians, Vietnamese, and Japanese), and their advice on health matters does not go unheeded. It is not uncommon for a grandparent, usually a grandmother, to introduce traditional remedies at the same time as Western medicines are being used, and family members may feel obliged to go along. Grandparents who take over the care of children when a couple goes out to work may have to manage a child's illness. They may decide whether to use traditional medicine and other traditional health practices or to combine traditional treatments with Western medicine.

Health professionals also need to keep in mind that a patient, though agreeing to treatment, may not follow directions if the family does not approve. Or, the treatment may be adjusted to include the use of traditional remedies. In some instances the dosage may be reduced out of concern that the medication is too strong for the patient. Dosage might also be reduced because the family does not have the money to buy the medication but is embarrassed to discuss this with the health professional. It is important to recognize that traditional beliefs, such as "hot" and "cold" equilibrium, and cultural practices, such as not drinking "cold" drinks after childbirth or drinking special soups to replenish blood loss, might be adhered to even after a family has lived in Canada for several generations. On the other hand, some newcomers, depending on their backgrounds, do not follow these cultural practices, while some traditions may cut across socioeconomic groups. The practitioner should therefore not make assumptions and be careful to assess each person individually.

Relationships with Children and the School System

Although male children are favoured in certain groups, it cannot be assumed that this is always the case. In some groups girls are equally favoured, and a high value is placed on all children. To Canadians, some immigrant families may appear overly indulgent of young children. A baby may not be allowed to cry, and may be cuddled either by grandparents, parents, or older siblings. On the other hand, older children may appear to be strictly controlled, as they are expected to show respect for their parents and other family members. Physical punishment, seen as in the child's best interest, may be used in some groups. Many immigrant families have put their hopes for the future in their children, and a good education is seen as the only way to get ahead. Parents may object to the time the child is expected to spend on non-academic activities. For example, field trips or sports may be seen as not contributing to their goals for the child. Children may be expected to stay home during the evenings to do their homework instead of socializing with other children. As well, the more liberal aspects of the school curriculum do not always meet with approval from immigrant parents. They may object to the inclusion of sex education as transgressing the boundaries of good etiquette.

As children become Canadianized, tensions may arise with their parents. Children are usually the first to learn English, and may become interpreters of the outside world for their parents. This gives them a source of power over parents, who become dependent upon them to communicate with authority figures within the larger Canadian society. Health professionals should be aware that using a child as an interpreter can undermine the parents' competence in the eyes of the child. Children should not be used in this capacity, especially when sensitive matters are being discussed.

Severe communication problems can arise when parents (especially mothers) do not acquire English-language skills while the child loses the language of the home country. Children who become rapidly socialized into Canadian society may not use their mother tongue outside the home. Communication between mother and child will be diminished if they feel that there is nothing left to talk about. Consequently, parents and children may find that they do not have a common language in which to communicate.

As children learn more about Canadian society, they may object to the forms of discipline used by parents. Forms of physical punishment of children seen as normal in some groups are not acceptable in Canada. Some immigrant parents may be seen as abusive by mainstream Canadians. As children learn about their rights they may report their parents to the authorities, a step that widens the gulf between the children and their families, who regard it as betrayal.

Health professionals should be cautious in their interpretation of what constitutes abuse and should take time to assess the situation carefully. To give appropriate care, they have to be aware of the problems that can arise from acculturation into a new society. Health professionals also need to be aware that a child is often caught between two value systems: peer pressure to conform to mainstream values against parental insistence on the values of the home country. Issues arising from dating, especially in the case of girls, may be worrisome for parents, as they may view North American standards as totally unacceptable for their child. This conflict can lead to depression and rebellion, particularly among teenagers.

The immigrant child needs family support, and every effort should be made to help the parents and child reconcile their differences. Leaving home, an appropriate measure in some mainstream Canadian families, can be devastating to an immigrant teenager caught between two worlds. In the long run it may serve the child's best interests to maintain ties with a stable ethnic community.

A frequent problem confronting many immigrant families in Canada is that children are sometimes mistakenly assessed as lacking the academic competence to succeed at school. Teachers and health professionals may underestimate the ability of a child who does not use the vocabulary of mainstream Canadian children. Speaking with an accent different from a Canadian accent may be interpreted as incompetence. The coping strategies of the child to deal with the upheavals of resettlement may be construed as lack of assertiveness. On the other hand, certain styles of assertiveness may be construed as belligerence. Those who work with children need to be culturally sensitive in assessing their potentialities, so that children are channelled into programs that fit their talents, whether academic or vocational. Professionals and teachers need to work collaboratively to recognize when apparent learning problems are associated with uprooting and resettlement.

Relationships with Elderly Family Members

The traditionally dominant position of elders may be weakened when they come to Canada if they become dependent on the children who sponsored them. In fact, some older parents sponsored by their children live in fear that the support could be withdrawn. Elderly immigrant parents tend to inherit household chores but lose control of the family, inverting their status in the home country when they had control and no chores.

A pressing problem for elderly immigrants in Canada is social isolation. Many have left their peers behind and now stay at home to look after their grandchildren. Unaccustomed to the way of life, bewildered by the transportation system, and often lacking English, many are afraid to venture outside on their own. The lack of English also bars them from using the resources available to other senior citizens.

In addition to dealing with the problems of adjusting to a new environment, many elderly immigrants find themselves in conflicts with their children. Their points of view may differ about how the routines of everyday life should be managed or how grandchildren should be raised. But perhaps the most worrisome concern for seniors is that, with all adults in the family working, no one will be at home to care for them in their old age. To be placed in an institution seems unacceptable and even an abandonment. Children, for their part, may feel guilty at being unable to meet traditional obligations to their parents. Health professionals need to be aware that placement in an institution is not always by choice and consensus. Both the elderly and their offspring may need help working through feelings of guilt, resentment, abandonment, and depression.

Dealing with Hospitalization

One of the most trying times for newcomers to Canada occurs when a family member is hospitalized. The patient and family members are usually bemused by the technical language and the overpowering environment of the modern hospital. They may be completely confused by the admitting procedures and the detailed medical examination, requiring them to remove their clothing for examination and to wear a hospital gown that barely covers them. Many immigrant patients are not used to this. On the basis of their past experience in the home country, some patients, such as Vietnamese, may be disinclined to remove more clothing than is absolutely necessary for a physical examination. Women may not be used to having a male physician examine them. It is important for health professionals to be aware of such issues, especially when people are admitted through the emergency department without the usual benefit of an orientation visit to the hospital and an opportunity to find out about hospital procedures.

Some hospitals now try to make the environment more welcoming to all patients. There may be a pre-admission visit to familiarize people with the surroundings and give them a sense of what will happen to them in the hospital. Upon admission, food preferences may be accommodated. Many hospital personnel now recognize that families from some parts of the world are concerned that their loved ones will be neglected if they are left alone in hospital and that some patients feel abandoned if their families are not with them. These families expect to be involved in the care of their loved ones, providing food and attending the sick person in hospital. So visiting hours are now more lenient in many hospitals, and arrangements can be made for parents to stay overnight, especially with child patients.

Tensions can still arise. Many family members may visit at the same time, or the noise level created by visitors may disturb other patients, or the presence of family members may interfere with the care of the patient. Health professionals become distressed when they believe that the family members are infringing on their ability to provide care to patients in a timely way. However, there is now generally greater negotiation between families and health care professionals around issues that used to be highly problematic. Many patients see health care providers as empathetic and trying to do their best under often difficult circumstances.

Language remains a critical problem, one so important that a special section is devoted to it at the end of this chapter. Suffice it to say that many patients in our research studies have experienced great distress because they were not able to communicate their needs to health professionals, especially older Punjabi-speaking and Cantonese-speaking patients. Many could not tell them about their pain or get the medications that would help them. Health professionals did not always draw on the interpreter resources available to them, often being too busy or moving on to deal with more urgent needs of other patients. We encourage health professionals to use interpreters and suggest how to do so later in the chapter.

Issues around the Transition from Hospital to Home

A source of distress for patients and their families is discharge from hospital. In an ever-changing health care system, families are expected to take on greater responsibility for the care of the ill person in the home. Hospital stays are shorter, and many patients go home needing treatment to continue. Families can be overwhelmed by the expectations to provide complex care, especially when they cannot fully comprehend the disease process, treatment procedures, and what they are supposed to do. Some believe that they are overloaded with "discharge teaching" – too much information given to them at a time when they can least cope with it. These experiences are usually aggravated by language barriers. Patients often feel that their concerns are not taken into account, or that they are being asked to do things that are totally inappropriate. While home care services are a source of assistance to families, if they are not put in place before the patient leaves the hospital the family may not know how to access them. And so the patient ends up in the hospital again, with wounds that have become infected, or pain that has become unbearable. Restructuring of health care is also putting new demands on families. Sometimes a family member has to take time off from work to care for the ill person, resulting in a loss of pay that the family can ill afford.

Nurses, physicians, and social workers, in particular, should be aware of the plight of immigrant families and try to involve them wherever possible in a patient's care. Given that language is such a major issue, especially with the rising expectation that families should be involved in the care of patients in the home, extra time is needed for clear interpretation to families who do not speak English or French fluently.

Newcomers' Expectations of Health Professionals

The health care system in Canada is so different from that of the countries from which people come that many immigrants and refugees, especially those coming from rural areas, need to learn how the system works. Many immigrants were accustomed to receiving all their care from a clinic, not from one physician on a long-term basis. The practice of detailed history-taking and lengthy diagnostic procedures may also be strange, and even seen as a lack of competence in the physician. Physicians may be expected to decide promptly what is wrong and immediately prescribe medications or specific treatment. It is important to explain to immigrant patients that histories are taken and tests conducted before a diagnosis is made and treatment prescribed.

Many immigrants are not familiar with the Canadian "medical examination." For example, many women from rural India, even those who have had several children there, have never had a pelvic or breast examination. For such women it is clearly very important to explain what is being done and more acceptable if it is done by a female physician with a female family member present.

Some wealthy newcomers, of course, have been accustomed to receiving high-quality health care in a timely way. Well-off immigrants from, for instance, Hong Kong, mainland China, Taiwan, or Iran may resent being put on a waiting list for months for treatment they could have received promptly in the home country. Not understanding the universal nature of Canadian health care, they expect to be able to get the services they need right away by paying for them.

While some patients assert their rights and engage with health professionals as equals, others are hesitant to ask questions and will appear very agreeable and compliant. However, their manner may reflect etiquette rather than agreement. Many immigrant cultures find it impolite to disagree. If an elderly Japanese man smiles and nods at medical directions, the health professional should regard this as an indication of politeness rather than of agreement. Furthermore, it should not be assumed that even patients who understand treatment directions will follow them. Compliance with medical regimens is affected by many factors, such as family priorities, traditional beliefs about illness and treatment, opinions of elders about prescribed medications, and economic pressures. Health professionals therefore need to take time to learn the patient's situation and the factors at home that might influence management of the illness. At the same time, sensitivity is required so as not to appear intrusive. It is well to remember that talking about family relationships with an outsider may seem to an immigrant patient not only threatening but also rude, since respect for family must always be shown and may in any case be much greater than the respect owed to some inquiring physician.

While doctors are highly respected in many of the countries from which patients come, nurses do not always have the same prestige. Unlike Canada, some countries have few professional schools of nursing. Most nurses are trained on the job and are considered as one of many parts of the "medical system." Nurses need to introduce themselves as professionals to newcomers to Canada, and explain their roles clearly. Once they have established their professional role and demonstrated their competencies, their status will be confirmed. Many immigrants have reported highly positive interactions with nurses, and quite clearly stereotypes about nursing change once immigrants become aware of the scope of nursing in Canadian society. Nurses, whether in community health or hospitals, are in a position of great value to immigrant patients, not only in providing care and health education but also more broadly in explaining how Canadian health care works.

An example of this is the role of social workers. Many immigrants are unfamiliar with social work services, which tend to be rare in their home countries. Interviews by social workers aimed at obtaining information about the person's individual situation not only may be seen as intrusive and rude, as described above for physicians, but also may feed a suspicion that social workers are really government agents. Furthermore, in the cultures from which many immigrants come, social services may seem a last resort, useful only in the failure of family support. Helping newcomers to understand how these services work is essential if they are to make use of them.

Guidelines for Clinical Practice

The main issues identified in this book have been used to develop guidelines for clinical practice. These guidelines are offered in recognition that health care professionals often work under significant time and resource constraints. A family doctor's eight- or ten-minute interview certainly sets limits on the number of questions that can be asked. These guidelines will alert the busy professional to the important issues to watch for. By listening carefully with these issues in mind to what the patient says, the professional can follow up with an insightful question or two, and in time develop a richer and much more useful understanding of the patient's situation. As shown in the guidelines, the primary aspects of intercultural health care are, first, assessment and, second, communication and language.

Assessment

Assessment is a clinical art that combines sensitivity, judgment, and scientific knowledge. One must know not only when to ask questions but also how to phrase them so that the patient does not find them offensive. The clinician should be alert to data that can be elicited without direct questioning. Yet there is also the need to guard against premature conclusions. Observations should be validated to avoid making incorrect assumptions. For example, if a woman wears traditional dress it should not be assumed that she subscribes to traditional medical beliefs. Only an interview can clarify her health beliefs and practices.

The process of assessment goes on over time. While certain data have to be obtained in an initial interview so as to deal with pressing health problems, patients should not be expected to share sensitive information until trust has been established. Patients may also be reluctant to reveal their beliefs about illness to the Western health professional for fear of being ridiculed. Once trust has been built information may be shared quite spontaneously. A community health nurse recalled an experience with a patient who turned out to be using herbal remedies instead of Western medicine. Only after the nurse had made several visits to the patient's home was this information volunteered by the patient. Health professionals can find out more by asking questions phrased in a non-judgmental way. For example, asking "Have you found anything else that has helped you?" is likely to be more effective than asking "Are you taking other medicines besides those prescribed by the doctor?"

The timing of such questions can be as important as the wording. Some patients expect doctors to know immediately what is wrong and what treatment is appropriate. They may see weakness and uncertainty in questions such as "What do you think has caused your illness?" or "What kind of treatment do you think you should receive?" Such questions should be held back until the professional has demonstrated clinical abilities beyond doubt.

A common problem is that the patient may not have English or French language competence. The central issue of communication and language is discussed below, with some concrete guidelines for practice.

From these general subjects, we move now to outline the main considerations in assessing patients from minority ethno-cultural groups.

Recognizing How One's Own Background Affects Interactions with Patients

Whatever background we come from, and regardless of our country of birth and first language, we *all* have personal values that are deeply embedded in our own histories, in our upbringing, and in the cultures that have shaped us. These personal values influence who we are as professionals and how we use professional knowledge. Patient evaluation, problem definition, and the formulation of possible solutions are not derived solely from impersonal, objective, scientific criteria but also from these personal values. For this reason we must always be self-reflective about what we bring to each health care encounter and how it shapes what we hear and see and how we interact with people.

Our goal as health professionals is to find a way to connect with each person, regardless of how different from us that person seems to be. We should remember that we are all connected in sharing a common humanity. When clients sense this connection, they will participate more openly in a dialogue that builds mutual understanding and goal-setting. This dialogue arises less from knowing the right questions to ask than from establishing a relationship of mutual respect that opens up space for negotiating between differences in perspective.

Differences and diversity fall along many lines, not just ethnicity and culture. We sense group affiliations based on gender, nationality, age cohort, religion, class, sexual orientation, and so forth. Some group affiliations offer us privilege in certain situations and disadvantages in others. These multiple roles contribute to our "identity," that is, who we are as a person in relation to other people. We can use some affiliations to connect with a person from whom we are separated by other affiliations. We might, for instance, share the feeling of being an "outsider" on some aspect of our own identity, such as if we ourselves are also immigrants. Women from very different backgrounds often connect with one another through the common experience of raising children or caring for elderly relatives. Young professionals may find that their age and recent student experience help them connect with younger patients. Of course there are limits to this: one must be careful not to presume a similarity the other might not recognize. To attempt to sympathize with a persecuted refugee by mentioning personal experiences of marginalization that are scarcely comparable will generate separation rather than connection. Sensitivity to such limits takes us in the direction of more thoughtful self-appraisal.

A first step in assessing a patient, therefore, is to recognize one's personal values and social background and consider how they may influence interactions with others who do not share them. To develop trust and connection, it is especially important to recognize potential areas of conflict between the values of the health professional and the patient. For example, in working with women from other countries, health professionals need to realize how far their Western values may frame their initial interpretation of a woman's situation so they can avoid recommending an unreflectively facile solution that is deeply inappropriate to her position as she sees it. Examples of questions that might help in this process of reflection include the following:

- What are my own beliefs about newcomers to Canada, and how might these enter into how I interact with this person?
- What assumptions am I making about this person? And about this particular cultural group?
- Why do I think this way?
- Where did I get my information?
- What might I learn if I talk to the person?
- What may we have in common?

Furthermore, the values of the health professional are not just personal but also reflect the values and demands of the current work environment. For example, efficiency has become highly valued in health care settings.

Although the "human side of interactions" is also valued, there may not seem enough time for the personal interactions needed for the health professional to assess the situation of a particular patient and family. In this spirit, however, the health professional should not ignore the possibility that more immediately effective care will also be more efficient in the long run.

Establishing the Patient's Beliefs about Illness

An ethnic group is always internally diverse. Not everyone will subscribe to the group's usual beliefs about health and illness. A second step in the assessment is therefore to discover the extent to which the patient shares certain health beliefs, practices, and experiences of illness with others in his or her ethnic group. To avoid ethnic stereotyping, the pattern of questioning in an initial interview should be directed at locating the patient's social position and relation to the group. Questions should put the patient at ease. Don't assume from appearances that the patient was born outside of Canada. Following are examples of crucial things health professionals can listen for to get a sense of the patient:

- Where the person was born – including urban/rural. (This might be standard information on the patient admission form.)
- If born outside Canada, how long the person has been in Canada, and whether there are family members here.
- Employment in country of origin, and whether there is downward employment mobility in Canada.
- Health services in country of origin, and help-seeking patterns.
- Expectations about health care in Canada.

Ascertaining this information will shed light on the patient's background and a number of other pertinent issues. An urban professional will quite likely have greater familiarity with Western health care than will patients from rural farming backgrounds. The patient's occupation in Canada may also alert the health professional to downward socioeconomic mobility and difficulties in adjusting to life in Canada.

Questions about level of education, although useful in placing a patient, must be handled with tact, because they can be humiliating for those with little schooling. The health professional has to decide when the timing is appropriate and whether this information would really be of use.

Professionals need to establish the kinds of medical systems patients have encountered in the past. Everyone coming into Canada will have had some contact with Western medicine for purposes of immigration, but these services may have been provided very differently. In some places there is no appointment system and no regular family doctor, and medical records are held by the patient, not the doctor. Some people might have used the traditional medicine of their homelands with some limited access to Western medicine. Hospitals may have been far away, and no prenatal care available. Where patients seem more familiar with traditional medicine, it is advisable to find out more about these beliefs and practices and detect any points of conflict with the professional's understandings, plans, and expectations.

The process of assessment continues over time. Many people are reluctant to reveal their beliefs and health practices to strangers. More time will have to be spent with patients who are reticent. Some topics, such as the experience of torture, may never be raised.

Determining Differences in Viewpoints of Patients and Clinicians: The Explanatory Model

Health professionals and patients quite often bring different ideas to the clinical encounter even when both come from the same backgrounds. As noted above, the priority for the health professional may be for the patient to buy and take a medication. For the patient, the priority may be buying food for the family. Kleinman (1980) refers to a perspective that is elaborated around and expresses a key priority as an "explanatory model." The explanatory model approach is to identify the key priority governing and explaining a whole perspective. The approach gives health professionals a method to explore with clients and their families the cultural and social meanings influencing the understanding of health and illness. The approach also prompts the professionals to reflect on the different explanatory models in their own culture – both personal and professional – which inform each encounter. In addition, the explanatory model helps us examine larger social issues, such as systemic discrimination, poverty, and access to resources, which profoundly influence life opportunities, health, and illness.

There may be, and often are, discrepancies between patients' and professionals' perspectives in the explanation of disease and illness, the expectations of how each should behave, and the interpretation of treatment results. This book has referred to various cultural meaning systems, including balance (e.g., "hot" and "cold" beliefs), family relationships, individual or collective world views, present or future orientations, and non-physical disease causation. A clash in perspectives can have devastating consequences for the treatment process if care is not taken to work through differences. Often the health professional is trying to do what seems best for the patient and family, but this may be entirely contrary to what they think will work for them or what they are able to do.

Health professionals must consciously find out the extent to which their own viewpoints differ from those of their patients. The issue here is not that viewpoints differ, but that these differences can lead to misunderstanding and affect the results of treatment. Health professionals therefore need to explore with patients their beliefs about illness, expectations of treatment, and how illness is managed in daily life. This exploration has to be done with sensitivity, as patients are sometimes hesitant to discuss their beliefs for fear of being ridiculed. Furthermore, many do not expect to be questioned about their views; they believe the physician should be able to tell what is wrong with them without excessive questioning. Timing is important in introducing questions; sensitivity is also needed in phrasing questions that are not judgmental. The line of questioning suggested here is not meant as a rigid prescription for a first interview. Rather, these are areas to be covered over several or many interviews. Patients may discuss their beliefs about illness only after they are convinced of the health professional's competence. Treatments of some sort may have to be prescribed simply to demonstrate to the patient that the physician knows what the illness is.

The following explanatory model questions suggested by Kleinman and used by some physicians and nurses in clinical practice have been found to be helpful in obtaining data about patients' understanding of their illness. In her insightful book, Fadiman (1997, 260) remarks that the first time she read these questions, she hardly noticed them; then, around the fifteenth time, she began to think that, "like many obvious things, they might actually be a work of genius." Fadiman says she began to see clearly how, if these questions had been used by health professionals caring for the child and family discussed in her book, the experience of the family and treatment outcomes could have been entirely different.

Here are the questions suggested by Kleinman (1980, 106). They may also be used, not as direct questions, but as "listening for" cues. In this case the professional does not ask them but listens for them, notices them, and perhaps follows them up with a question.

- What do you call your problem? What name do you give it?
- What do you think has caused your problem?
- Why do you think it started when it did?
- What does your sickness do to your body? How does it work inside you?
- How severe is it? Will it get better soon or take longer?
- What do you fear most about your sickness?
- What are the chief problems your sickness has caused for you (personally, in your family, and at work)?
- What kind of treatment do you think you should receive? What are the most important results you hope you will receive from the treatment? (Explore home remedies used, and judged to be helpful.)

From using these questions in our research, we have found that they give us rich insights into people's lives and help reveal differences between patients over what health means to them. These questions are intended not only for newcomers to Canada but also for a patient and family of any culture.

Kleinman cautions that the questions should not be presented as a list to the patient. The timing and phrasing of questions should be adapted to the individual. The questions are not posed in isolation from the rest of the interview but are woven into the interview and asked only when appropriate. They should be asked in such a way as to demonstrate the health professional's genuine interest in the answers.

Understanding the Social Context of Patients' and Families' Lives

For all patients, but especially for newcomers to Canada, it is very important for health professionals to get a sense of how they are managing with jobs, housing, child care, and financial resources. With families in Canada expected to take on greater responsibility for patient care in the home, the financial circumstances of the family will influence how they are able to do this. We have found that health professionals in hospitals are usually not familiar with patients' home environments, and may assume that a family has, for example, adequate space, laundry facilities, ownership of a car, and other domestic amenities that would help them care for a sick person at home.

It is a mistake to assume that family members will be able to take on the responsibility of care. This is often not the case for families struggling to make ends meet. For a family member to stay home from work to look after a sick relative may mean lost wages that the family cannot afford. Some families who come to Canada may be wealthy and able to afford assistance in the home, but others live in poverty. In fact, our research shows that it is the social circumstances of people's lives, rather than "traditional beliefs," that seem to have an impact on how they manage illness. Most immigrants to Canada want to make use of the resources that are here, negotiate care quite readily with health professionals, and make decisions based on what they see as the efficacy of care. But having to work long hours in a factory, and getting paid only for the hours worked, tends to give survival priority over health and illness management. Managing care for an ill person at home may be devastating to a family with few resources. In other words, for health professionals the priority may be illness management; for the patient and family the priority may be survival in a new country.

For the hospitalized patient about to go home, certain questions can help the health professional understand the home situation. Here are examples of questions that may be used as beginning probes to get a sense of the resources available to the person at home and what else needs to provided:

- Is there anything that stands in the way of your treatment at home?

- Who will be at home to help you out when you go home? (E.g., do the shopping, prepare meals, do the laundry?)
- What is the layout of your home like? (E.g., Bedroom upstairs? Access to bathroom?)
- What do you need at home to be able to manage?
- Do you have any difficulties with income? (This question is one that should be explored by the social worker, as families are often reluctant to talk about financial troubles.)

Identifying the Influence on Health Care of the Family and Social Support Networks

Family members play an important part in health care decisions, especially when they must care for an ill person at home. The likelihood that a patient will follow prescribed treatments often depends on how he or she is viewed by the family. Certain key family members may have the final say, and it is important to find out who they are.

The proximity of numerous relatives does not always mean that the patient feels supported by the family. Obligations or tensions within a family can foster isolation and loneliness among members even when an extended family shares a household. Family beliefs about a particular illness and its cultural meaning may have a profound impact on the kind of support the sick person receives. Mental illness can be especially difficult for some families to deal with. They may not accept a diagnosis of mental illness, and may therefore not believe that the medication is necessary. It is often better for the health professional to focus on what can be done to help the patient than on the diagnosis of the illness.

Dealing with HIV/AIDS may also be a source of great distress for some families. The ill person may be reluctant to divulge the diagnosis to others in the family.

Finding out about the structure and functioning of the family is therefore critical. The following areas could be included in the assessment:

- Do you live alone? Who is the closest person to you?
- Who else lives in your home? (Explore presence of extended family in household: grandmothers, grandfathers, older aunts and uncles.)
- Do you have family and friends living nearby who can give you a hand if you need it? (Explore support inside and outside the home; if the wife works, who helps at home.)
- Who is the first person you turn to for help? What kinds of things do you usually need help with?
- For elderly family members: What kinds of help do you need? Who do you usually turn to for help? Tell me about your day. What kinds of things do you do?

- Have you found any other medicines that have worked for you in the past? (Explore special remedies, those used in the home country and those used here.)
- Tell me about the children in the family. (Starting with questions about children usually puts people, especially mothers, at ease.) Find out how children are doing in school and at home.

Questions about family life should be approached with caution. Some people coming from other countries consider family life and problems as personal, and regard questions on the subject as intrusive. The health professional may be wise to hold the question for a cue from the patient or family.

Establishing Any Difficulties in Adjusting to Life in Canada

Uprooting from one's home country and settling in a new country are traumatic under the best of circumstances. In addition to this, most immigrants are challenged to find employment, cope with language problems, and manage on a tight budget. How a patient experiences and manages illness may be inextricably linked to the adjustment issues. Therefore, it is imperative that health professionals establish if there are difficulties in adjustment. These can be sensitive questions for the patient and family, so it is best to preface them with a statement such as this: "When people come to a new country, there are usually a lot of things that are new, that they may have difficulties with. I would like to find out if any of these are difficult for you, so we can talk about some of the resources that are available to people who are new to Canada."

Areas to explore include the following:

- English-language skills: assessed from moment of first contact, but the patient may discuss problems of getting a well-paid job.
- Are you working at the moment? Could you tell me a little about the job you now have? (Establish if there is downward mobility for both men and women.)
- Can you tell me how you came into Canada? (Explore whether the person is an immigrant or refugee, as physical, emotional, and social problems can be quite different for the two. If refugee, find out whether convention refugee or asylum seeker, as this will make a difference to the resources available to the person. This issue can be very sensitive, so it is better to weave these questions in as exploratory queries while discussing life in Canada rather than to ask them as direct questions.)
- Can you tell me about how well life has gone for you here? Are there any special things that you are worrying about at the moment, and that we may be able to provide some help with? (Gender-related issues might

surface here; trouble with adolescent children; financial support and how family is currently obtaining income. These questions indicate resources that may be made available to the person.)

Tact is needed in posing these questions so that the patient will not feel threatened. These are obviously not areas to explore early in the relationship. Patients usually give cues when they feel sufficiently at ease to discuss such matters with a physician, nurse, social worker, or other health professional.

Physical examinations and other diagnostic procedures are usually required to complete the assessment of a patient. Consideration has to be given to cultural variations in executing these procedures. For example, women coming from some countries may be reluctant to be examined by a male physician or be cared for by a male nurse, and older male patients may object to being examined by a young female physician. Sensitivity is required in dealing with these issues to ensure that the patient is not humiliated.

As well, some diagnostic procedures may be refused. A patient may refuse to give blood in the belief that the loss of blood will weaken and harm the body. Or may not: for the health professional this is not something to assume but to be prepared for and to find out about from the patient. It is important for health professionals to understand the patient's system of beliefs, past experience with home-country health care, and day-to-day issues, rather than writing off certain behaviour as "non-compliance."

Communication, Language, the Use of Interpreters, and Informed Consent

Health professionals often mistakenly look to the patient's family to offer assistance with translation. Instead they should turn to the professional interpretive services increasingly offered by hospitals and other health care organizations. This is especially critical at times when important exchanges are required with the patient (e.g., obtaining consent, assessments, pre-operative teaching, discharge teaching). Family members may be willing to translate, but there are often shortcomings with their fluency in English and particularly their understanding of key medical terminology. Family members may be placed in uncomfortable situations when asked to communicate personal information, or may only selectively relay information back to the patient. Children should *not* be used as interpreters. The professional's ability to communicate clearly with patients is foundational to knowing how they manage health and illness.

There is also a legal reason never to use a family member to interpret when important matters such as informed consent are to be discussed, or when complex diagnoses, medical procedures, or treatment outcomes are to be described. The practitioner can be legally liable if the patient or family sues. The practitioner must therefore be assured, without a doubt, that there is clear communication with the patient and family. The College of Physicians and Surgeons of British Columbia (1995) recommends the use of an independent interpreter if the person does not speak English and the physician is not fluent in the patient's language.

Apart from the steps required to find a professionally trained interpreter, the very process of communicating through an interpreter is complex and not without difficulty. For example, the interpreter may give a précis of what the patient says, grossly altering the meaning of the communication or omitting vital details. The clinician should be sure to ask the interpreter to translate verbatim (see guidelines below). The dialogue should be between the clinician and the patient, with the interpreter translating in the background. This facilitates the building of rapport with a patient in the absence of a common language.

Another problem can arise if the interpreter and patient are from different social classes. The interpreter may be embarrassed to discuss folk beliefs, wanting instead to portray the culture in a certain light. Therefore, the health professional should let the interpreter know that there is genuine interest in the patient's viewpoint, that the patient's opinions are legitimate and an essential part of the treatment plan.

When using an interpreter, it is important to follow certain guidelines:

- Meet with the interpreter prior to the session with the patient and family to ensure that the interpreter does not know them, given that they may be from the same ethno-cultural community. Although the professional interpreter understands issues of confidentiality, having someone from their community interpret may still be a source of great embarrassment to the patient or family and could lead to miscommunication of information.
- Explain what is expected, and also give the interpreter some idea about the information to be interpreted. Clarify words and meanings that may be ambiguous.
- Set out clear guidelines: the conversation should be between physician and the patient and family; seating should be arranged so that the physician looks at the patient and family and speaks directly to them; they should speak directly to the physician.
- The interpreter should translate verbatim everything that is said by everyone.
- Validate that the patient and family understand what is being interpreted. They should repeat back to the interpreter key points to show they understand (especially on issues such as informed consent), and the interpreter should convey this back to the physician, so there are no miscommunications.

Further to these specific guidelines for the use of interpreters, some expert health professionals have provided "tips" as to what works best for them in communicating with patients, sometimes across linguistic barriers.

- Find a point of connection with the patient, even if you can't communicate verbally. You may want to learn a few words in the patient's language to show respect for his or her language and your desire to communicate.
- Look directly at the person you speak to, talk slowly, and use simple English.
- Anticipatory planning is crucial. Foresee when you will need an interpreter (for example, to discuss a difficult diagnosis, to explain treatment options and outcomes) and get one. Most hospitals and other health care agencies now provide interpretion services. In situations where this is not available, AT&T telephone translation services can be used. Interpretation services in physicians' offices are not covered by the Medical Services Plan, so, when necessary, the patient has to bring an interpreter. In some instances a professional interpreter can be arranged through a social worker.
- When the patient does not speak English, ask the professional interpreter to help you to write down a few very clear instructions for simple tasks in the patient's language. (Make sure first that the patient is able to read.) Anticipate what is needed on a regular basis, and write this down, so that you will be able to communicate with the person if there is no one around to help out.
- Patients and their families can be very anxious in the hospital and may hear little of what you tell them. Write down instructions in English in a clear and concise way, in point form, in simple language, so the patient can take them home. Health professionals working in a clinic or a doctor's office can do likewise.
- Write down resources in the community that patient and family can use. A family member or friend may be able to read and explain the information to the person.
- If at all possible, a follow-up phone call by a home care nurse to the patient a few days after his or her discharge from hospital would make a lot of difference to the patient. Many patients don't anticipate what it will be like when they get home from the hospital and are completely bewildered, even when it seemed that they would have no difficulties. This means that hospital personnel should communicate clearly with the home care nurse about the patients that are being discharged home.
- Be aware that, for some groups, sexual matters, mental illness including dementia, and family issues are seen as extremely private, and open discussion can cause embarrassment. The family and patient may see it as

more appropriate to discuss such issues with a trusted relative or friend rather than a health professional. But in order to make sure the patient gets the help that is needed, you will have to use tact in finding a language to communicate with families so that the patient can get treatment.

- Be aware that some patients are very uncomfortable with joking relationships and feel more comfortable with a more formal approach. So it's important to act in a professional, respectful way with people, while at the same time conveying empathy.

Concluding Comments

Most immigrants and refugees recognize that Canadian health care is excellent and are eager to receive the best treatment that Western medicine has to offer. It is not their "traditional beliefs" that stand in the way of getting the help they need. Rather, the current organization of the health care system may be a barrier to care. Although hospitals in the past ten to fifteen years have become more welcoming to people from different cultural groups by making visiting hours more flexible, responding to dietary preferences, providing interpreter services, and the like, there are still gaps in care.

The restructuring of hospitals has meant increased workloads for staff, and a cutback in the in-service education needed for professionals to respond to an increasingly complex patient population. In many instances, health professionals on the front line of service do not use available resources, such as language services, which might facilitate the care of patients. "Not enough time" is usually given as the reason for not using these services, but clinical decision making may also be an issue. Health professionals may not be sufficiently aware of how crucial it is to communicate effectively with patients or of their legal liabilities if there is miscommunication.

Our research with people of different ethno-cultural backgrounds shows that language difficulties are, by far, the most pressing issue for non-English-speaking people. The story of one hospitalized South Asian woman exemplifies some of the issues in today's health care system:

> I know that because I did not speak English I had limited ways of telling them about my pain and where it is, and what kind of pain and other things that I wanted to say, and one cannot say or explain what I needed to tell them. I can only tell them pain, and they would give me pain medicine, but not all the nurses gave me the medication.

Patients seeking care in a physician's office may come up against similar language difficulties. Since physicians are not reimbursed for interpreter services by the Medical Services Plan, communication is a challenge when the patient and physician do not share a common language. In some instances, patients intentionally seek out physicians who speak their language, but this is not always possible. Immigrants from Laos or Cambodia may be hard pressed to find a physician who speaks their language. When there are urgent medical problems, especially issues requiring informed consent, it might be prudent for the physician to seek the assistance of a social service agency to obtain interpretation services.

Professionals still depend on families to interpret for them or else they call on other staff to help out. The anticipatory planning that is necessary to ensure adequate interpretation is often not put in place, which compromises the care of the patient.

Another concern involves the casual assumptions that health professionals sometimes make about their patients, based on "ethnicity." Some health professionals assume that all Asian patients have extended families to look after them when they return home from the hospital. Such assumptions are not benign; they have consequences for the allocation of resources. A referral to home care services may be based on a mistaken expectation about family support. There are also notions around entitlement to care. Stereotypes about some ethno-cultural groups feed a belief that some of them make extra demands on the health care system.

But there are other complex issues that confront us today. Health professionals themselves are increasingly members of ethno-cultural minority groups. The first edition of this book implicitly assumed that the professional was a mainstream Canadian and the patient an immigrant. This assumption can no longer be made. Many health professionals are immigrants with English as a second language, and some are people of colour. Tensions now arise when Anglo-European patients refuse the care of professionals who are people of colour. This opens up the issue of racism in the workplace, which must be addressed by hospital administrators to ensure a workplace free of discrimination for both patients and health professionals.

"Culturally responsive care" means that health professionals assess the issues for each patient and respond to these issues in a timely way. It means responding to the patient's cultural perspectives and social context. It means understanding the ways in which past experiences in the home country, as well as everyday life experiences in Canada, shape immigrant expectations of health care. The content of this book has provided background information that will help health professionals interpret what patients have to tell them. It does not replace the task of learning about every patient and family. Rather, it shows why culturally responsive care requires special efforts to understanding the unique perspective and life circumstances of every immigrant and refugee patient.

Recommended Reading

Fadiman, Anne. 1997. *The Spirit Catches You and You Fall Down: A Hmong Child, Her American Doctors, and the Collision of Two Cultures*. New York, NY: Farrar, Strauss and Giroux.

This very readable book captures many of the themes we deal with. Written by an anthropologist, it tells the story of the young daughter of Hmong refugees who falls ill with epilepsy. As the family seeks health care, the story highlights issues of language and communication and conflicting views of disease etiology, acculturation, and settlement, all within the larger sociopolitical history of the Hmong people and the culture of Western medicine. Fadiman helps the reader empathize with both health care providers and the patient and her family, and does much to promote intercultural understanding and negotiation. We highly recommend her book.

Further Reading

Anderson, J., J. Perry, C. Blue, A. Browne, A. Henderson, K. Khan, S. Kirkham, J. Lynam, P. Semeniuk, and V. Smye. 2003. "Re-writing cultural safety within the postcolonial and postnational feminist project: Toward new epistemologies of healing." *Advances in Nursing Science* 26: 196-214.

Citizenship and Immigration Canada. 2003. *Facts and Figures 2002: Immigration Overview*. Ottawa, ON: Minister of Public Works and Government Services. http://www.cic.gc.ca/english/pub/facts2002-temp/index.html

College of Physicians and Surgeons of British Columbia. 1995. *Policy Manual*. Vancouver, BC: College of Physicians and Surgeons of British Columbia.

Fadiman, Anne. 1997. *The Spirit Catches You and You Fall Down: A Hmong Child, Her American Doctors, and the Collision of Two Cultures*. New York, NY: Farrar, Strauss and Giroux.

Kleinman, A. 1980. *Patients and Healers in the Context of Culture*. Berkeley, CA: University of California Press.

Mojab, S. 1999. "De-skilling immigrant women." *Canadian Woman Studies* 19: 123-28.

Ramsden, I., and Kawa Whakaruruhau. 1993. "Cultural safety in nursing education in Aotearoa (New Zealand)." *Nursing Praxis in New Zealand* 8: 4-10.

About the Authors

Joan M. Anderson is the Elizabeth Kenny McCann Professor in the School of Nursing at the University of British Columbia and Research Director of the Culture, Gender and Health Research Unit. She studied at UBC and McGill Universities and received her PhD in Sociology from UBC. She has done research in Canada with people from different ethno-cultural communities, including Anglo-, Indo-, and Chinese Canadians.

Chansokhy Anhaouy was born in Phnom Penh, Cambodia, immigrated to Canada from a refugee camp in Thailand in 1981, and currently is a Multicultural Liaison Worker for the Vancouver School Board.

Shashi Assanand lived in Uganda and India before migrating to Canada. She is the Founder and Executive Director of the Vancouver and Lower Mainland Multicultural Family Support Services Society, which provides services to women who are in transition and facing family violence. As a Registered Social Worker, she has worked in immigrant communities for the past twenty-eight years and is actively involved in the areas of multiculturalism and women's issues locally, provincially, and nationally.

Afsaneh Behjati-Sabet is from Tehran, Iran, where she studied psychology. After coming to Canada, she completed an MA in Counselling Psychology at the University of British Columbia. For the past fifteen years she has worked as a therapist with Addiction Services (Vancouver Coastal Health) and in private practice in Vancouver and Richmond.

Natalie A. Chambers was born and raised in London, England. She did undergraduate studies at the University of East Anglia and completed her MA in Anthropology from Simon Fraser University. She has done cross-cultural and health behaviour research with immigrants and is the Research and Development Officer at Okanagan Families Society, British Columbia.

Maud Dias was born in that part of India which later became Pakistan. She is a Registered Social Worker, holds an MSW from Pakistan, and in Canada has worked in agencies serving the South Asian community. She is now retired.

Dai-Kha Dinh is a family physician who practised in Richmond, BC. He was born in Vinh-yen City in Vietnam, received his MD from the University of Saigon, and did further specialty training in France and Quebec.

Soma Ganesan was born and grew up in Vietnam, where he received his MD from the University of Saigon. He is a Clinical Professor as well as Director of the Crosscultural Psychiatry Programme in the Department of Psychiatry at the University of British Columbia and is Medical Director of the Department of Psychiatry at Vancouver General and UBC Hospitals.

Danica Gleave was born in British Columbia. She received a BA in Anthropology and an MD from the University of British Columbia and did her specialty training through McMaster University in Thunder Bay, Family Medicine North. She is a family physician in Victoria.

Carol Herbert is Dean of the Faculty of Medicine and Dentistry at the University of Western Ontario. She was born and brought up in Vancouver and received her MD and specialty training at the University of British Columbia. After joining the UBC Medical Faculty, she became head of the Department of Family Practice.

Sheryl Reimer Kirkham is an Associate Professor in Nursing and Leadership at Trinity Western University in Langley, BC, and an Investigator with the Culture, Gender and Health Research Unit at the University of British Columbia. She was born in Manitoba, studied at the University of Victoria, and received her MSN and PhD at UBC. She conducts research at the junctures of culture, religion, and health.

Karen Kobayashi is an Assistant Professor in Sociology and a Research Affiliate with the Centre on Aging at the University of Victoria. She received her PhD in Sociology from Simon Fraser University and held a Michael Smith Foundation Postdoctoral Fellowship in Population Health. She has done research on relationships between adult Japanese Canadian children and their parents.

Arturo S. Manes was born in Santiago, Chile, to parents who had migrated there from Germany. He did undergraduate studies in Santiago and received his MD and specialty training at the University of British Columbia. He is a family physician in Vancouver and has many Latin American patients.

Maureen Murphy, formerly with the UBC School of Nursing and the Vancouver Health Department, is now with Ottawa Public Health, where she manages Family and Community Health Services. She was born in Ontario and educated at the University of Western Ontario, where she received her MSN.

Teruko Okabe was born and brought up in Japan, where she studied sociology and received an MA in Educational Psychology in Kyoto. Since coming to live in British Columbia, she has become a Registered Social Worker and has been an instructor at the Centre for Continuing Education at the University of British Columbia.

Elizabeth Richardson was born and grew up in India, where her Canadian parents lived for many years. She was educated at the University of British Columbia and at McMaster University, from which she received an MA in Sociology, and has taught English in Japan. Currently she works as a social worker for the BC government in North and West Vancouver.

Kazuko Takahashi is a registered nurse, now retired, who was born in British Columbia and received a BSN from the University of British Columbia. Like many Canadian citizens of Japanese descent, she lived in government relocation camps during the Second World War.

Nancy Waxler-Morrison is Associate Professor, Emerita, in the School of Social Work and the Department of Anthropology and Sociology at the University of British Columbia. She was born and received her early education in Illinois and received her PhD in Sociology at Harvard. She has done research in the medical sociology field in Sri Lanka and India.

Ka-Ming Kevin Yue is a family physician who practises in Vancouver. He was born in Canton, China, grew up in Hong Kong, and received his MD and family physician specialty training at the University of British Columbia.

Index

Printed and bound in Canada by Friesens

Set in Stone by Artegraphica Design Co. Ltd.

Copy editor: Larry MacDonald

Proofreader: Deborah Kerr

Indexer: Christine Jacobs